基金项目：扬州大学卓越本科课程建设工程项目（2022ZYKCC-36）
扬州大学重点教材项目（2018-24）
扬州大学出版基金资助项目

病原生物学与免疫学实验教程

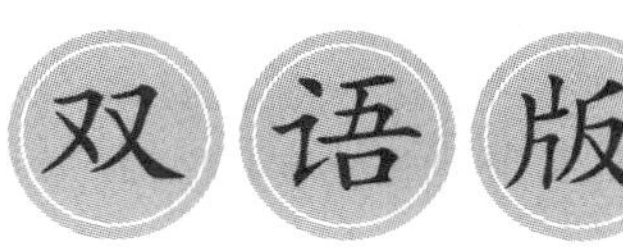

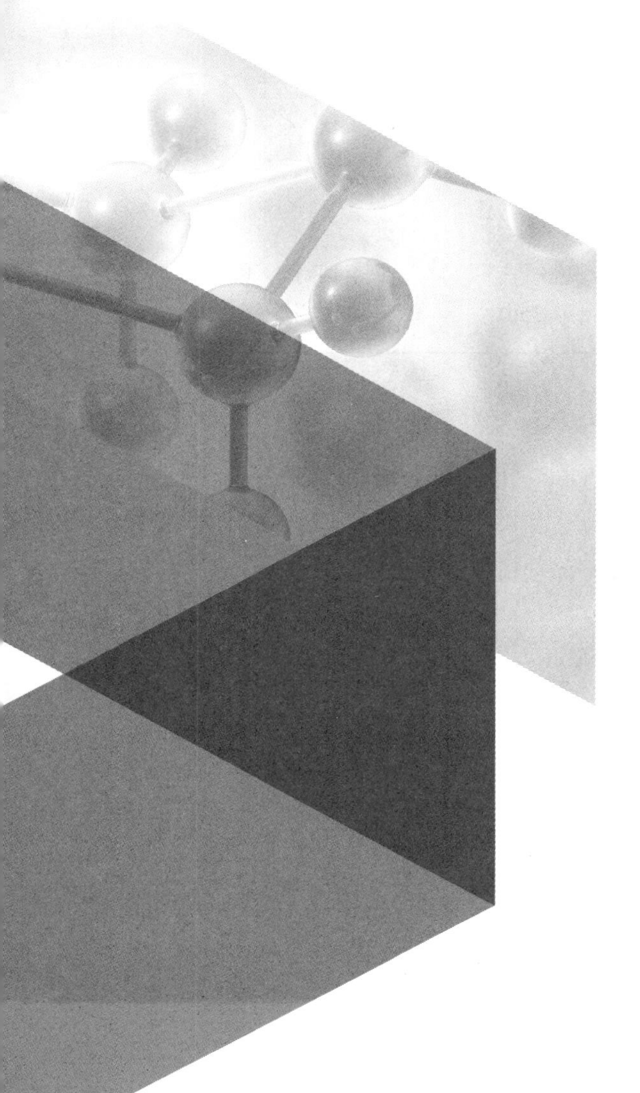

主　　编 ◎ 李国才　焦红梅　田　芳　潘兴元
参　　编（按姓氏笔画排序）
乌日汗　孔桂美　刘翠翠　阴银燕
陆　凤　段秋芳　钱　莉　高成凤
龚卫娟　蔡良良　蔺志杰
编者单位 ◎ 扬州大学医学院

華中科技大學出版社
http://press.hust.edu.cn
中国 · 武汉

内 容 简 介

本书为扬州大学卓越本科课程建设工程项目(2022ZYKCC-36)、扬州大学重点教材项目(2018-24)和扬州大学出版基金资助项目。

本书分为三篇共三十七个实验。第一篇为免疫学基础实验,包括血清总补体溶血活性(CH_{50})的测定等八个实验;第二篇为病原生物学基础实验,包括细菌的生理等二十二个实验;第三篇为综合性实验,包括多克隆抗体的制备及效价测定等七个实验。书后还有附录和部分实验结果的彩图。所有内容均用中文和英文两种语言编写。

本书不仅可作为高等医学院校临床医学、医学检验技术、中西医临床医学等专业学生的病原生物学与免疫学实验教材,还可作为医院、卫生防疫部门中从事病原生物学与免疫学工作的技术人员的参考书。

图书在版编目(CIP)数据

病原生物学与免疫学实验教程 :汉英对照 / 李国才等主编. -- 武汉 :华中科技大学出版社, 2024. 8.
ISBN 978-7-5772-1143-5

Ⅰ. R37-33;R392-33

中国国家版本馆 CIP 数据核字第 2024XR3289 号

病原生物学与免疫学实验教程(双语版)
Bingyuan Shengwuxue yu Mianyixue Shiyan Jiaocheng(Shuangyu Ban)

李国才　焦红梅
田　芳　潘兴元　主编

策划编辑:蔡秀芳
责任编辑:马梦雪　曾奇峰　丁　平
封面设计:廖亚萍
责任校对:刘小雨
责任监印:周治超

出版发行:华中科技大学出版社(中国·武汉)　电话:(027)81321913
武汉市东湖新技术开发区华工科技园　邮编:430223

录　排:华中科技大学惠友文印中心
印　刷:武汉市洪林印务有限公司
开　本:889mm×1194mm　1/16
印　张:14.75
字　数:500 千字
版　次:2024 年 8 月第 1 版第 1 次印刷
定　价:52.80 元

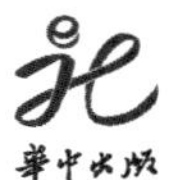

前　　言

病原生物学与免疫学实验是重要的医学实践课程，也是医学相关专业本科生必须掌握的专业基础课程。实施双语教学是我国高等教育国际化发展的必然趋势。为了适应“新医科”背景下卓越医学人才培养新格局及教育教学改革和创新的需要，本书遵循实用性、科学性、启发性和时代性的原则，将医学免疫学、医学微生物学和人体寄生虫学的主要实验内容整合，注重实验技能的培养、专业知识和课程思政元素的融合，并以中英双语的形式编写，有助于医学生掌握病原生物学和免疫学诊断的基本原理和相关实验技能，提高科技英文水平。中英文内容并不完全对应，旨在为不同语言背景的读者提供更灵活的学习资源。本书不仅可作为高等医学院校临床医学、医学检验技术、中西医临床医学等专业学生的病原生物学与免疫学实验教材，还可作为医院、卫生防疫部门中从事病原生物学与免疫学工作的技术人员的参考书。

本书的编写和出版得到了扬州大学卓越本科课程建设工程项目(2022ZYKCC-36)、扬州大学重点教材项目(2018-24)和扬州大学出版基金资助，对此我们表示衷心的感谢。

由于实验教学仍处于不断探索之中以及编者水平有限，书中不足之处在所难免，敬请广大读者提出宝贵意见。

编　者

Preface

The experiment of pathogenic biology and immunology is an important medical practical course and also a fundamental professional course that medical undergraduates must master. The implementation of bilingual teaching is a necessary development trend for the internationalization of higher education in China. In order to adapt to the new pattern of cultivating outstanding medical talents and the need for educational reform and innovation in the context of the "new medical science", this book follows the principles of practicality, scientificity, inspiration and modernity, integrating the main experimental contents of medical immunology, medical microbiology and human parasitology, emphasizing the cultivation of experimental skills, the integration of professional knowledge and curriculum ideological and political elements, and is written in both Chinese and English. It helps medical students master the basic principles and related experimental skills of pathogenic biology and immunological diagnosis, and improves their technical English proficiency. The Chinese and English parts are not completely corresponding, aiming to provide more flexible learning resources for readers with different language backgrounds. This book can not only serve as an experimental textbook for students of pathogenic biology and immunology in clinical medicine, medical laboratory technology, traditional Chinese and western clinical medicine and other majors in higher medical colleges, but also serve as a reference book for technical personnel engaged in pathogenic biology and immunology in hospitals and health and epidemic prevention departments.

The compilation and publication of this book are supported by the Excellent Undergraduate Course Construction Project of Yangzhou University (2022ZYKCC-36), the Key Textbook Project of Yangzhou University (2018-24) and the Publishing Foundation of Yangzhou University, for which we would like to express our heartfelt thanks.

Due to the continuous exploration of experimental teaching and the limitation of the authors' ability, this book inevitably has shortcomings. We kindly request valuable opinions from readers.

Authors

实验室基本规则

病原生物学与免疫学是实践性很强的学科，尤其微生物学实验材料中有些是病原微生物，因此必须树立生物安全意识，除了必须遵守国家和单位的相关实验室管理规范外，还必须遵循以下基本规则。

(1)进入实验室前须穿好工作服，与实验无关的物品(书包、衣物等)不得带入实验室，以免造成污染。

(2)严格遵循无菌操作原则，避免污染甚至感染事件的发生。

(3)遵循生物安全原则，禁止在实验室内进行饮食等行为。

(4)保持实验室安静、整洁，勿大声喧哗或随意走动。

(5)认真进行各项实验操作，实验中如发生意外，应立即报告老师，及时处理。

(6)实验完毕，应认真整理桌面，需培养的材料要标记组别、姓名等，并置于培养箱中培养。显微镜用后要擦净，各功能部件复位。其他用过的物品按要求放回原处，值日生认真清扫实验室，关好水、电及门窗后方可离开实验室。

Laboratory basic rules

Pathogenic biology and immunology is a highly practical subject, especially microbiological experiment, in which some materials are pathogenic microorganisms. Therefore, biosafety awareness should be established, and in addition to complying with relevant national and unit laboratory management norms, the following basic rules must be followed.

(1) To avoid contamination, one should wear work clothes when entering the laboratory and not bring items unrelated to the experiment (backpacks, clothing, etc.).

(2) Strictly adhere to aseptic operation principles to avoid contamination and the occurrence of infection incidents.

(3) Follow the principles of biosafety and prohibit behaviors such as eating and drinking inside the laboratory.

(4) Keep the laboratory quiet and tidy. Do not make loud noises or walk around at will.

(5) Carefully carry out various experimental operations. If any accidents occur during the experiment, immediately report them to the teacher and handle them in a timely manner.

(6) After the experiment is completed, the desktop should be carefully organized, and the materials to be cultivated should be labeled with groups, names, etc., and placed in an incubator for cultivation. After using the microscope, it should be wiped clean and all functional components should be reset. All other items used should be returned to their original places as required. The duty personnel should carefully clean the laboratory and close the water, electricity, doors and windows before leaving the laboratory.

目　　录

Contents

第一篇　免疫学基础实验

实验一　血清总补体溶血活性(CH_{50})的测定

[实验目的]

掌握 CH_{50} 测定实验的原理，熟悉其方法及意义。

[实验器材]

(1)待检人血清或豚鼠血清、2%绵羊红细胞(sheep red blood cell，SRBC)悬液、溶血素、pH 7.2～7.4 PBS、1.8%(*W*/*V*)NaCl 溶液、蒸馏水等。

(2)制冰机、水浴锅、离心机、分光光度计、容量瓶、15 ml 离心管、移液器、记号笔等。

[实验内容]

1. 溶血素的配制和灭活

(1)原理：商品化溶血素是干粉制剂，需要溶解后使用。由于溶血素本质上是兔抗 SRBC 抗体，其中含有大量兔源补体，可以裂解 SRBC，因此配制好的溶血素必须进行灭活，否则会影响实验结果。

(2)方法。

①10×溶血素母液的配制：取 0.5 ml 蒸馏水溶解商品化溶血素(4000 U/ml)，用 PBS 洗瓶 3 次并全部转移至 100 ml 容量瓶中，用 PBS 定容后充分混匀。

②1×溶血素工作液的配制：取 10 ml 10×溶血素母液移入 100 ml 容量瓶定容后充分混匀，配成 2 U/ml 溶血素工作液。

③56 ℃孵育 30～35 min 以灭活补体，每 10 min 轻轻摇动混匀 1 次。

2. 2% SRBC 悬液的配制

(1)原理：商品化 SRBC 悬液保质期很短，一般保存 3 周就会有明显的自发性溶血现象(离心后上清液发红)，所以实验前需要洗涤除去自发性溶血释放出来的血红素以及红细胞碎片等。

(2)方法。

①取适量商品化 SRBC 悬液分装至 50 ml 离心管中，2000 r/min 离心 10 min，轻轻倾倒弃去上清液。

②取 40 ml PBS 充分洗涤，2000 r/min 离心 10 min，弃去上清液。根据实际情况可以洗涤多次，直至上清液呈无色。

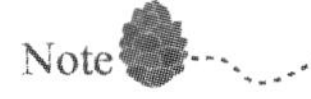

③用移液器吸取 1 ml 压积的红细胞，PBS 稀释 50 倍，轻轻摇动混匀，即成 2% SRBC 悬液。

3. 致敏 SRBC 悬液的配制

(1)于 50 ml 小烧杯中加入 6 ml 2% SRBC 悬液,逐滴加入 6 ml 2 U/ml 溶血素工作液,边加边轻柔摇动,充分混匀。

(2)37 ℃水浴保温 10 min,使 SRBC 充分致敏,然后立即放在冰上。

4. 50%溶血标准液的配制

(1)取一支 15 ml 离心管,加入 0.5 ml 2% SRBC 悬液和 2 ml 蒸馏水,室温放置 5 min,其间轻轻摇动数次,使 SRBC 全部低渗溶解。

(2)加入 2 ml 1.8% NaCl 溶液使校正为等渗溶液。

(3)加入 0.5 ml 2% SRBC 悬液,即为 50%溶血标准液。

5. 待检血清的配制

(1)方法一(人血清)。

①静脉抽血,室温放置 30 min,再 4 ℃放置 1 h,使血块收缩。

②4 ℃,3000 r/min 离心 10 min。

③取上清液,用 PBS 稀释 20 倍。

(2)方法二(豚鼠血清):血清中补体极不稳定,而获取临床样本需要多级审批,时间较长,所以用人血清作为本科生实验材料可能存在困难。可以用豚鼠血清模拟人血清,现配现用,以保证补体的活性。

①取 1 瓶商品化豚鼠血清冻干粉(100 U/ml),加 1 ml 蒸馏水溶解,冰上静置 10 min。

②将上述液体转移至 15 ml 离心管中,用 PBS 洗瓶 3 次,全部转移至同一容量瓶中,定容至 3 ml,即为 1∶3 稀释的豚鼠血清。

6. CH_{50} 测定实验

(1)原理:补体能使溶血素致敏的 SRBC 发生溶血,当致敏 SRBC 悬液浓度恒定时,在规定的反应时间内,溶血程度与补体含量和活性成正比。因此,将新鲜待检血清做不同倍数稀释后,与致敏 SRBC 悬液反应,测定溶血程度,可测知总补体溶血活性。待检血清的补体活性与溶血程度呈“S”形曲线,接近 50%溶血时,二者之间近似直线关系且斜率最大,此时,补体含量稍有变动就可对溶血程度产生很大影响,故以 50%溶血作为最敏感的判断终点,以引起 50%溶血所需的最小补体含量为 1 个 CH_{50} 单位,可计算出待检血清中总的补体溶血活性,单位以“U/ml”表示。CH_{50} 测定实验测定的血清中补体溶血活性可用以下公式表示:

$$CH_{50}=\frac{1}{\text{引起 50\%溶血的血清量(ml)}}\times\text{血清稀释倍数}$$

本实验主要反映补体经典活化途径的溶血活性,其结果与补体 C1～C9 各组分的量及活性均有关。

(2)方法。

①每组标记 11 支 15 ml 离心管,置于冰上预冷。

②在冰上按表 1-1-1 加入各试剂,轻轻混匀,10 号管为非溶血对照管。

③37 ℃水浴保温 30 min,2000 r/min 离心 3 min。

④肉眼比色,选与 50%溶血标准管(11 号管)颜色最接近的一管,按公式计算 CH_{50}。

表 1-1-1 CH_{50} 测定实验方法

离心管号	1	2	3	4	5	6	7	8	9	10	11
待检血清体积/ml	0.1	0.15	0.2	0.25	0.3	0.35	0.4	0.45	0.5	0	50%溶血标准液 2.5 ml
PBS 体积/ml	1.4	1.35	1.3	1.25	1.2	1.15	1.1	1.05	1	1.5	
致敏 SRBC 悬液体积/ml	1										
CH_{50}/(U/ml)	200	133	100	80	66.6	57.1	50	44.4	10	—	—

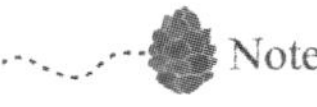
Note

(3)结果判定:10 号管是非溶血对照管,离心后上清液应无色透明,管底可见红细胞沉淀。11 号管是 50%溶血标准管,离心后上清液红色透明,管底可见较少的红细胞沉淀;其他管与 11 号管对比,可粗略判断样品中补体经典活化途径的溶血活性。本方法测定总补体溶血活性的正常值为 75～160 U/ml。

[注意事项]

(1)补体对热敏感,所有操作应尽可能在冰上进行,以保持补体活性。

(2)致敏 SRBC 悬液等各种试剂均应新鲜配制,若被细菌污染,可能导致溶血。

(3)实验所用玻璃器皿一定要保持清洁,酸、碱均会影响实验的准确性。

(4)补体的溶血活性与反应时缓冲液的 pH、离子强度、钙镁离子含量、SRBC 量、反应总体积及温度有一定关系,因此实验时需严格控制反应的各个环节,以保证实验的准确性与可重复性。

[临床意义]

补体活性增高常见于妊娠状态、糖尿病、各种急性炎症、组织损伤、心肌梗死和某些恶性肿瘤等;降低常见于各种免疫复合物病,如系统性红斑狼疮、急/慢性肾小球肾炎、类风湿性关节炎、强直性脊柱炎和自身免疫性溶血性贫血,也可见于严重肝病、营养不良、弥散性血管内凝血、蛋白丢失性肠病、严重灼伤、急性粒细胞白血病等。

[实验报告]

描述 CH_{50} 测定实验的原理、方法、结果与注意事项。

[思考题]

(1)什么样的患者需要进行 CH_{50} 测定?

(2)如果这是临床样本,根据你的实验结果给出诊断意见,列出患者可能罹患的疾病。

(3)补体活性检测方法还有哪些?试比较各种方法的优缺点。

(潘兴元　蔡良良)

实验二　人外周血单个核细胞的分离

[实验目的]

掌握用聚蔗糖-泛影葡胺(Ficoll-Paque)淋巴细胞分离液分离人外周血单个核细胞(peripheral blood mononuclear cells,PBMCs)的原理及方法。

[实验器材]

(1)人静脉血(肝素或者 EDTA 抗凝)。

(2)Ficoll-Paque 淋巴细胞分离液,pH 7.2～7.4 PBS 等。

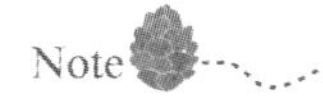

(3)离心机、15 ml 离心管、移液管等。

[实验内容]

1. 原理 外周血中各种血细胞的密度不尽相同,利用 Ficoll-Paque 淋巴细胞分离液进行密度梯度离心,使一定密度的细胞群按相应密度梯度分布,可以将各种血细胞加以分离。人 PBMCs 包括淋巴细胞与单核细胞,其密度为 1.075~1.090 g/ml,而血小板、粒细胞与红细胞的密度分别为 1.030~1.035 g/ml、1.092 g/ml、1.093 g/ml。因此,将血液轻轻加在密度为 1.076~1.078 g/ml 的 Ficoll-Paque 淋巴细胞分离液上,使成一界面,再经离心,即出现分层。最上面为血浆及血小板层,血浆与 Ficoll-Paque 淋巴细胞分离液界面处的一白色云雾状细胞层即为淋巴细胞和单核细胞,红细胞和粒细胞则沉于管底。

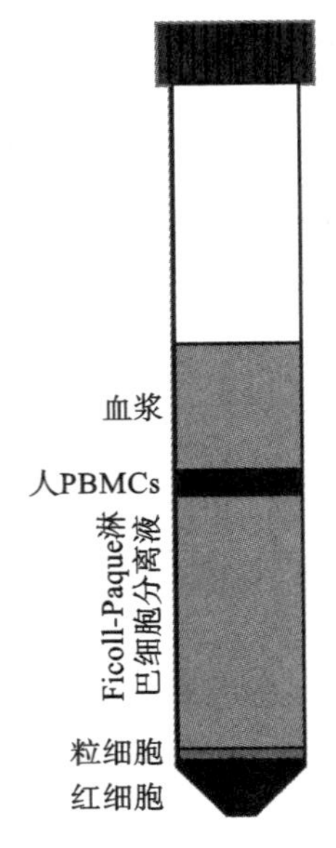

图 1-2-1 分离后的人外周血

2. 方法

(1)取一支 15 ml 离心管,将移液管直接伸入管底加入 2 ml Ficoll-Paque 淋巴细胞分离液(预先平衡到室温),以防分离液接触管壁。

(2)于另一支 15 ml 离心管中加入 2 ml 静脉抗凝血,再加入等量 PBS 以稀释血液,混合时要沿管壁吹匀,避免产生气泡。

(3)将稀释的血液沿管壁徐徐加入分离液离心管中,使之与 Ficoll-Paque 淋巴细胞分离液形成一界面,两者不能混合。

(4)室温下于 1500~2000 r/min 离心 20 min,注意离心机设置为“No break”,避免离心完成后因为急剧减速将已经分层的细胞层重新混合。

(5)离心结束后可见管内分为 5 层(图 1-2-1),用吸管轻轻穿过血浆层至白膜层,沿离心管周缘吸出白膜层细胞,即 PBMCs,置于新离心管中。注意宁缺毋滥,尽量减少血小板和 Ficoll-Paque 淋巴细胞分离液的污染。

(6)加入 5 倍以上体积的 PBS 充分洗涤人 PBMCs,室温下于 1500 r/min 离心 10 min。

(7)倾倒出上清液,用 PBS 补至 1 ml,重悬淋巴细胞,此时细胞密度为$(1\sim2)\times10^{6}$/ml,需要时可用细胞计数板进行精确计数。

3. 结果 每毫升静脉血能分离出$(0.5\sim1)\times10^{6}$个 PBMCs,用 7-ADD 或 PI 等荧光染料染色,流式细胞仪检测出的活细胞比例应大于 95%。

[注意事项]

(1)Ficoll-Paque 淋巴细胞分离液应适量,外周血应充分稀释。

(2)温度直接影响 Ficoll-Paque 淋巴细胞分离液的密度和分离效果。

(3)不同物种的淋巴细胞分离液密度不同,不能混用。

[实验报告]

描述 Ficoll-Paque 淋巴细胞分离液分离人 $PBMC_s$ 的原理、方法与注意事项。

[思考题]

分离产物中理论上会有哪些杂质?什么情况下需要继续分离纯化?有哪些方法?

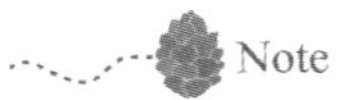
Note

(潘兴元　蔺志杰)

实验三　E 花环形成试验

[实验目的]

(1)掌握 E 花环形成试验的原理、方法和应用。
(2)熟悉光镜下 E 花环的形态和计数方法。

[实验器材]

(1)人 PBMCs(由本篇实验二制备)。
(2)pH 6.4～6.8 PBS、pH 7.2～7.4 PBS、1% SRBC 悬液、0.8%戊二醛、瑞氏-吉姆萨染液等。
(3)制冰机、离心机、水浴锅、显微镜、15 ml 离心管、移液器、载玻片等。

[实验内容]

1. 原理　T 细胞表面具有的能与 SRBC 表面 LFA-3 结合的受体被称为 E 受体(CD2 分子),已证实,E 受体是人类 T 细胞所特有的表面标志。当 T 细胞与 SRBC 混合后,SRBC 便黏附于 T 细胞表面,呈花环状(即 E 花环)(图 1-3-1)。通过 E 花环的形成检查 T 细胞的方法,称为 E 花环形成试验。根据 E 花环形成的多少,可测知 T 细胞的数目,从而间接反映机体细胞免疫功能状态。该试验广泛应用于肿瘤免疫、移植免疫及免疫性疾病的研究,可为某些疾病的诊断、防治、预后及药物疗效判断等提供免疫学方面的重要参考。

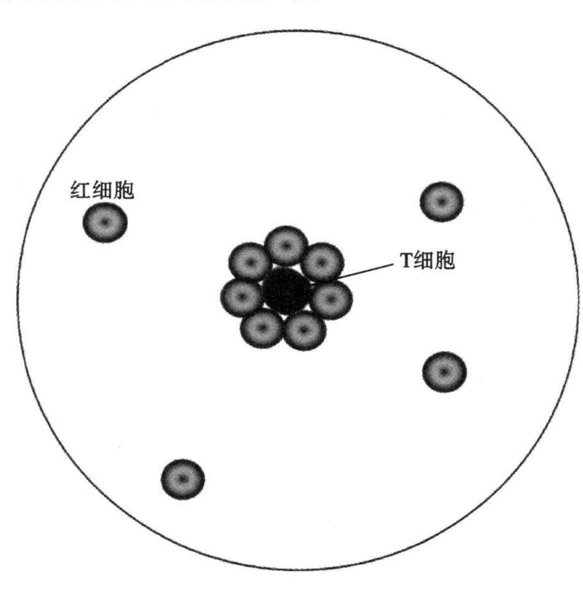

图 1-3-1　E 花环

T 细胞具有高度异质性,不同 T 细胞表面 CD2 分子的表达水平不同,与 SRBC 的亲和力不同,E 花环形成能力也不同。多数 T 细胞处于静止状态,CD2 分子表达水平较低,需要与 SRBC 在 4 ℃反应 2 h 以上(一般是过夜)才能形成花环,所形成的花环数代表被检标本中 T 细胞总数,这种花环形成试验称为总花环试验(total E-rosette test,Et 花环试验)。某些 T 细胞受到抗原刺

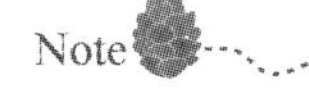

激后表达较高水平的 CD2 分子，与 SRBC 混合后无须经过 4 ℃孵育或只需要短暂孵育即可形成花环，称为活化花环试验(active E-rosette test，Ea 花环试验)，可反映活化 T 细胞数目，这部分 T 细胞的免疫学功能更能反映机体细胞免疫功能和动态变化。

2. 方法

(1)Ea 花环试验。

①在 0.1 ml PBMCs 悬液(约 10^6/ml)中加入等体积 1% SRBC 悬液(淋巴细胞与 SRBC 的比例为 1∶20 左右)，轻柔混匀。

②37 ℃水浴 5 min，其间轻轻摇动 2～3 次。注意：T 细胞和 SRBC 的结合并不牢固，所以后续操作中应尽量避免剧烈振摇。

③4 ℃，500 r/min 离心 5 min，置于冰上孵育 20 min。

④弃去大部分上清液，轻轻混匀，加入 1～2 滴 0.8%戊二醛(现配，15 min 内使用)固定 E 花形，混匀后置于冰上固定 15 min。

⑤轻轻旋转离心管，使沉淀细胞重悬，取 1 滴细胞悬液滴于事先浸在预冷蒸馏水中的载玻片上，使细胞悬液自然均匀铺开，用吹风机冷风吹干。

⑥滴加数滴瑞氏-吉姆萨染液，保证完全覆盖住细胞悬液，染色 2 min。滴加同样滴数的 pH 6.4～6.8 PBS，轻轻晃动使染液充分混匀，染色 5 min。

⑦用 pH 7.2～7.4 PBS 冲洗(勿倾斜载玻片冲洗，应水平冲洗)，干燥后在高倍镜下观察。

(2)Et 花环试验。

①取 0.1 ml PBMCs 悬液(约 10^6/ml)，再加入 0.5 ml 1% SRBC 悬液(淋巴细胞与 SRBC 的比例约为 1∶100)，混匀。

②37 ℃水浴 10 min，其间轻轻摇动 2～3 次。

③4 ℃，500 r/min 离心 5 min，置于冰上孵育 2 h 以上或者于 4 ℃过夜。

④后续步骤同 Ea 花环试验步骤④至步骤⑦。

3. 结果 高倍镜下观察，可见较多蓝色的淋巴细胞与单核细胞，淋巴细胞较小，单核细胞较大，很容易区分。大量 SRBC 呈红色，围绕淋巴细胞形成花环，凡表面黏附有 3 个或 3 个以上 SRBC 者为 E 花环形成细胞(即 E 阳性细胞)。计数 200 个淋巴细胞，算出 E 花环形成率，并推测 T 细胞百分率。

4. 正常值 Et 花环试验阳性的淋巴细胞比例为 60%～80%；Ea 花环试验阳性的淋巴细胞比例为 10%～40%。

[注意事项]

(1)NK 细胞也表达 CD2 分子，也能形成 E 花环，但 NK 细胞数量很少，且比 T 细胞大，很容易区分；单核细胞不表达 CD2 分子，没有形成 E 花环的能力。

(2)分离的 PBMCs 放置时间不得超过 4 h，否则 CD2 分子会自行脱落。同时 PBMCs 活细胞比例应不少于 95%。

(3)SRBC 的制备时间(新鲜程度)对本试验也有重要影响，一般不宜超过 2 周，否则，其与淋巴细胞的结合能力会下降。

(4)Ea 花环试验 SRBC 与淋巴细胞的比例以(10～20)∶1 为宜；Et 花环试验 SRBC 与淋巴细胞的比例以(100～200)∶1 为宜。

(5)温度对试验结果影响较大，样本从 4 ℃或冰上取出后应立即计数。

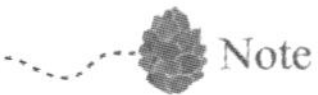

(6)计数前应将沉于管底的细胞重悬，但只宜轻缓旋转离心管，使细胞团块松开即可，不可强力吹打，否则 E 花环会消失或减少。

[实验报告]

(1)描述 E 花环形成试验的原理与方法。
(2)对试验结果进行讨论。

[思考题]

(1)何时需要检测 T 细胞功能?
(2)检测 T 细胞功能的方法还有哪些?

(潘兴元 蔺志杰)

实验四 中性粒细胞吞噬功能测定

[实验目的]

(1)掌握中性粒细胞吞噬功能测定的原理及方法。
(2)通过本实验加深对机体非特异性免疫机制的理解。

[实验器材]

(1)人静脉血(枸橼酸钠抗凝),白色葡萄球菌。
(2)肉汤培养基、碱性美蓝染液、甲醇、pH 7.2~7.4 PBS 等。
(3)离心机、15 ml 离心管、滴管等。

[实验内容]

1. 原理 中性粒细胞是外周血和免疫系统中含量最丰富的免疫细胞,具有变形与吞噬能力,在抵抗疾病和保护机体方面起着非常重要的作用。中性粒细胞可以黏附于大静脉内皮细胞表面,在感染和应激时可被快速动员,具有趋化、吞噬和杀菌等多种生物学功能,是机体固有免疫系统的重要组成部分。将白细胞悬液与细菌混合一段时间后,取样、涂片、染色、镜检,可以测定中性粒细胞吞噬百分率和吞噬指数,判断中性粒细胞的吞噬功能。

2. 方法

(1)菌液的制备:将白色葡萄球菌接种于肉汤培养基中,放于 37 ℃温箱内培养 12 h 左右,置于水浴(100 ℃)中加热 10 min 以杀死细菌,用无菌 PBS 稀释成约 6×10^8/ml 备用。

(2)取 50 μl 抗凝血与 50 μl 稀释菌液混合,轻轻摇匀,37 ℃水浴 30 min,其间振摇 1 次。

(3)作用完毕,用吸管将混合血液吹匀后,滴 1 滴于载玻片上,推成薄片。

(4)自然晾干后,用甲醇固定 4~5 min,碱性美蓝染液染色 2~3 min,置于油镜下观察。

(5)随机计数 100 个中性粒细胞,分别记录吞噬和未吞噬细菌的中性粒细胞个数,以及每个中性粒细胞所吞噬的细菌个数。

3. 结果

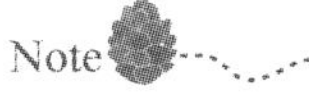

(1)吞噬百分率指中性粒细胞中吞噬细菌的中性粒细胞所占的百分比,正常参考值在 60%~

70%。

(2)将100个中性粒细胞所吞噬的细菌总个数除以100,得到每个中性粒细胞吞噬细菌的平均个数,即吞噬指数。

[注意事项]

(1)EDTA作为抗凝剂会影响细胞吞噬功能,肝素可能会影响某些染色方法(如瑞氏染色法)的效果,故选用枸橼酸钠抗凝剂可能比较合适。

(2)涂血片时不宜过厚,否则不易观察结果。

(3)由于不同标本的年龄和健康状况不同,其吞噬能力也有差别。

(4)同一个体对不同病原体的吞噬百分率和吞噬指数不同。

[实验报告]

(1)描述中性粒细胞吞噬功能测定的原理、方法与注意事项。

(2)报告并讨论实验结果所反映的患者的健康状况。

[思考题]

中性粒细胞是数量最多的白细胞,其生物学意义可能有哪些?

(潘兴元　蔡良良)

实验五　双向琼脂扩散试验

[实验目的]

(1)理解和掌握双向琼脂扩散试验的原理与方法。

(2)通过这个经典的血清学实验,加深对抗原-抗体结合的原理与特点的理解。

[实验器材]

(1)健康体检者血清、pH 7.2~7.4 PBS、兔抗人IgG抗血清等。

(2)温箱、微波炉、巴斯德吸管、锥形瓶、湿盒、载玻片等。

[实验内容]

1.原理　双向琼脂扩散试验利用琼脂凝胶为介质,通过扩散作用使分处两处的抗原和相应抗体相遇,形成抗原-抗体复合物,在比例合适处形成沉淀线。

根据沉淀线的有无、形态和位置可分析抗原或抗体的存在与否、两者的相对含量和相对分子质量、抗原的性质、抗原或抗体的纯度,以及进行粗略的抗体效价滴定。

双向琼脂扩散试验简单易行,用途广泛,但存在敏感性低、出结果慢、不能精确定量等缺点,属于经典的沉淀反应试验。

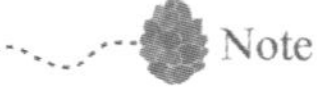

2. 方法

(1)用 PBS 配制 1%～1.5%的琼脂溶液,于微波炉内加热促溶。待琼脂溶液冷却至 50～60 ℃时,用巴斯德吸管吸取溶液,从载玻片中间开始滴加,直至胶厚度达到 2 mm 左右,保证抗原/抗体的加样量能达到 10 μl。

(2)室温静置数分钟,待其充分凝固后,用滴管在琼脂板上打梅花孔(图 1-5-1),孔间距为 5～8 mm。打完孔后将载玻片在酒精灯上过几次火,以封闭孔底,防止加入的抗原/抗体溶液通过孔底渗漏,影响试验结果。

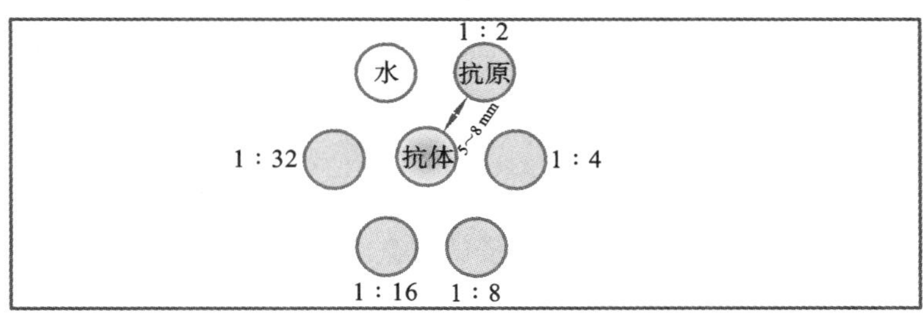

图 1-5-1 双向琼脂扩散试验梅花孔

(3)于中心孔加入 10 μl 兔抗人 IgG 抗血清,周围 5 个孔加入 10 μl 倍比稀释的健康体检者血清,留 1 个孔加水作为阴性对照。

(4)将载玻片放在垫有潮湿吸水纸的湿盒中,做好标记,置于 37 ℃温箱中孵育过夜,第 2 天查看结果。

[注意事项]

(1)倒板时速度要快,避免琼脂溶液在凝集时出现不均匀的现象。

(2)过火时间不能过长,否则琼脂凝胶会熔化。

[实验报告]

(1)简述双向琼脂扩散试验的原理与方法。

(2)画出试验结果,包括沉淀线的位置、形状和粗细。

(3)判断抗原、抗体的相对浓度和相对分子质量。

[思考题]

(1)相比于单向琼脂扩散,双向琼脂扩散有何优势?

(2)如何加快双向琼脂扩散试验的速度?

(潘兴元 蔺志杰)

实验六 PCR-SSP 法检测 HLA-A*02 基因

[实验目的]

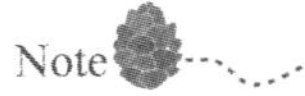

(1)掌握 PCR-SSP 法检测 HLA-A*02 基因的原理与方法。

(2)通过实验结果,加深对人类白细胞抗原(HLA)多态性的理解。

[实验器材]

(1)引物(表 1-6-1)。

表 1-6-1　引物序列及产物长度

引物	序列	产物长度
HLA-A* 02 特异性 5′ 端引物	5′-TCCTCGTCCCCAGGCTCT-3′	813 bp
HLA-A* 02 特异性 3′ 端引物	5′-GTGGCCCCTGGTACCCGT-3′	
内参 5′ 端引物	5′-ATGATGTTGACCTTTCCAGGG-3′	256 bp
内参 3′ 端引物	5′-ATTCTGTAACTTTTCATCAGTTGC-3′	

(2)健康体检者外周血、全血样本直接 PCR 试剂盒、TAE 缓冲液、GoldView Ⅱ型核酸染色剂(索莱宝)、DNA 分子量标准(marker)等。

(3)PCR 仪、离心机、JY-SPDT 水平电泳槽、移液器、一次性 PE 手套等。

[实验内容]

1. 原理　HLA 系统是人体多态性最高的系统,其对人体的疾病易感性以及器官移植结果有重要影响。随着技术的进步,已鉴定出的 HLA 类型越来越多,传统的血清学检测技术无法满足临床的需求,目前 HLA 分型主要采用 PCR 技术。

HLA-A* 02 在汉族人群中出现的比例很高,是肿瘤和器官移植研究的热点之一。本实验采用最基础的低分辨率 PCR-SSP 分型技术检测人群中 HLA-A* 02 等位基因的比例,而在临床和科研中往往需要进行更加精细的 PCR 分型。

2. 方法

(1)PCR 反应体系(25 μl):如表 1-6-2 所示。

表 1-6-2　PCR 反应体系

组分	体积/μl
血液样本(外周血)	3
5′端引物(10 μmol/L)	1
3′端引物(10 μmol/L)	1
2×PCR 缓冲液	12.5
DNA 聚合酶	0.5
水	7

(2)PCR 条件:95 ℃预变性 5 min,然后 95 ℃变性 30 s,60 ℃退火 30 s,72 ℃延伸 90 s,共 30 个循环。

(3)PCR 产物检测:用 1×TAE 缓冲液配制含 0.02% GoldView Ⅱ型核酸染色剂的 2%琼脂糖凝胶,将 PCR 反应产物于 1000g 离心 2 min 以沉淀血细胞碎片,取 15 μl 上清液点样,5 V/cm 稳压电泳 25 min。

[注意事项]

(1)吸血样时避免吸取血液凝块。

(2)本实验涉及人源血液成分，应严格遵守污染物处理程序。

[实验报告]

(1)简述 PCR-SSP 法检测 HLA-A* 02 基因的原理与方法。
(2)粘贴电泳图，报告样品是否呈 HLA-A* 02 基因阳性。

[思考题]

(1)HLA 数据对国家安全有何意义?
(2)该实验有可能出现假阴性结果吗？请每个小组推荐一个合适的阳性对照。
(3)汇总全班的数据，推算扬州地区人群中 HLA-A* 02 等位基因频率。

(潘兴元　蔡良良)

实验七　利用 SPA 亲和层析法分离纯化 IgG 抗体

[实验目的]

(1)掌握 SPA 亲和层析法的原理与方法。
(2)从人血清中分离纯化出高纯度的 IgG 抗体。

[实验器材]

(1)SPA-琼脂糖凝胶 4B、健康体检者血清、生理盐水、pH 3.2 甘氨酸-盐酸缓冲液、0.1 mol/L $NaHCO_3$溶液、7 mol/L 尿素溶液、PBS 等。

(2)2 cm×10 cm 层析柱、751 分光光度计、蠕动泵、通用电源、小型垂直电泳槽等。

[实验内容]

1. 原理　亲和层析是利用生物高分子与配体可逆结合的原理，将配体通过共价键牢固结合于载体上而制得的层析系统。利用抗原、抗体之间高特异性的亲和力进行分离的方法称为免疫亲和层析，它通常只需经过一步处理即可使某种待提纯的蛋白质从很复杂的蛋白质混合物中分离出来，而且纯度很高。

琼脂糖凝胶 4B 是一种常用于亲和层析的琼脂糖凝胶过滤填料，分离范围为 6 万～200 万 Da，工作 pH 为 4～9，适用于多种生物大分子的分离纯化。SPA 是一种分离自金黄色葡萄球菌的细胞壁蛋白质，主要通过 Fc 片段与哺乳动物 IgG 结合，而不影响 Fab 片段与抗原的结合，其与不同 IgG 亚类的结合力存在差异，改变 pH 及离子强度可洗脱结合于层析柱上的 IgG 或不同的 IgG 亚类。偶联有 SPA 的琼脂糖凝胶 4B 可直接纯化血清或小鼠腹水中的 IgG 抗体，并获得高纯度产物。

2. 方法

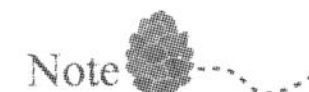

(1)装柱：将充分溶胀的 SPA-琼脂糖凝胶 4B 倒入 2 cm×10 cm 层析柱中，自然沉降后用 10 倍以上柱体积的生理盐水充分平衡。

(2)上样:用生理盐水将血清稀释5倍,按25～30 mg IgG/g湿胶比例加样,室温作用15 min。用生理盐水洗脱,流速为20 ml/h。SPA将IgG吸附在层析柱上,其他蛋白质随洗脱液流出,洗脱至洗脱液的$OD_{280}<0.02$为止。

(3)洗脱:用pH 3.2甘氨酸-盐酸缓冲液进行洗脱,将洗脱下来的蛋白液迅速用0.1 mol/L $NaHCO_3$溶液中和至pH 7,此即为提纯的IgG。

(4)纯度鉴定:取10 μl纯化的IgG进行SDS-PAGE电泳,以稀释血清作为对照检查纯化效果。

(5)再生:用10倍柱体积的7 mol/L尿素溶液洗柱后,再用10倍柱体积的生理盐水洗涤,最后用PBS平衡。

[注意事项]

(1)SPA-琼脂糖凝胶4B较为昂贵,必要时样品可以先离心以除去杂质,再用0.22 μm滤膜过滤,以保护层析柱。

(2)装柱前要使凝胶充分悬浮,一次性装柱,避免多次装柱形成截痕,影响纯化效果。

(3)凝胶再生后加入终浓度为0.02%的NaN_3溶液于4 ℃储存,可反复使用10～20次。

(4)本实验涉及人源血液成分,应严格遵守污染物处理程序。

[实验报告]

(1)写出SPA亲和层析的原理与方法。

(2)粘贴电泳图并分析纯化效果。

[思考题]

SPA亲和层析在疫苗研发中有何作用?

(潘兴元　蔡良良)

实验八　人血清总IgE检测

[实验目的]

掌握用ELISA法定量检测血清中总IgE的原理与方法。

[实验器材]

(1)阴性和阳性对照、标本稀释液、酶结合物、标准品(10 IU/ml、50 IU/ml、100 IU/ml、200 IU/ml、400 IU/ml)、30×浓缩洗液、显色液(A/B)、终止液(2 mol/L H_2SO_4溶液)等。

(2)预包被反应板、酶标仪、振荡器、吸水纸等。

[实验内容]

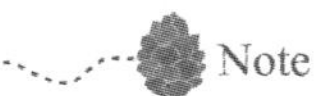

1. 原理　IgE在血清中的浓度极低,约占免疫球蛋白的0.02%,主要存在于皮肤、黏膜中,一

般认为由鼻咽、扁桃体、支气管、胃肠道黏膜基底的浆细胞产生，能与肥大细胞及血液中的嗜碱性粒细胞结合。过敏原与结合在细胞上的 IgE 发生作用后，就会促使细胞脱颗粒，释放组胺，从而引发变态反应，如血清病、季节性过敏性鼻炎等。IgE 增高常见于过敏性哮喘、寄生虫感染、药物过敏、IgE 型骨髓瘤、肝脏疾病、系统性红斑狼疮、类风湿性关节炎等。IgE 降低则常见于共济失调毛细血管扩张症、无丙种球蛋白血症、非 IgE 型骨髓瘤、慢性淋巴性白血病、免疫功能不全等。

本实验采用双抗夹心 ELISA 法，利用亲和素将生物素化的抗人 IgE 单克隆抗体 A 预包被在反应板上，最大限度保持抗体 A 的免疫学活性，配以 HRP 标记的抗人 IgE 单克隆抗体 B 作为标志物，可以定量检测人血清总 IgE 水平。加入底物 TMB 显色后在 450 nm 波长处测各孔 OD 值，OD_{450} 值与待检抗体含量成正比。

2. 方法

(1)加样：先在各反应孔中加入 80 μl 标本稀释液，再加入 20 μl 不同浓度的标准品及待检标本。设置阴性及阳性对照孔（每孔 100 μl，不稀释）和空白孔（加入 100 μl 标本稀释液）各 1 孔。

(2)37 ℃温育 60 min。甩去孔内液体，用洗涤液洗板 3 次并在吸水纸上拍干。

(3)加入酶结合物：每孔加入 2 滴（或 100 μl），混匀后置于 37 ℃温育 30 min。同上法洗涤 3 次并在吸水纸上拍干。

(4)显色：每孔各加入 1 滴（或 50 μl）显色液 A 和 B，轻拍混匀（或振荡器混匀）后置于 37 ℃温育 10 min。

(5)测定吸光度：每孔加入 1 滴（或 50 μl）终止液，混匀后于 450 nm 下测定各孔 OD 值。

(6)以 5 支标准品的 OD 值为纵坐标，浓度（10 IU/ml、50 IU/ml、100 IU/ml、200 IU/ml、400 IU/ml）为横坐标，绘标准曲线。待检标本的 OD 值在标准曲线上所对应的浓度即为该标本中 IgE 的实际含量。

3. 参考值 本方法测得的正常人外周血血清中总 IgE 含量为 20～200 IU/ml。待检标本中总 IgE 含量大于 200 IU/ml 表示总 IgE 升高，与过敏有关；小于 200 IU/ml 表示总 IgE 在正常范围内。

[注意事项]

(1)滴加试剂前，应将滴瓶翻转数次混匀，滴加试剂时保持瓶身垂直。

(2)洗板时每孔均须加满洗涤液，以防孔内的游离酶无法被洗净。

(3)建议标准品做双孔，取 OD 值均值。

(4)待检标本的总 IgE 含量大于 400 IU/ml 时呈非线性，需要对标本进行适当稀释才能获得准确值。

(5)本实验涉及人源血液成分，应严格遵守污染物处理程序。

[实验报告]

(1)写出用 ELISA 法定量检测血清中总 IgE 的原理与方法。

(2)根据标准曲线，计算样品中 IgE 的含量。

[思考题]

有些人的血清 IgE 水平远高于正常人，你知道任何可能的免疫学机制吗？

Note

（潘兴元　蔺志杰）

第二篇　病原生物学基础实验

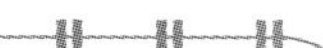

实验一　细菌的生理

[实验目的]

(1)掌握不同培养基中细菌的接种方法。

(2)熟悉常用细菌培养基的配制方法及细菌在不同培养基中的生长现象。

(3)了解细菌常用生化反应及其在细菌鉴定过程中的意义。

[实验器材]

(1)平板、斜面、固体、半固体、液体等细菌培养基。

(2)细菌的琼脂斜面培养物。

(3)葡萄糖发酵管、乳糖发酵管、蛋白胨水培养基、醋酸铅培养基、尿素培养基、普通琼脂平板培养基等。

(4)吲哚试剂(柯氏试剂)、甲基红试剂、VP 试剂。

(5)无菌棉拭子、接种环、接种针、生理盐水、酒精灯、恒温培养箱等。

[实验内容]

1. 细菌培养基的配制

(1)肉汤/液体培养基:可用于一般细菌培养或增菌培养,也可用于制备糖发酵管及琼脂培养基。

①分别称取 3～5 g 酵母粉、10 g 蛋白胨、5 g 氯化钠溶于 900 ml 蒸馏水中,搅拌使其充分溶解。

②调节 pH 至 7.4～7.6,定容到 1000 ml。

③分装于适当容器内,于 121 ℃、103 kPa 高压灭菌 20 min,无菌检测后,存放于 4 ℃冰箱备用。

(2)普通琼脂培养基:可用于一般细菌分离培养,也可用作无糖培养基。

①称取 4.5 g 琼脂粉溶于 1000 ml 肉汤培养基中。

②调节 pH 至 7.6,于 121 ℃、103 kPa 高压灭菌 20 min。

③待琼脂冷却到 50～60 ℃,若将其分装于无菌试管内,倾斜放置,凝固后即制备成琼脂斜面培养基;若倒入无菌培养皿内,待其凝固后即制备成琼脂平板培养基。无菌检测后,置于 4 ℃冰箱备用。

注意:琼脂平板培养基需倒置存放,既便于取放,又可避免水分蒸发和保持无菌状态。

(3)半固体琼脂培养基:可用于保存一般菌种或菌种的短途运输,也可用于检测细菌的动力。

①称取 0.25～0.5 g 琼脂粉溶于 100 ml 肉汤培养基中。

②于 121 ℃、103 kPa 高压灭菌 20 min。

③在琼脂凝固前分装于试管内，直立放置，待琼脂凝固后即成半固体琼脂培养基。无菌检测后，置于 4 ℃冰箱备用。

(4)血琼脂培养基：用于培养和分离营养要求较高的病原菌。

①取 100 ml 高压灭菌后的普通琼脂培养基(pH 7.6)冷却至 50～55 ℃，以无菌操作技术加入 8～10 ml 无菌脱纤维羊血或兔血(临用前置于 37 ℃培养箱中预温 30 min)，轻轻摇匀(防止产生气泡)，倾注于灭菌培养皿内或分装于试管内，制备成血琼脂平板培养基或血琼脂斜面培养基。

②待培养基凝固后，随机选取部分培养基于 37 ℃无菌培养 18～24 h，培养基上无细菌生长即可使用或保存于 4 ℃冰箱备用。

2. 细菌的接种方法 细菌在自然界及人体中分布广、种类多，因此在临床上检测各种标本中是否存在某种病原菌时，须先对不同细菌进行分离，以获得某种病原菌，此过程称为细菌的分离培养。

(1)平板分区划线法：该方法主要用于含菌量较多的标本，如粪便、脓液等标本的分离与纯化。

①右手持接种环(握铅笔/毛笔样姿势)，用酒精灯外焰烧灼接种环和金属杆，待接种环冷却后(判断接种环是否冷却的方法：等待 3～5 s，先用接种环触碰平板培养基的边缘空白处，若琼脂未熔化，则提示接种环已冷却)，用接种环轻轻触碰待测标本。

②左手托起琼脂平板，在靠近酒精灯火焰处打开；右手持沾菌的接种环，使接种环面与琼脂平板表面成 30°～40°角；在琼脂平板上来回密集划线，线与线之间无交叉。划线时以指力在平板面上做轻快的滑移，接种环不应嵌入培养基内。

③烧灼接种环，杀灭接种环上残留的细菌，待接种环冷却后进行第二区划线，接种环与第一区接触 1～2 次，先连续划线再单独划线，划线面积占平板总面积的 1/5～1/4；第二区划线完毕后，用火焰烧灼接种环灭菌，再以同样的方法进行第三区、第四区划线。

④划线完毕，将接种环灭菌后放回原处，盖上平板盖。做好标记后将平板倒置(避免培养过程中凝结水自平板盖滴下而冲散菌落)放入 37 ℃培养箱中培养。

⑤培养 18～24 h 后取出，观察琼脂平板表面形成的各种菌落，注意观察其大小、形状、边缘、透明度、颜色等性状。

平板分区划线法示意图见图 2-1-1。

(2)平板连续划线法：该方法主要用于含菌量较少的标本，如咽拭子标本、脑脊液标本等。

①右手持接种环(握铅笔/毛笔样姿势)，用酒精灯外焰烧灼接种环和金属杆，待冷却(等待 3～5 s)，用接种环轻轻触碰待测标本。

②左手托起琼脂平板，在靠近酒精灯火焰处打开。将标本涂布于培养基的 1/5 处，然后用接种环或直接用咽拭子在平板上连续划线并逐渐下移，直至划满平板表面。

平板连续划线法示意图见图 2-1-2。

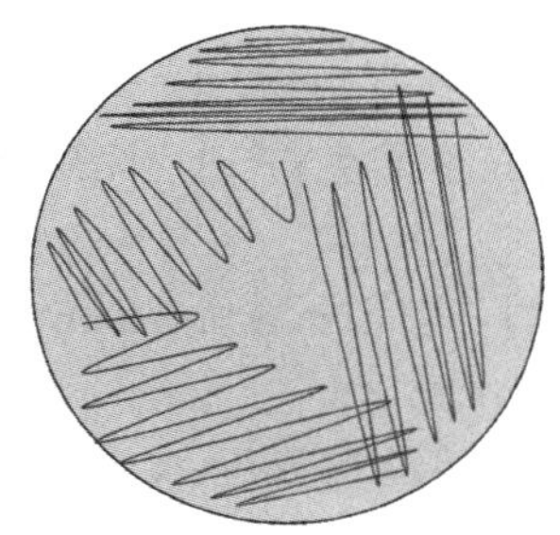

图 2-1-1 平板分区划线法示意图

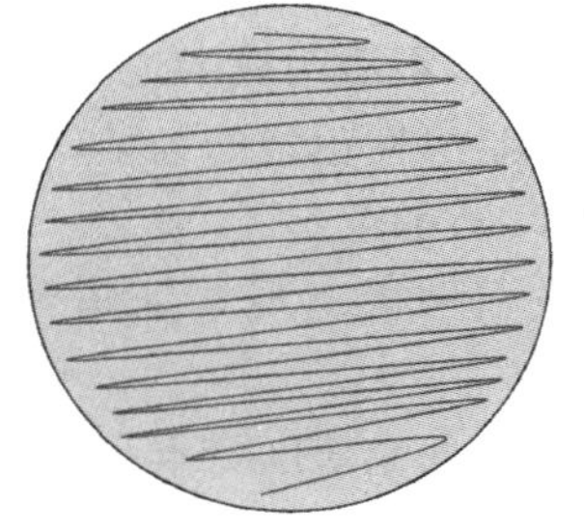

图 2-1-2 平板连续划线法示意图

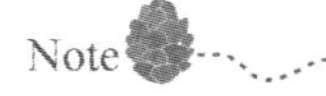

(3)斜面培养基接种法:该方法主要用于纯种培养、菌种保存等。

①用左手拇指和食指、中指和无名指分别握持菌种管与待接种的培养基管,使菌种管位于左侧、培养基管位于右侧。培养基斜面向上,勿成水平位,以免管底凝结水浸润培养基表面,甚至沾湿胶塞。

②右手拇指和食指分别拧松两试管的胶塞,以便于接种时拔取。

③右手持接种环,将欲伸入试管内的接种杆部分迅速通过酒精灯火焰 2～3 次,以杀灭表面的杂菌。灭菌过的接种环勿再碰及他物。

④以右手手掌与小指、小指与无名指分别拔取并夹持两试管的胶塞,将两试管管口迅速通过酒精灯火焰数次进行灭菌。

⑤将接种环伸入菌种管,从斜面上挑取少许菌苔后缓慢退出菌种管,再伸进待接种的培养基管,自斜面底部向顶端轻轻划一直线,再由底部向上蜿蜒划线。注意操作过程中勿划破培养基表面,沾菌的接种环进出试管时,勿触及试管内壁。

⑥接种完毕,将接种环灭菌后放回原处;将两试管管口迅速通过酒精灯火焰 2～3 次,塞回胶塞,将培养基管置于 37 ℃培养 18～24 h 后观察细菌生长情况。

(4)半固体培养基接种法(穿刺接种法):该方法主要用于动力试验、菌种保存等。

①左手同斜面培养基接种法握持菌种管及半固体琼脂培养基管。

②右手握接种针,灭菌冷却后将其伸入菌种管挑取少量菌苔后退出,再垂直刺入待接种的半固体琼脂培养基管的中心直至接近管底(勿触及管底),然后沿原路退出。

③接种完毕,将接种环灭菌后放回原处;塞好胶塞,将半固体琼脂培养基管放于 37 ℃培养 18～24 h 后观察细菌生长情况。

(5)液体培养基接种法:该方法主要用于纯种培养、生化试验等。

①左手同斜面培养基接种法握持菌种管及液体培养基管。

②右手握接种环,灭菌冷却后将其伸入菌种管挑取少量菌苔后退出,再伸入待接种的液体培养基管;在接近液面的管壁上轻轻磨研,可蘸取少许液体培养基调和,使细菌混合于液体培养基中。

③接种完毕,将接种环灭菌后放回原处;塞好胶塞,将液体培养基管放于 37 ℃培养 18～24 h 后观察细菌生长情况。

3. 细菌培养性状的观察

(1)细菌在固体培养基上的培养特征。

在固体培养基上,细菌经分裂增殖后形成的细菌集团称为菌落。菌落融合在一起形成菌苔。不同细菌的菌落各有特点,观察菌落时应注意如下几点。

①大小:以直径(mm)表示,1 mm 左右为小菌落,2～3 mm 为中等大小菌落,3 mm 以上为大菌落。

②形状:圆形及不规则形。

③边缘:整齐或不整齐。

④表面:凸起、凹陷、平坦、光滑、粗糙、干燥、湿润等。

⑤透明度:透明、不透明或半透明。

⑥颜色:产生脂溶性色素的细菌,菌落本身有颜色,培养基无色;产生水溶性色素的细菌,菌落及周围培养基均有颜色。

⑦溶血性:在血平板上观察细菌对红细胞的溶解作用,有完全溶血、不完全溶血及不溶血之分。

⑧菌落类型:根据菌落的特点可分为光滑型菌落(S 型)、粗糙型菌落(R 型)和黏液型菌落(M 型)。光滑型菌落呈圆形,表面光滑、湿润,边缘整齐、透明,粗糙型菌落则相反;黏液型菌落表面湿润,有黏性。

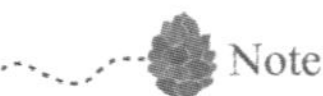

(2)细菌在半固体培养基中的培养特征。

半固体培养基可用于观察细菌有无动力:无动力细菌经穿刺培养后,细菌沿穿刺线生长,培养基清亮,此为线状生长;有动力的细菌沿穿刺线向外散开生长,故穿刺线模糊不清,培养基变混浊,此为混浊生长。

(3)细菌在液体培养基中的培养特征。

①混浊生长:培养基呈均匀混浊或颗粒混浊,如葡萄球菌、大肠埃希菌等。

②表面生长:培养基表面有平滑或皱褶状的菌膜,或呈"钟乳石"状下沉等,如枯草杆菌、结核分枝杆菌等。

③沉淀生长:培养基澄清,试管底部有菌体沉淀等现象,如链球菌等。

4. 生化试验结果观察

(1)糖发酵试验。

①原理:不同种类细菌含有发酵不同糖(醇、苷)类的酶,因而对各种糖(醇、苷)类的代谢能力不同,其代谢产物也不同。该试验根据细菌分解培养基中糖(醇、苷)后产酸,或产酸、产气的能力鉴定细菌种类。在培养基中加入一定量的指示剂并放入一支倒置的试管,糖的终浓度为0.5%～1%。接种细菌并孵育一段时间后,若该细菌具有分解某种糖的酶,则其分解糖产酸就会使指示剂变色。指示剂为甲基红则变成红色,为溴甲酚紫则呈黄色。若有气体生成,则倒置的试管中有气泡生成。绝大多数细菌能利用糖类作为碳源和能源,但是它们在分解糖的能力上存在很大差异:有些细菌能分解多种糖类产酸并产气,有些只产酸不产气。例如,大肠埃希菌能分解乳糖和葡萄糖产酸并产气;伤寒杆菌能分解葡萄糖产酸但不产气,不能分解乳糖;普通变形杆菌能分解葡萄糖产酸并产气,不能分解乳糖。

②方法:将伤寒杆菌、大肠埃希菌和普通变形杆菌分别接种于两种糖发酵管中,37 ℃培养18～24 h后观察结果。

③结果:培养基未变色,倒置的试管内无气泡,表明不产酸不产气,糖未被分解,实验结果以"－"表示;培养基变红(或黄),倒置的试管内无气泡,表明产酸不产气,实验结果以"＋"表示;培养基变红(或黄),倒置的试管内有气泡,表明产酸产气,实验结果以"⊕"表示。

(2)VP试验。

①原理:某些细菌分解葡萄糖产生丙酮酸,丙酮酸进一步脱羧生成中性的乙酰甲基甲醇,后者在碱性条件下可被氧化成二乙酰,二乙酰与蛋白胨中精氨酸的胍基作用,生成红色化合物,即VP试验阳性。

②方法:将大肠埃希菌和伤寒杆菌分别接种于蛋白胨水培养基中,37 ℃培养18～24 h后分别加入VP试剂,混匀后静置观察。

③结果:试剂呈红色为VP试验阳性,试剂呈黄色或类似铜色为VP试验阴性。

(3)甲基红(MR)试验。

①原理:某些细菌分解葡萄糖产生丙酮酸,丙酮酸进一步分解成甲酸、醋酸、乳酸等,使培养基pH＜4.5,甲基红指示剂呈红色;若丙酮酸进一步脱羧生成中性的乙酰甲基甲醇,则培养基pH＞5.4,甲基红指示剂呈橘黄色。

②方法:将大肠埃希菌和伤寒杆菌分别接种于蛋白胨水培养基中,37 ℃培养18～24 h后分别加数滴甲基红指示剂,观察培养液颜色变化。

③结果:培养液呈红色为阳性结果,呈橘红色为弱阳性结果,呈橘黄色为阴性结果。试验结果若呈阴性,应继续培养细菌4～5 d后再次进行试验。

(4)吲哚(indole)试验。

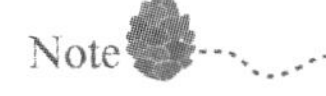

①原理:有些细菌具有色氨酸酶,能分解蛋白胨中的色氨酸形成吲哚。吲哚无色,不易直接观察,若加入柯氏试剂,试剂中的对二甲氨基苯甲醛与吲哚作用后可形成红色的玫瑰吲哚。

②方法:将大肠埃希菌和伤寒杆菌分别接种于蛋白胨水培养基中,37 ℃培养 18～24 h;每管中加入数滴柯氏试剂,使之于液面上形成一薄层,轻轻摇动试管观察颜色变化。

③结果:表层试剂呈红色为阳性结果,呈黄色为阴性结果。

(5)硫化氢试验。

①原理:某些细菌能分解培养基中的含硫氨基酸生成硫化氢;硫化氢遇亚铁离子(如硫酸亚铁)或铅离子(如醋酸铅),则形成黑褐色的硫化亚铁或硫化铅沉淀物;黑褐色沉淀物越多,表明生成的硫化氢越多。硫化氢试验使用的培养基中含有硫代硫酸钠,它是一种还原剂,能保持还原环境而使形成的硫化氢不再被氧化。

②方法:分别贴着试管内壁穿刺接种大肠埃希菌、普通变形杆菌于醋酸铅培养基中,37 ℃培养 18～24 h 后观察穿刺线处颜色变化。

③结果:穿刺线处呈黑褐色为阳性结果,无黑褐色为阴性结果。

(6)尿素酶试验。

①原理:具有尿素酶的细菌可分解尿素产生氨,在培养基中形成碳酸铵,使培养基呈碱性,酚红指示剂在此环境下变成红色。

②方法:将大肠埃希菌、普通变形杆菌分别接种于尿素培养基上,37 ℃培养 18～24 h 后观察培养基颜色变化。

③结果:培养基变成红色为阳性结果,变成黄色为阴性结果。

(7)枸橼酸盐试验。

①原理:某些细菌利用枸橼酸盐作为唯一碳源,可分解枸橼酸盐生成碳酸盐,并分解培养基中的铵盐生成氨,使培养基呈碱性,溴麝香草酚蓝指示剂在该环境中由淡绿色变为深蓝色。

②方法:将大肠埃希菌和产气肠杆菌分别接种于枸橼酸钠琼脂斜面上,37 ℃培养 24～48 h 后观察培养基颜色变化。

③结果:培养基变为深蓝色为阳性结果;若培养 7 d 后,培养基仍不变色,则为阴性结果。

(8)数码分类鉴定系统。

①原理:a. 数据库,由许多细菌条目组成,每个条目代表一个细菌种或一个细菌生物型。b. 编码,将细菌生化反应模式转换成数字模式,将生化反应结果快速转录成数字(编码),经查阅编码检索本或计算机分析系统又可将数字转化成相应的细菌名称。c. 查码,在编码检索本内查找数码信息,如菌名、鉴定结果评价、生化结果、阳性百分率、必须增加的补充试验项目、注意事项等。d. 解释,如果一个编码只对应一种细菌,无论概率大小,则为该种细菌的可能性(ID%)均为 99.99%。如果一个编码对应两种或两种以上种类的细菌,应计算每种细菌出现的可能性。如 ID%≥99%,为该种细菌的可能性非常大;如 90%≤ID%<99%,为该种细菌的可能性较大;如 80%≤ID%<90%,为该种细菌的可能性也较大,但需做补充试验进一步确证;如 ID%<80%,则一般无法准确区分菌种,必须增加多个补充试验才可得出准确结果。

②组成:a. 鉴定卡,常用的生化反应有发酵试验、同化试验、同化或发酵抑制试验、酶试验等。b. 添加试剂,有些试验经孵育后需添加试剂才能呈现颜色变化;添加的试剂可以是配套试剂盒,也可以是单种试剂。c. 检索工具,由计算机自动处理并报告。

(9)自动化细菌鉴定系统。

自动化细菌鉴定系统是将光电技术、计算机技术和细菌数码鉴定相结合的系统。该系统大大改进了传统的细菌检测方法,为临床提供较传统人工检测更翔实的检测数据。自动化细菌鉴定系统有 MicroScan、Vitek-AMS 和 PHOENIX™100 等。现以 MicroScan 自动化细菌鉴定系统为例,进行简要介绍。

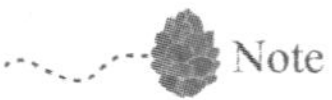

①原理:采用光电比色法测定细菌分解底物导致 pH 改变而产生的不同颜色;利用 8 进位制细菌数码鉴定原理,经矩阵分析获得最后的鉴定结果;部分鉴定系统因使用荧光技术而使鉴定速

度提高 4～8 倍。MicroScan 是目前普遍使用的鉴定系统，可鉴定近 500 种细菌，且有良好的计算机界面，为感染性疾病的诊断和治疗提供了准确和方便的检验方法；它还可以利用软件的统计功能，统计不同标本菌株的检出率、每月病房分离菌株的趋势，以及不同菌株的分离率等。

②方法：采用平板分区划线法将待检标本接种于适当的培养基后进行革兰染色和镜检。用定量取菌针采集 1～3 个菌落加入菌种稀释液中；将稀释好的菌悬液倾注于分注槽内；用真空接种器安装好 96 孔接种板，从分注槽内吸取菌悬液；将菌悬液加入相应反应板；将反应板置于主机内反应板位。仪器可自动保温、加试剂、判读和处理结果。

③结果：系统可自动打印报告。当结果中产生异常情况时，可启动提示系统，重要提示将会出现在报告中，供临床医生和检验医生参考。

[实验报告]

(1)画出细菌在平板、斜面、半固体、液体培养基中的培养结果。
(2)写出生化代谢原理并画出不同细菌生化代谢的结果。

[思考题]

(1)配制不同培养基时应注意哪些问题？如何从含有大量杂菌的标本中分离出可疑的病原菌？
(2)用不同方法接种时，如何更好地保证菌种不被污染？接种后的平板为什么要倒置培养？
(3)常用哪些生化试验来鉴定大肠埃希菌与产气肠杆菌？
(4)所有细菌都可以成功培养吗？所有病原菌都可以被分离和培养吗？

（孔桂美　高成凤）

实验二　细菌分布及外界因素对细菌的影响

[实验目的]

(1)掌握常用消毒灭菌方法。
(2)掌握纸片琼脂扩散法检测细菌对药物的敏感性的步骤。
(3)掌握药物最低抑菌浓度和最低杀菌浓度检测方法。
(4)了解细菌分布情况及其检查方法，树立无菌操作观念。

[实验材料]

(1)LB 琼脂平板、LB 液体培养基、庆大霉素。
(2)金黄色葡萄球菌、沙门菌。
(3)酒精灯、接种环、镊子、药敏纸片、无菌黑纸片、紫外线灯等。

[实验内容]

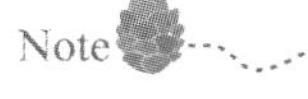

1. 空气及手指皮肤的细菌检查

(1)原理：空气和人体表寄生着大量微生物，采集样本经培养后可以长出菌落，而经过消毒后的样本,菌落数量显著减少。

(2)方法。

①取 5 个无菌 LB 琼脂平板,分别放置于 10 m^2 房间的四个角及中间,打开皿盖放置 30 min 后盖好皿盖,于 37 ℃培养 24 h 后观察细菌生长情况。

②取 2 个无菌 LB 琼脂平板,将未经消毒的手指在其中 1 个 LB 琼脂平板表面进行涂抹,然后用 2%碘酊棉球消毒该手指,再用 75%酒精脱碘,然后在另 1 个 LB 琼脂平板表面进行涂抹,37 ℃培养 24 h 后观察结果。

(3)结果:培养基表面生长有多种大小、形态及颜色不同的菌落。注意区分手指消毒前、后的细菌生长情况。

2. 紫外线杀菌试验

(1)原理:波长为 210～310 nm 的紫外线具有杀菌能力,其中以 260 nm 紫外线的杀菌能力最强。紫外线可通过诱导胸腺嘧啶二聚体的形成,抑制细菌 DNA 的复制,从而发挥杀菌作用。

(2)方法。

①用接种环蘸取金黄色葡萄球菌菌液,在 LB 琼脂平板上连续划线。

②打开皿盖,用无菌镊夹取无菌黑纸片放置在 LB 琼脂平板中间,将平板放置在距紫外线灯 1.2 m 的范围内照射 30 min。然后用无菌镊揭去黑纸片并烧毁,盖好皿盖,37 ℃培养 24 h 后观察细菌生长情况。

(3)结果:黑纸片遮盖的培养基表面有细菌生长,而未遮盖的培养基表面无细菌生长,表明细菌已被杀死。

(4)注意事项。

①紫外线穿透力不强,仅适用于无菌室、手术室内的空气及物体表面的灭菌。

②紫外线灯距离被照射物不可超过 1.2 m。

3. 纸片琼脂扩散法检测细菌对药物的敏感性

(1)原理:将含有定量抗菌药物的药敏纸片贴在已接种细菌的琼脂平板上,药敏纸片中所含的药物被琼脂中的水分溶解后,在药敏纸片周围会形成递减的药物浓度梯度。在纸片周围的抑菌浓度范围内,细菌的生长受到抑制,从而形成抑菌圈。抑菌圈的大小可反映细菌对抗菌药物的敏感性。

(2)方法。

①取琼脂平板 2 个,在底部注明金黄色葡萄球菌及沙门菌。

②将两种菌液分别连续划线接种于上述琼脂平板表面。

③用无菌镊夹取药敏纸片,分别贴于涂有细菌的琼脂平板表面。

④置 37 ℃培养 18～24 h 后,观察药敏纸片周围抑菌圈的情况,并比较抑菌圈的大小,判断细菌对药物的敏感性。

(3)结果:用游标卡尺测量抑菌圈直径。查表 2-2-1 和表 2-2-2 即可得出该菌对药物的敏感性,即敏感(S)、中度敏感(I)、耐药(R)。

表 2-2-1　肠杆菌科细菌的抑菌圈直径判读标准

抗生素	每张药敏纸片含药量/μg	抑菌圈直径/mm		
		耐药	中度敏感	敏感
氨苄西林	10	≤13	14～16	≥17
链霉素	10	≤11	12～14	≥15
庆大霉素	10	≤12	13～14	≥15

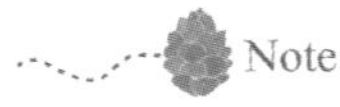

续表

抗生素	每张药敏纸片含药量/μg	抑菌圈直径/mm		
		耐药	中度敏感	敏感
四环素	30	≤11	12～14	≥15
卡那霉素	30	≤13	14～17	≥18
氯霉素	30	≤12	13～17	≥18
磺胺类药	250/300	≤12	13～16	≥17

表 2-2-2　葡萄球菌科细菌的抑菌圈直径判读标准

抗生素	每张药敏纸片含药量/μg	抑菌圈直径/mm		
		耐药	中度敏感	敏感
苯唑西林	30	≤21	—	≥22
庆大霉素	10	≤12	13～14	≥15
红霉素	15	≤13	14～22	≥23
四环素	30	≤14	15～18	≥19
氯霉素	30	≤12	13～17	≥18
磺胺类药	250/300	≤12	13～16	≥17

(4)意义：药敏试验适用于了解病原微生物对各种抗生素的敏感性，以指导临床合理用药。

(5)注意事项：不同细菌对同一种抗生素的敏感性的判定标准不同。

4. 检测药物最低抑菌浓度和最低杀菌浓度

(1)原理：用液体培养基对药物进行倍比稀释，依次装入 1.5 ml EP 管中，然后将细菌接种到 EP 管中，培养 24 h 后，观察各 EP 管中细菌生长情况，得出药物最低抑菌浓度(minimum inhibitory concentration，MIC)。

(2)方法。

①取 12 个无菌 EP 管，标记为 1～12(第 11 管为无菌阴性对照，第 12 管为有菌阳性对照)。

②每管各加入 500 μl LB 液体培养基。

③第 1 管中加入 500 μl 800 μg/ml 庆大霉素，混匀后吸取 500 μl 至第 2 管，依次稀释至第 11 管。

④第 1～10 管和第 12 管，每管各加入 500 μl LB 液体培养基和 50 μl 浓度为 5×10^5 CFU/ml 的沙门菌液。

⑤37 ℃培养 18～24 h 后观察结果。

(3)结果：试验正常时，第 11 管应无菌生长，第 12 管应有菌生长，观察其他 EP 管中细菌生长情况。

最低抑菌浓度的判定：培养 18～24 h 后，EP 管中培养基澄明，摇匀后仍澄明，则认为该管无菌生长；若 EP 管中培养基浑浊，则表明该管有菌生长。EP 管中无菌生长的最低药物浓度即为最低抑菌浓度。

最低杀菌浓度的检测：当药物浓度略高于最低抑菌浓度时，药物的抑菌作用是不可逆的，称为杀菌作用。依次从未见细菌生长的 EP 管中吸取 0.1 ml 培养物接种于琼脂平板上，37 ℃培养 18～24 h，以平板上菌落数小于 5 个的最大稀释度的药物浓度为最低杀菌浓度。

(4)注意事项。

①最低抑菌浓度和最低杀菌浓度的单位以 μg/ml 表示。

②最低抑菌浓度与最低杀菌浓度可以相同，也可以不同。

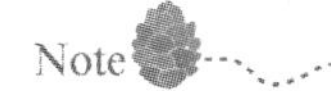

[实验报告]

(1)画出空气和手指细菌检测结果。
(2)画出紫外线杀菌结果。
(3)画出药敏试验结果。
(4)写出最低抑菌浓度和最低杀菌浓度。

[思考题]

(1)紫外线杀菌的主要原理是什么?操作过程中应注意哪些问题?有何实际意义?
(2)药敏试验的主要原理是什么?操作过程中应注意哪些问题?有何实际意义?
(3)最低抑菌浓度和最低杀菌浓度的判定标准是什么?
(4)你认为抗菌药物使用中可能存在哪些问题?这些问题与细菌耐药性之间的关系是怎样的?
(5)细菌耐药性及耐药机制的研究策略有哪些?

(阴银燕　刘翠翠)

实验三　细菌形态结构的检查

[实验目的]

(1)熟悉细菌的基本形态及结构特点。
(2)掌握革兰染色法的原理与方法。

[实验材料]

(1)示教片。
球菌:葡萄球菌涂片标本。
杆菌:大肠埃希菌涂片标本。
弧菌:霍乱弧菌涂片标本。
荚膜:肺炎球菌荚膜标本。
鞭毛:变形杆菌鞭毛标本。
芽孢:破伤风梭菌芽孢标本。
(2)葡萄球菌、大肠埃希菌琼脂斜面培养物(18～24 h)。
(3)革兰染色试剂:结晶紫、鲁氏碘液、95%酒精和石炭酸复红稀释液。
(4)接种环、载玻片、生理盐水、酒精灯和光学显微镜(油镜)等。

[实验内容]

1. 细菌形态及特殊结构的观察

(1)用油镜观察葡萄球菌、大肠埃希菌和霍乱弧菌的基本形态,比较其形状、大小、排列及染色性。

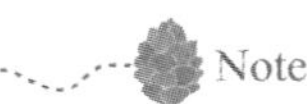

(2)用油镜观察细菌特殊结构：肺炎球菌荚膜的大小、颜色及其与菌体的关系；破伤风梭菌芽孢的形态、位置；变形杆菌鞭毛的形态、数目及位置。

2. 革兰染色法

(1)原理：革兰染色法是1884年由丹麦医师Gram创立的，是细菌学中重要的染色方法之一。该方法可以根据不同的染色特点，将细菌分为革兰阳性菌和革兰阴性菌两大类。一般认为，革兰染色的原理与细菌细胞壁的成分和结构有密切关系。通过结晶紫初染和鲁氏碘液媒染后，细菌细胞壁内形成了不溶于水的结晶紫-碘复合物。革兰阳性菌（如金黄色葡萄球菌）的等电点（pI 2～3）比革兰阴性菌（如大肠埃希菌）的等电点（pI 4）低。在相同pH条件下，革兰阳性菌所带负电荷比革兰阴性菌多，故与带正电荷的结晶紫结合得较牢固；鲁氏碘液中的碘在细菌体内与结晶紫结合后又与革兰阳性菌体内的核糖核酸镁盐-多糖复合物结合，使已着色的细菌不易脱色。革兰阳性菌的细胞壁肽聚糖网层次较多且交联紧密，而脂类物质含量低，当用酒精处理时，由于脱水而引起网状结构的孔径变小、通透性降低，使结晶紫-碘复合物被保留在细菌体内而不易脱色，因此，呈现蓝紫色；革兰阴性菌的细胞壁中肽聚糖含量低，而脂类物质含量高，当用酒精处理时，脂类物质溶解，细胞壁的通透性增加，结晶紫-碘复合物易被酒精抽出而脱色，在下一步复染过程中被染上复红的颜色，呈现红色。

(2)方法。

①涂片标本的制作：取洁净载玻片1张，分为两区，各加入1滴生理盐水，分别加入葡萄球菌和大肠埃希菌少许，混匀。

②初染：加结晶紫2～3滴于涂片上，室温下孵育1 min后，用细流水冲洗，甩干。

③媒染：加鲁氏碘液数滴于涂片上，室温下孵育1 min后，用细流水冲洗，甩干。

④脱色：加95%酒精数滴，轻轻晃动，倾斜涂片，至流下的酒精无紫色为止（时间约30 s），用细流水冲洗，甩干。

⑤复染：加石炭酸复红稀释液数滴。作用30 s后，用细流水冲洗，甩干。

⑥观察：用吸水纸吸干涂片上的水分或自然干燥后，在涂片上加一滴香柏油，用显微镜的油镜（10×100）观察。

(3)结果：染色反应呈紫色者称为革兰阳性菌，染色反应呈红色者称为革兰阴性菌。葡萄球菌为革兰阳性球菌，成堆或呈葡萄串状排列；大肠埃希菌为革兰阴性杆菌，不规则分散排列。

[注意事项]

(1)细菌涂片量适中，涂片不宜太厚或太薄，使菌体分散均匀。

(2)固定时避免菌体过分受热而破坏其形态。

(3)脱色是革兰染色是否成功的关键，脱色时间要根据涂片厚薄灵活掌握，脱色不够易造成假阳性结果，脱色过度易造成假阴性结果。

[实验报告]

(1)画出油镜下你所观察到的细菌基本形态及特殊结构。

(2)画出油镜下你所观察到的两种细菌革兰染色结果。

[思考题]

(1)革兰染色的主要原理是什么？操作过程中应注意哪些问题？有何实际意义？

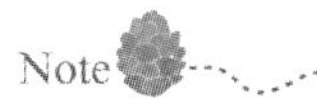

(2)当你对某一未知菌株进行革兰染色时，怎样确证你的染色结果正确？

(3)哪些细菌可通过形态与结构特点进行初步检查?分别可以鉴定到分类单元中的哪一级层次?

(4)病原菌形态学检查的临床意义有哪些?

(焦红梅　乌日汗)

实验四　化脓性球菌

[实验目的]

(1)掌握化脓性球菌的形态及染色特性。
(2)掌握化脓性球菌的培养特性。
(3)熟悉血浆凝固酶试验和抗链球菌溶血素 O 试验。

[实验材料]

(1)示教片:葡萄球菌、链球菌、肺炎球菌、脑膜炎奈瑟菌及淋病奈瑟菌革兰染色标本片,肺炎球菌荚膜染色标本片。

(2)金黄色葡萄球菌、表皮葡萄球菌、腐生葡萄球菌的普通琼脂平板培养物,甲型溶血性链球菌、乙型溶血性链球菌、丙型链球菌和肺炎球菌的血琼脂平板培养物。

(3)兔血浆、生理盐水、待检标本(含葡萄球菌模拟标本)或葡萄球菌琼脂斜面培养物。

(4)载玻片、移液管、显微镜等。

(5)待检血清、微量反应板、ASO 胶乳试剂等。

[实验内容]

1. 在光学显微镜下观察化脓性球菌的形态和染色特性

(1)葡萄球菌:菌体呈球形或略呈椭圆形。革兰染色阳性。典型的葡萄球菌排列成葡萄串状;在脓汁中,常呈双球状或短链状。其衰老、死亡或被中性粒细胞吞噬后常常转为革兰阴性菌。在青霉素等药物影响下,可诱导成 L 形。

(2)链球菌:菌体呈球形或椭圆形。革兰染色阳性。链状排列,长短不一。临床标本中以成对、短链排列多见;在液体培养基中形成较长的链。多数菌株在培养早期可形成透明质酸荚膜,随着培养时间的延长,细菌产生的透明质酸酶使荚膜消失;在陈旧培养基或脓液标本中或被吞噬细胞吞噬后常呈革兰染色阴性。

(3)肺炎球菌:菌体呈矛头状,常成双排列,钝端相对,尖端相背。在痰标本、脓液标本、病变肺组织中可呈单个存在或短链状。其在机体内或含血清的培养基中能形成荚膜,荚膜需特殊染色才可见。

(4)脑膜炎奈瑟菌:革兰阴性双球菌,菌体呈肾形或豆形,两菌接触面平坦或略向内陷。人工培养后可呈卵圆形或球状,排列较不规则,单个、成双或 4 个相连等。在患者脑脊液涂片标本中,其常位于中性粒细胞内,形态典型。新分离菌株大多有荚膜和菌毛。

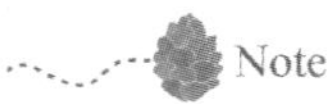

(5)淋病奈瑟菌:形态和染色特性与脑膜炎奈瑟菌相似,为革兰阴性双球菌,常成双排列。两

菌接触面平坦，形似一对咖啡豆。在脓液标本中，其常位于中性粒细胞内，分布不规则。慢性病患者中其多分布在细胞外。有荚膜和菌毛。

2. 化脓性球菌培养特性观察

（1）葡萄球菌：金黄色葡萄球菌、表皮葡萄球菌、腐生葡萄球菌在普通琼脂平板上孵育 24～48 h 后，形成中等大小、圆形、隆起、表面光滑、湿润、边缘整齐、不透明、脂溶性色素较明显的单个菌落。菌落初呈白色，随后因产生的色素不同，金黄色葡萄球菌呈金黄色，表皮葡萄球菌呈白色，腐生葡萄球菌大多呈柠檬色。三种葡萄球菌在血琼脂平板上出现的菌落类似于它们在普通琼脂平板上出现的菌落，但金黄色葡萄球菌菌落周围有明显溶血环，而表皮葡萄球菌和腐生葡萄球菌菌落周围无溶血环。

（2）链球菌：在血琼脂平板上菌落呈灰白色针尖状，菌落周围可出现不同的溶血情况。甲型溶血性链球菌菌落周围可见较窄的草绿色溶血环（不完全溶血，即 α 溶血）。乙型溶血性链球菌菌落周围可见界限分明、宽而透明的溶血环（完全溶血，即 β 溶血）。丙型链球菌不产生溶血素，菌落周围无溶血环。

（3）肺炎球菌：在血琼脂平板上菌落细小、灰白色、圆形略扁、半透明，有草绿色溶血环（α 溶血），与甲型溶血性链球菌很相似。随着培养时间的延长，细菌产生的自溶酶裂解细菌使菌落中央凹陷、边缘隆起，呈“脐状”。

（4）脑膜炎奈瑟菌：在巧克力（色）血琼脂平板上形成无色、圆形、光滑、透明、边缘整齐、似露滴状的菌落。

（5）淋病奈瑟菌：在巧克力（色）血琼脂平板上经 37 ℃培养 48 h 后，形成圆形、凸起、无色或灰白色、直径 0.5～1.0 mm 的光滑型小菌落。

3. 血浆凝固酶试验

（1）原理：血浆凝固酶试验是鉴定葡萄球菌致病性的重要试验。大多数致病性葡萄球菌能产生血浆凝固酶，而非致病性菌株一般不产生。致病性葡萄球菌产生的血浆凝固酶有两种：一种是游离凝固酶，是分泌至细菌体外的蛋白质，可被人或兔血浆中的协同因子激活为凝血酶样物质，使液态的纤维蛋白原变为固态的纤维蛋白，从而使血浆凝固；另一种是结合凝固酶，为细菌表面的纤维蛋白原受体，可直接作用于血浆中的纤维蛋白原，使其发生沉淀，包围于细菌外面而凝聚成块。

（2）方法。

玻片法：用于结合凝固酶的测定。

①取洁净的载玻片 1 张，分左、右两区，在左、右两区各加 1 滴生理盐水。

②用灭菌的接种环挑取金黄色葡萄球菌和表皮葡萄球菌琼脂斜面培养物少许，分别混悬于玻片上的生理盐水内，研磨均匀。

③于左、右两区的细菌悬液内分别加入未稀释的兔血浆 1 滴，混匀。

④数秒后观察结果，若细菌呈颗粒状凝集，则为血浆凝固酶试验阳性；若无颗粒状凝集，则为血浆凝固酶试验阴性。

试管法：用于游离凝固酶的测定。

①取试管 3 支，每管加入稀释 4 倍的新鲜兔血浆 0.5 ml。在第 1、2 管中分别加入 0.5 ml 金黄色葡萄球菌菌液和表皮葡萄球菌菌液，第 3 管中加入培养基作为对照。

②置 37 ℃水浴，每 30 min 观察 1 次结果，一般连续观察 3 h。

③若试管内血浆呈胶冻状，则为血浆凝固酶试验阳性；若试管内血浆仍能流动，则为血浆凝固酶试验阴性。

（3）结果：金黄色葡萄球菌能产生血浆凝固酶，试验呈阳性；表皮葡萄球菌不能产生血浆凝固酶，试验呈阴性。

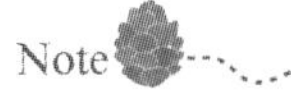

4. 耐热 DNA 酶测定

（1）原理：致病性的金黄色葡萄球菌产生一种耐热的 DNA 酶，能分解 DNA，而非致病性的表皮葡萄球菌和腐生葡萄球菌虽也能产生DNA酶,但均不耐热。因此,耐热DNA酶测定可作为鉴定致病性葡萄球菌的一种方法。

(2)方法。

玻片法:在甲苯胺蓝核酸琼脂上打孔,孔径为3~5 mm,每孔分别加入经沸水浴处理15 min的金黄色葡萄球菌、表皮葡萄球菌或腐生葡萄球菌培养物各1滴,37 ℃放置3 h,观察结果。

平板法:在有金黄色葡萄球菌菌落的平板上,选择试验菌落并标记,置于60 ℃干燥热力灭菌器内2 h,取出平板,倾注10 ml熔化的甲苯胺蓝核酸琼脂,37 ℃放置3 h,观察结果。

(3)结果:产生耐热DNA酶的金黄色葡萄球菌菌落周围有粉红色圈。

5. 抗链球菌溶血素O试验(抗"O"试验,ASO试验)

(1)原理:本试验的ASO胶乳试剂由溶血素"O"和聚苯乙烯胶乳交联而成,将ASO胶乳试剂的灵敏度调整至200 IU/ml,超过上述含量即出现肉眼可见的凝集颗粒。使用该试剂时血清标本不需要稀释即可直接测定。本试验可辅助诊断由链球菌引起的风湿热、肾小球肾炎等疾病。

(2)方法:在微量反应板上加1滴待检血清(可同时做阴性、阳性血清对照),再分别加1滴ASO胶乳试剂,轻轻摇动使其充分混匀,2 min后观察结果。

(3)结果:出现凝集现象可判断样本中ASO含量>200 IU/ml,阳性;无凝集现象出现可判断样本中ASO含量<200 IU/mL,阴性。

[注意事项]

(1)试剂在使用前应预先放置使之达室温并摇匀。

(2)试剂盒应储存于2~10 ℃,切勿冻存。

(3)加试剂和阴性、阳性血清对照时,应保证液滴大小一致。

[实验报告]

(1)画出化脓性球菌的镜下形态和染色特性。

(2)简述血浆凝固酶试验的原理、方法和结果。

[思考题]

(1)常见的化脓性球菌有哪些?它们的形态、染色及培养有何特点?

(2)如何区别致病性与非致病性葡萄球菌?

(3)ASO试验的原理是什么?如何解释结果?

(4)病原性球菌的耐药性现状和发展趋势如何?

(焦红梅　乌日汗)

实验五　肠道杆菌

[实验目的]

(1)熟悉致病性肠道杆菌的分离与鉴定方法。

(2)掌握肥达试验的原理、方法及结果分析。

[实验材料]

(1)大肠埃希菌、伤寒杆菌、痢疾杆菌、变形杆菌的革兰染色示教片。

(2)接种肠道杆菌的 SS 琼脂平板;分别接种大肠埃希菌、伤寒杆菌、乙型副伤寒杆菌、痢疾杆菌及变形杆菌的双糖铁、靛基质、半固体、尿素培养基。

(3)患者粪便(模拟)标本、SS 琼脂培养基干粉、蒸馏水、烧杯、玻璃棒、微波炉、灭菌平皿、肠道杆菌斜面培养物、肠道杆菌诊断血清等。

(4)伤寒患者血清(1∶10 稀释)、生理盐水、伤寒沙门菌 O 抗原诊断菌液、伤寒沙门菌 H 抗原诊断菌液、甲型及乙型副伤寒沙门菌诊断菌液、微量反应板、微量移液器及滴头、振荡器、恒温箱等。

[实验内容]

1. 主要的肠道杆菌

(1)形态及革兰染色特性:油镜下观察大肠埃希菌、伤寒杆菌、痢疾杆菌、变形杆菌的基本形态,比较其形状、大小、排列及染色特性。

(2)肠道杆菌的分离培养。

①原理:SS 琼脂培养基为分离肠道杆菌的强选择性鉴别培养基。培养基中除含有营养物质外,还含有胆盐、煌绿、硫代硫酸钠和枸橼酸钠等化学试剂。这些物质能抑制非致病菌(如大肠埃希菌)生长,而胆盐又有促进沙门菌、痢疾杆菌生长的作用。此外,SS 琼脂培养基中还加有乳糖和中性红指示剂(酸性时呈红色,碱性时呈黄色)。致病性肠道杆菌不分解乳糖,所以在 SS 琼脂平板上生长的菌落为无色或微黄色光滑型小菌落;变形杆菌、乙型副伤寒杆菌、鼠伤寒沙门菌能产生H_2S,形成的菌落中心呈黑色;大肠埃希菌在 SS 琼脂平板上一般不生长,但如果粪便标本接种量大,其中大肠埃希菌量大,SS 琼脂平板上仍可见其生长。因为大肠埃希菌能发酵乳糖产酸,所以在 SS 琼脂平板上形成红色、较大的光滑型菌落,很容易与致病菌区分。现在多用商品化的 SS 琼脂培养基干粉制备 SS 琼脂平板。

②制备 SS 琼脂平板:称取 SS 琼脂培养基干粉 48 g 置于烧杯中,加蒸馏水 1000 ml,将烧杯置于微波炉中加热 1～2 min(注意不要煮沸),取出烧杯用玻璃棒搅拌后放回微波炉中继续加热,重复上述操作直至培养基干粉完全溶解。将完全溶解的培养基于室温中稍冷后,倾注于无菌平板中(每个平板 15～20 ml),待琼脂凝固后即可用于细菌分离培养。

③标本接种:用无菌接种环挑取少量患者粪便(模拟)标本(注意接种环灭菌后要冷却才可取样),分四区划线接种于 SS 琼脂平板上;平板上注明标本编号、班级、姓名及接种日期等。将平板倒置后于 37 ℃培养 18～24 h,观察菌落特征。

(3)主要肠道杆菌的生化反应(示教):肠道杆菌生化反应活泼,能分解多种糖类和蛋白质,形成不同的代谢产物,常用生化反应来区别不同菌属和菌种。几种主要肠道杆菌的生化反应结果见表 2-5-1。

表 2-5-1 几种主要肠道杆菌的生化反应结果

细菌	克氏双糖铁			靛基质	半固体(动力)	尿素
	上层乳糖	下层葡萄糖	H_2S			
大肠埃希菌	⊕	⊕	−	+	+	−
伤寒杆菌	−	+	−/+	−	+	−
甲型副伤寒杆菌	−	⊕	−	−	+	−

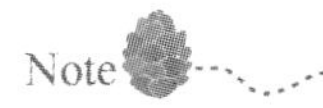

续表

细菌	克氏双糖铁			靛基质	半固体(动力)	尿素
	上层乳糖	下层葡萄糖	H_2S			
乙型副伤寒杆菌	−	⊕	+	−	+	−
痢疾杆菌	−	+	−	−	−	−
变形杆菌	−	⊕/+	+/−	+/−	+	+

注:①“−”表示不发酵,“+”表示产酸,“⊕”表示产酸产气。

②克氏双糖铁培养基用酚红作为指示剂,酸性时呈黄色,碱性时呈红色。细菌如能发酵乳糖而产酸产气,则培养基斜面与底层均呈黄色,且有气泡。如果细菌只发酵葡萄糖而不发酵乳糖,因葡萄糖含量较少(占乳糖量的 1/10),所生成的酸较少,接触空气后氧化挥发。细菌因生长繁殖,利用含氮物质生成碱性化合物,使培养基斜面部分变成红色,底层由于在缺氧状态下,细菌发酵葡萄糖所生成的酸类物质不被氧化挥发而仍保持黄色。如果细菌分解蛋白质产生硫化氢(H_2S),则与硫酸亚铁作用生成黑色的硫化铁,使培养基变黑。

(4)肥达试验(Widal test)。

①原理:用已知伤寒沙门菌菌体(O)抗原和鞭毛(H)抗原,以及甲、乙型副伤寒沙门菌 H 抗原的诊断菌液,与不同稀释度的待检血清做定量凝集试验,测定待检血清中有无相应抗体及其效价,以辅助临床诊断伤寒及副伤寒。

②方法。

a. 取微量反应板 1 块,本次实验使用其中 40 个孔(10×4)。

b. 稀释血清:按照表 2-5-2 所示,首先用微量移液器吸取 50 μl 生理盐水加入微量反应板每行的第 1~10 孔中,共 4 行;再吸取 1∶10 稀释的伤寒患者血清 50 μl 分别加入各行的第 1 孔中,吸吹混匀后,吸出 50 μl 加入第 2 孔中,混匀后再吸出 50 μl 至第 3 孔中,以此类推,直至每行第 9 孔,第 9 孔混匀后弃去 50 μl;第 10 孔不加血清,只加 50 μl 生理盐水作为阴性对照。

c. 按表 2-5-2 所示加入各种成分,振荡 3~5 min,放于 37 ℃恒温箱中孵育 1 h(注意孵育期间勿振荡微量反应板,以免凝块摇散)。观察结果:先观察阴性对照孔,应无凝集现象,即孔内液体均匀混浊或在孔底有一整齐的圆团;然后自第 1 孔开始依次观察至第 9 孔,根据凝集反应的强弱,分别以“++++”“+++”“++”“+”“−”符号记录。

表 2-5-2　肥达试验抗体稀释方法

50

项目	1	2	3	4	5	6	7	8	9	10
生理盐水体积/μl	50	50	50	50	50	50	50	50	50	50
血清(1∶10)体积/μl	50	—	—	—	—	—	—	—	—	—
诊断菌液体积/μl	50	50	50	50	50	50	50	50	50	50
血清稀释度	1∶40	1∶80	1∶160	1∶320	1∶640	1∶1280	1∶2560	1∶5120	1∶10240	阴性对照

注:所加诊断菌液分别为伤寒沙门菌 O 抗原诊断菌液、伤寒沙门菌 H 抗原诊断菌液、甲型副伤寒沙门菌 H 抗原诊断菌液和乙型副伤寒沙门菌 H 抗原诊断菌液。

③结果:“++++”,上层液澄清,细菌凝块全部沉于孔底;“+++”,上层液轻度混浊,凝块沉于孔底;“++”,上层液中等混浊,孔底有明显的凝集物;“+”,上层液混浊,孔底仅有少量凝集物;“−”,孔内液体与阴性对照孔相同,呈均匀混浊,无凝集现象。

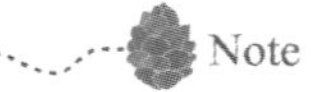
Note

④效价判断:以能出现“++”凝集现象的血清最高稀释度为该血清的凝集效价。

⑤结果分析:对肥达试验结果的解释必须结合临床表现、病程、病史以及地区流行病学情况,

须注意以下几点。

a. 正常值：正常人由于隐性感染或预防接种，血清中可含有一定量的抗体，其效价因地区不同而有差异。一般情况下伤寒沙门菌 O 抗体凝集效价≥1：80、H 抗体凝集效价≥1：160，甲、乙型副伤寒沙门菌 H 抗体凝集效价≥1：80 才有诊断价值。

b. 动态观察：抗体一般在患者发病 1 周左右出现，且随病程进展而增加；有时单次某一抗体凝集效价增高不能定论，可在病程中逐周复查。效价递增或恢复期效价增高 4 倍或 4 倍以上，才有诊断意义。

c. O 与 H 抗体在诊断上的意义：人患伤寒、副伤寒或预防接种后，O 与 H 抗体在体内的出现及消失情况不同。IgM 型的 O 抗体出现早、持续时间短，消失后不易受非特异性刺激而重新出现；IgG 型的 H 抗体出现较晚，维持时间长达数年，消失后易受非沙门菌等病原体刺激而短暂地重新出现（非特异性回忆反应）。因此，如 O、H 抗体凝集效价均超过正常值，则感染伤寒或副伤寒的可能性大；若两者均低，则感染伤寒或副伤寒的可能性小；若凝集效价 O 不高 H 高，有可能是预防接种或非特异性回忆反应（隔一段时间重复试验，若抗体效价不升高，则为非特异性回忆反应）；如凝集效价 O 高 H 不高，则可能是感染早期或与伤寒沙门菌 O 抗原有交叉反应的其他沙门菌（如肠炎沙门菌）感染，见表 2-5-3。

表 2-5-3 肥达试验效价判断

试验结果	临床意义
O<1：80 & H<1：160	正常值
O≥1：80 & H≥1：160	感染伤寒沙门菌
O≥1：80 & PAH≥1：80	感染甲型副伤寒沙门菌
O≥1：80 & PBH≥1：80	感染乙型副伤寒沙门菌
O≥1：80 & H<1：160，或 O≥1：80 & PAH/PBH<1：80	感染伤寒早期或者甲、乙型副伤寒早期，或与伤寒沙门菌 O 抗原有交叉反应的其他沙门菌感染
O<1：80 & H≥1：160，或 O<1：80 & PAH/PBH≥1：80	预防接种或非特异性回忆反应

注：O 表示伤寒沙门菌 O 抗体凝集效价；H 表示伤寒沙门菌 H 抗体凝集效价；PAH、PBH 分别表示甲、乙型副伤寒沙门菌 H 抗体凝集效价。

d. 其他：有少数伤寒、副伤寒病例，在整个病程中，肥达试验结果始终在正常范围内。其原因可能是早期使用抗生素治疗，或患者免疫功能低下等。

［实验报告］

（1）简述肥达试验的原理、方法、结果判断与分析。

（2）画出肠道杆菌在 SS 琼脂平板上的菌落特征与玻片凝集试验的结果。

（3）记录大肠埃希菌、伤寒杆菌、痢疾杆菌、变形杆菌在双糖铁、靛基质、半固体、尿素培养基上的生化反应结果。

［思考题］

（1）进行肥达试验过程中需要注意哪些问题？怎样保证结果判断的准确性？

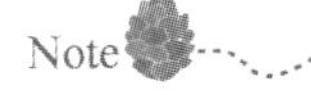

（2）肥达试验中伤寒沙门菌 O 抗体凝集效价为 1：160，患者一定感染伤寒沙门菌吗？原因是什么？

(3)致病性肠道杆菌分离培养中如何降低或排除正常菌群的影响?

(孔桂美　高成凤)

实验六　厌氧性细菌

[实验目的]

(1)掌握破伤风梭菌、产气荚膜梭菌、肉毒梭菌的形态及培养特性。

(2)熟悉厌氧培养的原理和方法。

[实验材料]

(1)菌种:破伤风梭菌、产气荚膜梭菌、肉毒梭菌的肉渣培养物。

(2)细菌形态观察:破伤风梭菌、产气荚膜梭菌、肉毒梭菌的革兰染色示教片。

(3)棉花、无菌纱布、10% NaOH 溶液、固体石蜡、载玻片、无菌滴管等。

[实验内容]

1. 观察破伤风梭菌、产气荚膜梭菌、肉毒梭菌的革兰染色示教片

(1)油镜下观察破伤风梭菌、产气荚膜梭菌、肉毒梭菌的形态、大小及位置。

(2)观察细菌特殊结构:破伤风梭菌和肉毒梭菌芽孢的形态、位置;产气荚膜梭菌荚膜的大小、颜色。

2. "汹涌发酵"试验

(1)原理:产气荚膜梭菌能迅速分解牛乳中的乳糖,产生大量酸、凝固酪蛋白,从而将培养基表面的凡士林冲至试管口棉塞处,称为"汹涌发酵"现象。一般培养 6～12 h 可以观察到此现象。

(2)方法。

①溴甲酚紫牛乳培养基的配制:将 0.1 ml 浓度为 16 g/L 的溴甲酚紫溶液加入 100 ml 新鲜脱脂牛乳中,以每管 5 ml 进行分装,在表面加已熔化的凡士林,厚度约 5 mm。行间歇蒸汽灭菌:第一天 75 ℃、30 min;第二天 80 ℃、30 min;第三天 85 ℃、30 min。

②将产气荚膜梭菌接种到溴甲酚紫牛乳培养基中,37 ℃培养 12～24 h,观察。

(3)结果:细菌分解乳糖产酸产气,酪蛋白凝固并形成海绵状碎块。

3. 庖肉培养基厌氧培养法

(1)原理:庖肉培养基不含饱和脂肪酸,氧化时能够消耗氧气而形成厌氧环境,故适用于培养厌氧性细菌。

(2)方法。

①庖肉培养基配制:取 0.5 g 牛肉渣,装于 15 mm×150 mm 的试管中,再加入 7 ml pH 7.6 的肉汤培养基,上面加入 3～4 mm 厚的熔化的凡士林,高压蒸汽灭菌备用。

②将破伤风梭菌接种至庖肉培养基,37 ℃培养 24～48 h,观察结果。

(3)结果:培养基混浊,肉渣被消化,变黑,稍有臭味。

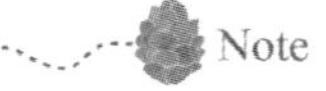

[实验报告]

画出油镜下破伤风梭菌、产气荚膜梭菌和肉毒梭菌的形态。

[思考题]

(1)厌氧培养的原理是什么？厌氧培养的方法有哪些？
(2)厌氧培养中应注意哪些生物安全问题？

(阴银燕　刘翠翠)

实验七　分枝杆菌

[实验目的]

(1)掌握结核分枝杆菌的形态、染色特性。
(2)掌握抗酸染色的方法。

[实验材料]

(1)结核分枝杆菌抗酸染色示教片。
(2)结核病患者痰液(模拟)标本。
(3)抗酸染色液：石炭酸复红稀释液、3%盐酸酒精溶液、吕氏美蓝液(配制见附录 A)。
(4)载玻片、接种环、酒精灯和显微镜等。

[实验内容]

1. 结核分枝杆菌的形态及染色特性观察　结核分枝杆菌细长、略弯曲，呈单个或分枝状排列，革兰染色阳性，但一般不进行革兰染色，常用抗酸染色法染色。抗酸染色后结核分枝杆菌呈红色，非抗酸性细菌和涂片中的其他成分均被染成蓝色。在陈旧的病灶和培养物中，结核分枝杆菌形态常不典型，可呈颗粒状、串珠状、短棒状等。

2. 结核分枝杆菌培养特性观察　将结核分枝杆菌接种于改良罗氏固体培养基中，于 37 ℃培养，每周观察 1 次。结核分枝杆菌生长缓慢，一般培养 2～4 周后长成肉眼可见的菌落。菌落干燥、坚硬，表面呈颗粒状，颜色为乳白色或米黄色，表面凸起，形似花菜。其在液体培养基中呈表面生长，形成粗糙皱纹状菌膜。

3. 抗酸染色(齐-内(Ziehl-Neelsen)染色)

(1)原理：结核分枝杆菌的细胞壁内含有大量类脂(如分枝菌酸)，一般不易着色。在加温染色或延长染色时间的条件下，分枝菌酸与石炭酸复红牢固结合，并能抵抗强脱色剂(3%盐酸酒精溶液)的脱色，故名抗酸染色。当经吕氏美蓝液复染后，结核分枝杆菌仍然呈红色，为抗酸染色阳性，而其他微生物和组织细胞呈蓝色，为抗酸染色阴性。

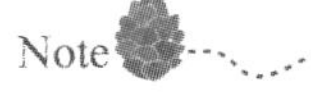

(2)方法。

①用接种环取痰液，均匀涂成厚膜涂片，自然干燥后经火焰固定。

②用玻片夹夹持涂片，将石炭酸复红稀释液加满于涂片部分，于火焰高处徐徐加热，当有蒸气冒出时即暂时离开火焰(不可煮沸)，若染液蒸发减少，应补加染液，以免干涸，如此维持 3～5 min，待标本冷却后水洗。

③加入 3%盐酸酒精溶液，脱色 1 min，脱色时轻轻晃动涂片，脱至无红色酒精流下为止，水洗。

④加入吕氏美蓝液，复染 1 min，水洗，用吸水纸吸干后在油镜下观察。

(3)结果：在油镜下，结核分枝杆菌散开分布、呈细长或稍弯曲的杆状，被染成红色，即抗酸染色阳性，非抗酸性细菌和其他成分均被染成蓝色。

[注意事项]

为了提高检出率，可采用厚涂片法(即普通涂片的 5 倍厚)。脱色时间需根据涂片厚薄而定，厚片可适当延长脱色时间，至无红色酒精流下为止。

[实验报告]

(1)画出在油镜下观察到的结核分枝杆菌的形态和染色特性。

(2)简述抗酸染色的原理、方法、结果及意义。

[思考题]

(1)若怀疑某患者患有肺结核，应如何进行微生物学检查？

(2)结核分枝杆菌感染的筛查方法有哪些？试述各方法的原理。

(3)结核分枝杆菌检测技术和防治技术的发展历程中体现了哪些科学精神？如何培养创新意识和科学态度？

(焦红梅　乌日汗)

实验八　其 他 细 菌

[实验目的]

(1)掌握放线菌“硫黄样颗粒”的形态特征。

(2)熟悉布鲁氏菌、炭疽芽孢杆菌、鼠疫耶尔森菌、放线菌及“四体”的形态及培养特性。

(3)熟悉梅毒螺旋体的血清学试验。

[实验材料]

(1)布鲁氏菌、炭疽芽孢杆菌、鼠疫耶尔森菌、放线菌及“四体”的示教片。

(2)梅毒螺旋体血清学试验的试剂。

[实验内容]

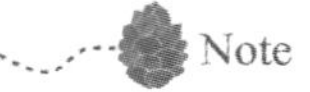

1. 布鲁氏菌

(1)通过示教片观察布鲁氏菌的形态：革兰阴性小杆菌。

(2)观察布鲁氏菌在双相肝浸液培养基上的菌落形态:微小、透明、无色素的光滑型菌落。

2. 炭疽芽孢杆菌

(1)通过示教片观察炭疽芽孢杆菌的形态:革兰阳性大杆菌,呈竹节状排列,有荚膜,芽孢呈椭圆形且位于菌体中央。

(2)观察无毒类炭疽芽孢杆菌在血琼脂平板和普通琼脂平板上的菌落,并进行比较。普通琼脂平板上,炭疽芽孢杆菌的菌落为扁平、灰白色、干燥、不透明、无光泽的粗糙菌落,菌落边缘呈卷发状。血琼脂平板上,菌落呈灰白色、表面粗糙隆起、无光泽、边缘不整齐;培养时间过长时,有轻度溶血现象。

3. 鼠疫耶尔森菌

(1)通过示教片观察鼠疫耶尔森菌的形态:蓝色卵圆形短粗杆菌(美蓝染色),两端浓染。

(2)普通琼脂平板上,菌落周边菲薄、中央隆起;在肉汤培养基中最初为混浊生长,逐渐形成絮状沉淀,48 h 后形成菌膜,继续静置培养 4～5 d,可见丝状物从液面薄膜下垂,呈钟乳石状,此特征具有鉴别意义。

4. 放线菌 放线菌“硫黄样颗粒”:将“硫黄样颗粒”制成压片,在显微镜下可见放射状的菌丝,直径为 1 μm。菌丝末端肥大呈棒状,菊花样。

5. 肺炎支原体 肺炎支原体没有细胞壁,呈多形态。其营养要求高,生长缓慢,培养 5 d 后,形成“油煎蛋”样菌落。不同支原体菌落形成的时间不同,故应连续观察 8 d,如未见菌落,方可报告阴性。

6. 衣原体 衣原体具有独特的发育周期,光镜下可见到两种不同的颗粒结构:一种是小而致密的颗粒,称为原体,圆形,吉姆萨(吉氏,Giemsa)染色后呈紫色,有感染性;另一种是大而疏松的颗粒,称为网状体,圆形或椭圆形,Giemsa 染色后呈红色,无感染性。

Giemsa 染色法如下所示。

(1)Giemsa 染色液的配制:见附录 A。

(2)用甲醇固定标本 5 min,将缓冲液与 Giemsa 染色液按 20∶1 的比例混匀后,染色 10～30 min,冲洗,油镜下观察。衣原体核质呈红色,胞质呈蓝色,色素颗粒呈褐色。

7. 立克次体 斑疹伤寒立克次体经 Giemsa 染色后呈紫色或蓝色,常有两极浓染;经 Macchiavello 染色后呈红色。

8. 螺旋体

(1)钩端螺旋体形态及染色特性:钩端螺旋体经 Fontana 镀银染色后呈棕褐色,菌体一端或两端弯曲,呈“C”“S”或“8”字形。

Fontana 镀银染色法如下所示。

①涂片干燥。

②用固定液固定 2 min。

③用无水酒精冲洗。

④加媒染剂加温孵育 2 min。

⑤水洗后,加银液加温孵育 2 min。

⑥水洗后镜检。

(2)梅毒螺旋体的形态及染色特性。

①采用镀银染色法检查梅毒螺旋体:将梅毒患者的生殖器分泌物涂片后进行镀银染色,可观察到有 8～14 个细密螺旋的螺旋体,两端尖直。螺旋体呈棕褐色,组织呈棕黄色。

②梅毒螺旋体血清学试验:梅毒螺旋体血清学试验常用的抗原有两种,一种是正常牛心肌的心脂质,另一种是螺旋体抗原。目前国际上通用的初筛梅毒的试验是快速血浆反应素(rapid plasma reagin,RPR)试验。

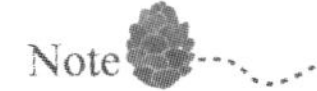

原理:将标准的心脂质抗原吸附在活性炭颗粒上,这种含碳抗原与患者血清混合在一起后,可以与血清中抗梅毒螺旋体抗体发生反应,在白色卡上形成肉眼可见的黑色凝集颗粒。通过该试验还可以对抗体水平进行半定量测定。

方法:a. 试验前 5 s,用 0.2 ml 生理盐水溶解冻干的阳性对照血清。b. 吸取 50 μl 待测血清滴加在卡片圈内。c. 将 RPR 抗原滴加在每个待检血清圈和阳性对照血清圈内,每圈 1 滴。d. 轻轻混匀,8 min 后观察结果。

结果:反应完成后,3 min 内按以下标准判断结果。

阳性反应,可见中等或大的黑色凝集块;弱阳性反应,可见散在的小的黑色凝集块;阴性反应,无颗粒凝集,或仅见粗糙碳颗粒聚集在中间。

[实验报告]

画出油镜下所观察到的炭疽芽孢杆菌、钩端螺旋体、梅毒螺旋体、放线菌“硫黄样颗粒”的形态。

[思考题]

(1)何谓 RPR 试验?简述其原理及应用。
(2)梅毒螺旋体感染的精准诊断对梅毒的防治有什么意义?

(阴银燕　刘翠翠)

实验九　病　　毒

[实验目的]

(1)了解病毒在电镜下的形态特征。
(2)认识病毒 CPE 和包涵体。
(3)掌握 ELISA 的原理和结果判定方法。

[实验材料]

(1)病毒形态的电镜照片、病毒包涵体示教片和显微镜。
(2)待测血清、ELISA 检测 HBsAg 试剂盒、37 ℃恒温箱。

[实验内容]

1. 观察病毒形态的电镜照片和病毒包涵体示教片

(1)病毒的基本形态。
①球形(近似球形):如多数人和动物病毒。
②杆形(丝状):如植物病毒。
③弹形:如狂犬病毒。
④砖形:如痘病毒。
⑤蝌蚪形:如细菌病毒(噬菌体)。

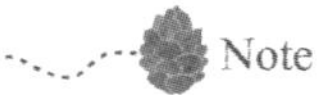

(2)病毒 CPE 和包涵体:部分病毒(如肠道病毒)感染细胞后使细胞变圆、聚集、坏死、溶解或脱落等。部分病毒(如麻疹病毒、巨细胞病毒等)导致细胞形成多核巨细胞(或称融合细胞),但各个细胞核能分辨清楚。狂犬病毒在培养细胞中形成包涵体(内氏小体):位于神经元胞质内,嗜酸性,呈圆形或椭圆形。

2. ELISA 检测 HBsAg

(1)原理:采用双抗体夹心法检测 HBsAg。用抗-HBs 包被板条,以 HRP 标记的抗-HBs 为酶标记物,以四甲基联苯胺(TMB)和过氧化物为底物。当标本中存在 HBsAg 时,HBsAg 与抗-HBs 结合并与抗 HBs-HRP 结合形成抗-HBs-HBsAg-抗-HBs-HRP 复合物,加入底物后发生显色反应,反之则无显色反应。在试验结束时,有颜色变化则提示有 HBsAg 存在,无颜色变化或颜色变化微弱则提示不存在 HBsAg。

(2)方法。

①在包被有抗-HBs 反应板条的孔内,加待检样品 50 μl,同时做一孔阴性对照、一孔阳性对照、一孔空白对照。

②每孔加酶标记物(酶标抗-HBs)50 μl(空白对照孔不加)。

③充分混合后将即时贴撕开,覆盖在反应板上,置 37 ℃保温 30 min。

④弃去即时贴及孔内反应物,用洗涤液洗板 5 次,吸干孔内液体。

⑤各孔(包括对照孔)加底物 A 液 50 μl、B 液 50 μl,置 37 ℃保温 10 min。

⑥各孔加终止液 50 μl 终止反应。目测或上机比色。

(3)结果。

①目测结果:可于白色背景上直接用肉眼观察结果,反应孔内颜色越深,阳性程度越强,阴性反应呈无色或极浅颜色,依据所呈颜色的深浅,以"+""-"表示。

②上机比色结果:将反应板置 ELISA 检测仪中,设波长为 450 nm,调零后测各孔 OD 值。若样品 OD 值大于判断值(阴性对照平均 OD 值×2.1)则为阳性,小于判断值则为阴性。

[实验报告]

简述 ELISA 检测 HBsAg 的原理、方法和结果。

[思考题]

(1)采集病毒标本有哪些原则?和细菌标本采集有何不同?

(2)检测病毒的常用方法有哪些?各有何优缺点?

(3)如果发生某种疑似新型病毒感染,如何精准、快速地确定感染的病原体种类?

(焦红梅　乌日汗)

实验十　真　　菌

[实验目的]

(1)掌握常见真菌的形态和培养特点。

(2)熟悉真菌不染色标本直接检查的制片技术。

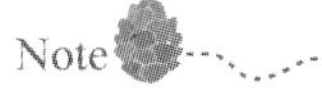

[实验材料]

(1)白念珠菌、新生隐球菌、皮肤癣菌,以及酵母菌的孢子、菌丝示教片。

(2)白念珠菌、新生隐球菌、皮肤癣菌斜面培养物。

(3)乳酸酚棉蓝染色液、优质墨汁、真菌荧光染色液等。

(4)小镊子、盖玻片、载玻片、显微镜等。

[实验内容]

1. 真菌形态及染色特性观察 白念珠菌的菌体呈圆形或卵圆形,有些菌的细胞有芽生孢子,出芽延长产生假菌丝;革兰染色阳性(着色不均匀)。新生隐球菌的菌体呈圆形或卵圆形,菌体外有一层宽厚的荚膜。用墨汁负染后镜检,可见圆形或卵圆形的菌体外包裹宽厚的空白带。皮肤癣菌是多细胞真菌,可见孢子、菌丝。

2. 真菌不染色标本的直接检查

(1)方法:用小镊子取甲屑或皮屑少许或病发一根,置于载玻片中央,滴加 10% KOH 溶液 1~2 滴。盖上盖玻片,将载玻片放在火焰上方微加热,使组织或角质溶解,但切勿过热,以免产生气泡或烤干。冷却后,压紧盖玻片使溶解的组织分散并使其透明,驱逐气泡,并吸去周围溢液,避免沾污盖玻片。先用低倍镜检查有无真菌菌丝或孢子,再以高倍镜检查菌丝、孢子的特征。镜检时用稍弱的光线以使视野稍暗。

(2)结果:低倍镜下,菌丝呈折光性较强、绿色纤维分枝丝状体;高倍镜下,菌丝分隔,有时菌丝末端有较粗短关节孢子。镜检时若见菌丝或孢子,即可初步诊断,但一般不能确定其菌种。

3. 真菌的染色

(1)乳酸酚棉蓝染色法。

①原理:乳酸酚棉蓝染色液能与真菌反应而使真菌着色(呈蓝色),乳酸对真菌有杀灭作用。该方法常用于真菌的染色与观察。

②方法:于载玻片中央滴加 2~3 滴乳酸酚棉蓝染色液,用灭菌接种环取一小块有颗粒或颜色部分酵母菌菌落,放入染色液中混匀。加上盖玻片,轻轻按压制片(加热或不加热),在低倍镜、高倍镜或油镜下观察。

③结果:酵母菌的细胞、菌丝和孢子等可被染成亮蓝色,背景为暗淡的蓝色。

(2)墨汁负染法。

①原理:新型隐球菌的荚膜较厚,一般不易着色,同时菌体折光性较强,用墨汁负染法可在黑色背景下看到透亮的菌体。

②方法:取 1 滴优质墨汁于载玻片上与被检材料混合,盖上盖玻片,在显微镜下观察。

③结果:新型隐球菌经墨汁负染后在镜下可见宽厚荚膜。

(3)真菌荧光染色。

①原理:绝大多数真菌含有几丁质,真菌荧光染色液中的重组几丁质酶可与真菌细胞壁成分几丁质结合,使荧光显微镜下 340~380 nm 波长处真菌菌丝及孢子发出明亮的蓝绿色荧光,从而实现真菌的快速检测。

②方法:将细胞培养物或碎屑置于载玻片上,滴入染色 A 液和 B 液,盖上盖玻片后直接观察。

③结果:单细胞或真菌菌丝和孢子在荧光显微镜下呈现蓝绿色荧光。

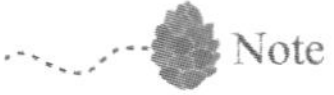
Note

4. 真菌的培养方法

(1)平板培养法:接种方法与细菌的接种方法相似。这是大多数实验室采取的方法,主要用于酵母菌及类酵母菌的分离培养。

(2)斜面培养法:接种方法与细菌的接种方法相似。主要用于临床标本的初代培养、丝状真菌的次代培养和菌种保藏。最常用于霉菌培养。

(3)小培养法:这是观察丝状真菌结构的最好方法,主要用于丝状真菌的鉴定。①用接种刀将培养基中的固体培养琼脂按 1 cm^3“井”字划线,取一块置于无菌载玻片中央;②在琼脂方块的四边中间位置点接种待检菌,盖上无菌盖玻片,放入无菌平板中的 U 形玻璃棒上,平板中加入少量无菌水保湿孵育;③待菌落生长后,揭下盖玻片,在载玻片上滴加一滴乳酸酚棉蓝染色液进行染色,将盖玻片盖在染色液上,用吸水纸吸去周边溢出的多余染色液,于镜下观察菌丝、孢子特征并进行鉴定。

5. 观察真菌的菌落

(1)新生隐球菌菌落属于酵母型菌落,呈圆形,光滑,湿润,乳白色或奶油色,有时呈黏液状。

(2)白念珠菌菌落属于类酵母型菌落,表面光滑、湿润、乳白色,但有营养菌丝伸入培养基中,对光观察可见菌落周围呈羽毛状。

(3)絮状表皮癣菌菌落为丝状菌落,菌落表面大量菌丝组成疏松,似棉絮状、绒毛状或粉末状,中央有皱褶,外周有放射状沟,常导致培养基裂开,菌落背面呈茶褐色。

[实验报告]

(1)画图说明不染色标本中真菌菌丝或孢子的形态。
(2)记录你所观察到的真菌菌落特点。

[思考题]

(1)为什么有时需要做真菌的小培养?
(2)浅部感染真菌与深部感染真菌的培养温度是否相同?为什么?
(3)试述真菌感染的快速检测方法及相应应用范围。

(焦红梅　乌日汗)

实验十一　内毒素检测(鲎试验)

[实验目的]

(1)掌握药物中细菌内毒素的检测方法。
(2)熟悉鲎试验的原理。

[实验材料]

鲎试剂、细菌内毒素标准品、细菌内毒素检查用水、无热原玻璃试管、1 ml 无热原注射器、针头、试管架、涡旋混合器、恒温培养箱、封口膜、酒精棉球、砂轮、供试品(注射用水)等。

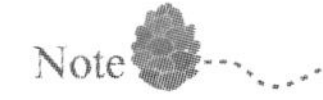

[实验内容]

1. 原理 鲎试剂是从栖息于海洋的节肢动物鲎的蓝色血液中提取的变形细胞溶解物经低温冷冻干燥而成的生物试剂,专用于细菌内毒素检测。凝胶法鲎试验是一种定性或定量检测微量细菌内毒素的体外检测方法。此方法中的鲎试剂含有能被微量细菌内毒素激活的凝固酶原,因此在适宜条件下,鲎试剂可以与细菌内毒素发生凝聚反应形成凝胶。生物制品类、注射用药剂、化学药品类、放射性药物、抗生素类、疫苗类、透析液等制剂以及医疗器械类(如一次性注射器、植入性生物材料)必须经过细菌内毒素检测合格后才能使用。

2. 方法

(1)细菌内毒素阳性对照溶液的制备:用细菌内毒素检查用水将细菌内毒素标准品稀释制成浓度为 4λ 和 2λ 的细菌内毒素标准溶液,备用。

例如:细菌内毒素标准品浓度为每支 10 EU,鲎试剂的灵敏度 λ 为 0.125 EU/ml,制备细菌内毒素标准溶液的步骤如下。

①取细菌内毒素标准品 1 支,用酒精棉球消毒瓶颈后开启,加细菌内毒素检查用水 1 ml,用封口膜封口,放置于涡旋混合器上混匀 15 min。此时细菌内毒素浓度为 10 EU/ml。

②取 3 支试管,标记后放置于试管架上。参照表 2-11-1 所示稀释方法制备浓度为 4λ 和 2λ 的细菌内毒素标准溶液。

表 2-11-1 细菌内毒素阳性对照溶液的制备方法

项目	标准溶液	1	2	3
细菌内毒素	1 支(10 EU)	0.2 ml	1.0 ml	1.0 ml
细菌内毒素检查用水	1 ml	1.8 ml	1.0 ml	1.0 ml
浓度/(EU/ml)	10	1.0	0.5(4λ)	0.25(2λ)

(2)供试品溶液的制备:供试品溶液最大有效稀释倍数(MVD)的计算公式为 $MVD=cL/\lambda$。式中,c 为供试品溶液的浓度;L 为供试品细菌内毒素的限值,单位以 EU/ml、EU/mg、EU/U 表示。当 L 的单位以 EU/ml 表示时,c 为 1 ml/ml;当 L 的单位以 EU/mg、EU/U 表示时,c 的单位为 mg/ml 或 U/ml(注意:当 L 的单位以 EU/ml 表示时,c 的值不是样品的浓度,就是 1)。EU 为细菌内毒素单位;λ 为鲎试剂的标示灵敏度。

举例:若供试品为注射用水,其细菌内毒素限值 L 为 0.25 EU/ml(《中华人民共和国药典》(2020 年版)规定:每 1 ml 注射用水中含细菌内毒素的量应小于 0.25 EU)。

所用鲎试剂的灵敏度 λ 为 0.125 EU/ml,则 $MVD=cL/\lambda=1\times0.25/0.125=2$。

故将原供试品进行 2 倍稀释,作为供试品溶液,即注射用水 0.5 ml+检查用水 0.5 ml。

(3)供试品阳性对照溶液的制备:取浓度为 4λ 的细菌内毒素标准溶液,加入同体积的供试品溶液,混合均匀。例如:对于注射用水,制备供试品阳性对照溶液时,用浓度为 4λ(0.5 EU/ml)的细菌内毒素标准溶液 0.5 ml,加入 0.5 ml 的注射用水,混合均匀即得。

(4)鲎试剂的准备:取规格为每支 0.1 ml 的鲎试剂安瓿 8 支,做好标记。轻弹瓶壁使粉末落入瓶底,先用砂轮在瓶颈轻轻划痕,再用 75%酒精棉球擦拭瓶颈后开启备用,开启时注意防止玻璃屑落入瓶内。每支分别加入 0.1 ml 液体,轻轻转动安瓿,使内容物充分溶解,不要剧烈振动,避免产生气泡。

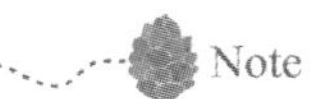

(5)加样和孵育:在每支鲎试剂安瓿中按表 2-11-2 所示加入不同试剂;加样完毕,用封口膜密封安瓿口,37 ℃孵育约 60 min 后观察结果。

表 2-11-2 鲎试验加样方法 单位:ml

试剂	阳性对照管(A)		阴性对照管(B)		供试品阳性对照管(C)		供试品管(D)	
	1	2	1	2	1	2	1	2
细菌内毒素阳性对照溶液(3号管)	0.1	0.1						
细菌内毒素检查用水			0.1	0.1				
供试品阳性对照溶液(5号管)					0.1	0.1		
供试品溶液(4号管)							0.1	0.1

(6)结果判断。

①判断试验是否有效:将各管轻轻取出,缓慢倒转180°观察。如表2-11-3所示,当阳性对照管(A)两个平行管中结果呈阳性,阴性对照管(B)两个平行管中结果呈阴性,供试品阳性对照管(C)两个平行管中结果呈阳性时,则试验有效。

表 2-11-3 鲎试验结果有效性判断

管号	观察现象		结果判断
A	+	+	试验有效
B	−	−	
C	+	+	

②判断供试品试验结果:如表2-11-4所示,供试品管(D)两个平行管中结果呈阴性,结果判断为符合规定;供试品管两个平行管中结果呈阳性,判断为不符合规定;一管阳性,另一管阴性,则需要复试,复试时需做4管供试品(注:复试的4管均呈阴性时,结果判断为符合规定;否则为不符合规定)。

表 2-11-4 鲎试验结果判断

管号	观察现象				结果判断
D	−		−		符合规定
	+		+		不符合规定
	+		−		复试
复试(4管)	−	−	−	−	符合规定

(7)注意事项。

①操作过程中应防止微生物和细菌内毒素的污染;试验前,须用肥皂洗手,并用75%酒精棉球消毒。

②玻璃试管、注射器、针头等应洗涤干净,再用蒸馏水反复冲洗3遍以上,最后用干烤法(250℃、30 min)除热原后方可使用。

③由于凝胶反应是可逆的,所以恒温反应过程中及观察结果时,注意不要使试管受到振动,以免凝胶破碎而产生假阴性结果。

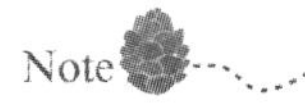

④溶解鲎试剂及混匀供试品和鲎试剂时,不要剧烈振动,以免产生气泡。

[实验报告]

(1)描述待测标本中细菌内毒素检测的方法和原理。

(2)写出供试品的细菌内毒素检测结果及结果分析。

[思考题]

(1)为什么生物制品类和医疗器械类产品需要进行细菌内毒素检测?进行细菌内毒素检测的过程中需要注意哪些方面?

(2)被细菌内毒素污染的样品应该怎样处理?常用的去除细菌内毒素的方法是什么?

(孔桂美　高成凤)

实验十二　寄生关系及寄生虫演化

[实验目的]

了解寄生关系及寄生虫演化过程。

[实验材料]

示教标本。

[实验内容]

1. 自生生活　如蝗虫,运动器官及感觉器官均发达,口器为咀嚼式的。

2. 共栖生活　如海洋中较小的鲫鱼用背鳍演化成的吸盘吸附在大型鱼类体表,从而被携带至各处觅食,对大鱼无利也无害,但对鲫鱼有利。

3. 互利共生生活　如海葵生活在寄居蟹甲壳的表面,寄居蟹可以携带海葵走动,使海葵觅食范围扩大了,同时海葵用其刺器官和其分泌物保护寄居蟹,两者均受益。

4. 寄生生活　为了适应寄生生活,寄生虫在形态结构和生理功能上发生相应改变,如:

(1)体形改变:血吸虫寄生在血管内,虫体细长;跳蚤为了在毛隙间活动,虫体两侧扁平。

(2)器官变化:如寄生在消化道的猪肉绦虫,头节有四个吸盘和小钩,附着能力很强,可防止被宿主排出;其通过体壁吸收营养,消化器官完全退化;但为了增加生存机会,其生殖器官发达,雌雄同体。

[实验报告]

简述生物与生物间的三种关系。

Note

(田　芳　陆　凤)

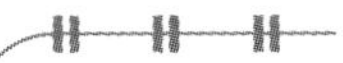

实验十三 吸 虫

[实验目的]

(1)了解吸虫的发育过程。熟悉华支睾吸虫(肝吸虫)、布氏姜片吸虫(肠吸虫)、卫氏并殖吸虫(肺吸虫)、日本血吸虫(血吸虫)各发育阶段的主要形态特征。

(2)掌握华支睾吸虫、布氏姜片吸虫、卫氏并殖吸虫及日本血吸虫成虫和虫卵的形态特征。

(3)了解华支睾吸虫、卫氏并殖吸虫、布氏姜片吸虫和日本血吸虫的中间宿主的形态特征。

(4)熟悉华支睾吸虫、卫氏并殖吸虫、布氏姜片吸虫和日本血吸虫在人体的寄生部位及引起的病理改变。

[实验材料]

示教标本(片)、显微镜、香柏油、二甲苯、擦镜纸等。

[实验内容]

一、示教内容

(一)吸虫的发育阶段

1. 虫卵 除日本血吸虫虫卵以外均有卵盖,内容物为已发育的毛蚴或未发育的卵黄细胞和卵细胞(华支睾吸虫虫卵标本)。

2. 毛蚴 梨形,周身被有纤毛,在水中运动活泼,必须进入螺体才能进一步发育(日本血吸虫毛蚴染色标本)。

3. 胞蚴 由钻入螺体的毛蚴发育而成。未发育成熟时为卵圆形囊状构造,以后逐渐变为长袋状,体内可见不同发育程度的胚细胞团(日本血吸虫胞蚴染色标本)。

4. 雷蚴 发育成熟的雷蚴为长椭圆形的囊状构造,一端有一明显肌肉性的咽及一不长的原始消化道,常见原始消化道有黑色物。雷蚴内含成熟或未成熟的尾蚴(华支睾吸虫雷蚴染色标本)。

5. 尾蚴 尾蚴从螺体逸出,分为体、尾两个部分,借尾部摆动在水中寻找第二中间宿主或终宿主。其形态因虫种不同而异(华支睾吸虫尾蚴染色标本)。

6. 囊蚴 多寄生于第二中间宿主,有明显的囊壁将蚴体包裹。活体囊蚴可见黑色排泄囊,其形状因虫种不同而异(华支睾吸虫囊蚴玻片标本)。

7. 成虫 观察寄生于人体的四种主要吸虫瓶装大体标本:华支睾吸虫(肝吸虫)、布氏姜片吸虫(肠吸虫)、卫氏并殖吸虫(肺吸虫)、日本血吸虫(血吸虫)。

(二)华支睾吸虫(肝吸虫)

1. 成虫大体标本(肉眼观察) 虫体体形狭长,扁薄半透明,外形似葵花子。前端稍窄,后端较钝圆,长 1～2 cm,隐约可见子宫、睾丸、卵黄腺。

2. 成虫染色玻片标本(低倍镜观察)

(1)口吸盘位于虫体顶端,腹吸盘位于虫体前 1/5 处,口吸盘大于腹吸盘。

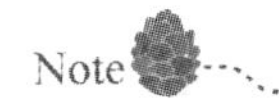

(2)睾丸 2 个,呈分枝状前后排列,位于虫体后 1/3 处。

(3)卵巢1个,浅分叶状,位于睾丸之前;子宫盘绕向前开口于生殖腔。

(4)椭圆形的受精囊及劳氏管清楚易见;卵黄腺呈滤泡状,位于虫体中部两侧。

(5)排泄囊为"S"形的长袋状结构,位于虫体后1/3中部。

3. 虫卵玻片标本(低倍镜及高倍镜观察) 肝吸虫卵是寄生蠕虫卵中最小的一种,大小为(27～35) μm×(12～20) μm,黄褐色,形似芝麻。用高倍镜观察,可见其卵盖周围的卵壳增厚形成肩峰,后端宽而钝圆,有一个小疣,卵内含有成熟的毛蚴。

4. 人工消化液消化囊蚴新鲜标本(低倍镜观察) 椭圆形,有两层囊壁,囊内可见到明显的呈黄褐色的排泄囊和口、腹吸盘。

5. 第一中间宿主(肉眼观察) 纹沼螺、长角涵螺等,呈卵圆锥形或短圆锥形,活时螺壳为青灰色,死后变为灰白色。

6. 第二中间宿主(肉眼观察) 淡水鱼、淡水虾等。

(三)布氏姜片吸虫(肠吸虫)

1. 成虫大体标本(肉眼观察) 寄生于人体的吸虫中最大的一种,大小为(20～75) mm×(8～20) mm×(1～3) mm,虫体扁平多肉,体表有皮棘。活时为肉红色,固定后为灰白色,可清楚见到口、腹吸盘,腹吸盘明显大于口吸盘。

2. 成虫染色玻片标本(肉眼或放大镜观察)

(1)口吸盘位于虫体顶端,腹吸盘呈漏斗状,比口吸盘大4～5倍,两吸盘相距很近。

(2)肠管呈波浪状弯曲。

(3)睾丸2个,高度分支,呈珊瑚状前后排列,占虫体后部的大半。

(4)卵巢位于虫体中部,分3瓣,每瓣再分支;子宫盘曲于腹吸盘与梅氏腺之间。

(5)无受精囊,卵黄腺呈滤泡状,分布于虫体两侧。

3. 虫卵玻片标本(低倍镜观察) 肠吸虫卵是蠕虫卵中最大者,大小为(130～140) μm×(80～85) μm,淡黄色,椭圆形,卵壳薄,卵盖小且不明显,卵内含1个卵细胞和20～40个卵黄细胞,卵细胞在已固定的标本中常不易见到。

4. 雷蚴染色玻片标本(高倍镜观察) 长袋形,具口、咽、原胚细胞团。

5. 尾蚴染色玻片标本(高倍镜观察) 体部无眼点,尾长,无膜包裹。

6. 囊蚴染色玻片标本(高倍镜观察) 有两层囊壁,外壁易破,内壁坚韧,囊中含幼虫,其排泄囊内含有折光颗粒,不规则地排列在囊的两侧,易于鉴别。

7. 中间宿主(肉眼观察) 扁卷螺,螺壳扁平盘曲,淡黄色,半透明。

8. 植物媒介 红菱、荸荠、茭白等。

(四)卫氏并殖吸虫(肺吸虫)

1. 成虫大体标本(肉眼观察) 虫体椭圆形,背部隆起,腹面扁平,大小为(7.5～12) mm×(4～6) mm×(1～3) mm,形如半粒黄豆。活时为棕红色,固定后为砖灰色,虫体腹面中部是充满黄色虫卵的子宫。

2. 成虫染色玻片标本(放大镜观察)

(1)口、腹吸盘大小几乎相等,口吸盘位于虫体前端顶面,腹吸盘位于虫体中横线之前。

(2)肠管位于虫体两侧,呈波浪状弯曲。

(3)睾丸和卵巢呈分叶状,2个睾丸并列于虫体后部,卵巢与子宫并列于虫体中部。

(4)卵黄腺呈繁枝状,遍布虫体两侧。

(5)排泄囊呈长裂隙状,自咽部直伸向末端开口。

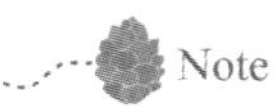

Note

3. 虫卵玻片标本(低倍镜及高倍镜观察) 肺吸虫卵大小为(80～118) μm×(48～60) μm,金黄色,椭圆形,卵壳厚薄不均,后端更厚。虫卵前端较宽,有一大而倾斜的卵盖,卵内含1个卵细胞和 10 余个卵黄细胞。

4. 雷蚴染色玻片标本(低倍镜观察) 圆柱形,前端有口、咽和原肠,其内含胚细胞团和短尾蚴。

5. 尾蚴染色玻片标本(高倍镜观察) 圆形或椭圆形,全身有细棘,前端有一小刺,尾极短,呈球状。

6. 囊蚴染色玻片标本(低倍镜观察) 球形,囊壁明显。囊内幼虫呈螺旋状弯曲,可见口、腹吸盘及大而明显的排泄囊。

7. 第一中间宿主(肉眼观察) 川蜷螺,为大型螺类,棕黄色,塔形,壳顶常因与溪石碰撞而磨损不全。

8. 第二中间宿主(肉眼观察) 石蟹、溪蟹和蝲蛄,石蟹、溪蟹生长于山区溪流,蝲蛄则多见于我国东北地区,均为甲壳动物。

9. 病理标本 肺吸虫感染人体后造成肺或脑部的病理改变,注意其表面有结节状隆起,成虫寄生于囊内,周围形成纤维性厚壁。

(五)日本血吸虫(血吸虫)

1. 成虫大体标本(肉眼观察) 虫体圆柱形,雄虫大小为(10～20) mm×(0.5～0.55) mm,乳白色,自腹吸盘后,虫体两侧略向腹面卷曲形成抱雌沟;雌虫大小为(12～28) mm×0.3 mm,灰褐色,较雄虫细长,尤其虫体前半部更为纤细,雌雄成虫常呈合抱状态。

2. 成虫染色玻片标本(低倍镜观察) 雄虫口吸盘较小,在虫体最前端。腹吸盘较大,位于离口吸盘不远的腹面,突出呈杯状。睾丸 7 个,椭圆形,呈串珠状或簇状排列,位于腹吸盘后方背侧。口开口于口吸盘中,无咽,下连一较短的食道,肠管先分为 2 支,在体后部再汇合成 1 支盲管。雌虫吸盘在虫体前端,较小而不明显,虫体中部略后处,有一染色较深的椭圆形卵巢。从其后方通出 1 根输卵管向前与卵黄管相通进入卵模,再向前即为子宫,内含 50～100 个虫卵,卵黄腺布满虫体后部,消化系统同雄虫。

3. 虫卵玻片标本(低倍镜及高倍镜观察) 血吸虫卵大小为(70～106) μm×(50～80) μm,淡黄色,椭圆形,壳薄无卵盖,一侧有一小棘,但常因虫卵的位置特殊或被卵壳上的黏附物遮盖而不易见到。成熟虫卵内含有一梨形的毛蚴。

4. 毛蚴

(1)毛蚴染色玻片标本(高倍镜观察):梨形,前端稍突起,体外的纤毛可能在制作的过程中脱落。体前部有原肠及 1 对头腺,体后部有胚细胞。

(2)活体毛蚴(肉眼或放大镜观察):自成熟虫卵孵化而出。观察时将含毛蚴的三角烧瓶放置在明亮处,使光源从侧前方射入,以深色物作为背景,主要看瓶颈部。毛蚴在水中为白色拉长的小点,做直线游动。

5. 胞蚴染色玻片标本(低倍镜观察) 从感染的钉螺肝脏内取出制片而成,有第一代与第二代之分。观察第二代胞蚴的示教标本,注意其长袋状构造,缺咽、肠,含有不同成熟度的尾蚴及胚细胞团。

6. 尾蚴

(1)尾蚴染色玻片标本(低倍镜观察):分体部和尾部,体部长圆形,有口、腹吸盘,腹吸盘两侧有 5 对穿刺腺;尾部末端分叉。

(2)活体尾蚴(放大镜观察):体部浮贴于水面,尾部悬于水面下并向前弯曲,虫体稍呈逗点状,活动时以其尾部扭曲摆动。注意观察时,勿用手去接触,以防感染。

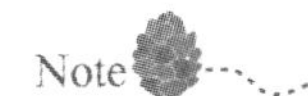

7. 中间宿主(肉眼观察) 钉螺:长约 1 cm,螺壳塔形,有 6～7 个螺旋,右旋,有厣。山区型螺壳较滑,平原型螺壳粗糙(有纵肋),褐色深浅不一。

8. 病理标本

(1)成虫寄生的肠系膜:合抱成虫在肠系膜静脉寄生,黑色的雌虫部分深入肠壁血管。

(2)虫卵沉积的兔肝:布满虫卵结节。

(3)健康兔肝:表面光滑无病变。

二、自己镜检

(1)观察华支睾吸虫、布氏姜片吸虫、卫氏并殖吸虫成虫及日本血吸虫的雌雄成虫玻片标本。

(2)观察华支睾吸虫、布氏姜片吸虫、卫氏并殖吸虫、日本血吸虫的虫卵玻片标本。

(3)观察吸虫卵混合滴片标本。

(4)观察日本血吸虫感染兔肝组织压片、日本血吸虫感染兔肠黏膜组织压片。

(5)观察日本血吸虫感染兔解剖标本,观察成虫寄生部位,肝、肠病变及虫卵结节。

三、录像片

观看日本血吸虫录像片。

[实验报告]

绘制华支睾吸虫、布氏姜片吸虫、卫氏并殖吸虫、日本血吸虫的虫卵图并注明其构造。

[思考题]

(1)华支睾吸虫、布氏姜片吸虫、卫氏并殖吸虫、日本血吸虫在生活史上的异同点有哪些?推断其防治措施上的异同。

(2)日本血吸虫成虫与虫卵在形态上与其他三种吸虫有哪些主要不同点?

(3)为什么能用粪便沉淀孵化法来诊断日本血吸虫病?

(4)肠黏膜活组织检查发现了日本血吸虫卵,是否就可以肯定是现症日本血吸虫病患者?如何进行分析?

(田　芳　陆　凤)

实验十四　绦　　虫

[实验目的]

(1)掌握带绦虫成虫、虫卵、囊尾蚴的形态特征和带绦虫病的诊断方法。

(2)熟悉棘球蚴和微小膜壳绦虫卵的形态构造。

(3)了解细粒棘球绦虫成虫、微小膜壳绦虫成虫及曼氏迭宫绦虫的成虫、裂头蚴和虫卵的形态特点。

[实验材料]

示教标本(片)、显微镜、香柏油、二甲苯、擦镜纸等。

[实验内容]

一、示教内容

(一)链状带绦虫(又称猪带绦虫)

1. 成虫大体标本(肉眼观察) 乳白色带状，背腹扁平，分节，长 2～4 m。虫体分为头节、颈部、链体三个部分。头节细小，直径约 1 mm，较细窄的颈部紧接其后，颈部后为链体，由 700～1000 个节片组成。与颈部接近的节片，宽度大于长度，为幼节；中部节片近正方形，为成节；远端节片长度大于宽度，为孕节。这三种节片是逐渐发育形成的，没有绝对的分界线。

2. 头节染色玻片标本(低倍镜观察) 圆球形，上有 4 个杯状吸盘，顶部有一向前突出的顶突。上有两圈小钩，小钩共 25～50 个。

3. 成节染色玻片标本(放大镜观察) 近正方形，节片内部为雌、雄生殖器官，其卵巢为三叶，卵巢后方是滤泡状构造的卵黄腺。其间向上伸出的一直管状的子宫是不开口的盲管。在节片两侧分散着许多滤泡状构造的睾丸，生殖孔开口于节片的侧缘。

4. 孕节染色玻片标本(放大镜观察) 经染色或从生殖腔中注射染液后封片制成。节片呈长方形，子宫纵贯节片中央并向两侧分支，每侧有 7～13 个分支，分支不整齐。

5. 囊尾蚴瓶装标本(肉眼观察) 黄豆大小，乳白色。半透明，囊内充满液体，囊壁内面的一白色小点是头节。活囊尾蚴放在胆汁中经加热后，头节翻出，染色后其形态与成虫头节相同。

6. 病理标本 囊尾蚴寄生于猪肉内，呈白色，水泡状，周围包以结缔组织纤维膜。

(二)肥胖带绦虫(又称牛带绦虫)

1. 成虫大体标本(肉眼观察) 形态与猪带绦虫成虫相似，但链体肥厚，虫体可长至 4～8 m，有 1000～2000 个节片。

2. 头节染色玻片标本(低倍镜观察) 头节略呈方形，上有 4 个杯状吸盘，无顶突和小钩。

3. 成节染色玻片标本(放大镜观察) 卵巢仅分左、右两叶，其余与猪带绦虫基本相同。

4. 孕节染色玻片标本(放大镜观察) 子宫分支较整齐，每侧有 15～30 个分支。

5. 病理标本 囊尾蚴寄生在牛肉中。

6. 带绦虫卵玻片标本(低倍镜及高倍镜观察) 无法区别两种绦虫卵，故统称带绦虫卵。虫卵呈圆形或椭圆形，直径 31～43 μm，卵壳薄而无色透明，易脱落，胚膜较厚，呈黄褐色并有放射状条纹。内有六钩蚴，直径 14～20 μm，6 个小钩常不易同时见到，或因虫卵保存时间过久、脱落而不能见到。

(三)细粒棘球绦虫(包生绦虫)

1. 成虫染色玻片标本(低倍镜观察) 虫体很小，长 2～7 mm，头节呈梨形，有 4 个吸盘，伸缩力很强的顶突上有两圈小钩，共 28～48 个。链体通常只有 1 个幼节、1 个成节和 1 个孕节，成节的结构与带绦虫相似，孕节的子宫向两侧形成袋状分支，内含虫卵 200～800 个。

2. 病理标本 棘球蚴寄生在人及动物肝脏内，其外层是宿主的组织包膜，内层是棘球蚴的囊壁。囊壁又可分为两层，外层角皮层较厚，状如粉皮，内层为生发层(胚层)，很薄。囊内充满无色或微黄色液体，称棘球液(囊液)。子囊、生发囊及原头蚴脱落后均可悬浮在囊液中，称棘球蚴砂。

3. 原头蚴染色玻片标本(低倍镜观察) 椭圆形，可见吸盘及缩入的顶突小钩。由于吸盘重叠，常仅见 2 个吸盘。1 个原头蚴在终宿主体内可发育为 1 个虫体。

4. 虫卵 与带绦虫卵基本相同，在普通光学显微镜下难以区别。

(四)微小膜壳绦虫(短膜壳绦虫)

1. 成虫大体标本(肉眼观察) 乳白色，长 5～80 mm，有 100～200 个节片，均宽度大于长度。

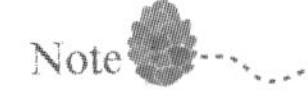

2. 成虫染色玻片标本(低倍镜观察)

(1)头节:菱形或圆形,4 个吸盘,1 个可伸缩的顶突,上有一圈小钩,小钩共 20～30 个。

(2)成节:椭圆形,3 个睾丸沿横线排列;卵巢两叶,位于中央,下有卵黄腺。

(3)孕节:子宫囊状,充满虫卵,虫卵数为 80～180 个。

3. 虫卵玻片标本(低倍镜及高倍镜观察) 圆形或椭圆形,无色透明,中间含 1 个六钩蚴。六钩蚴外被以胚膜,胚膜外有很薄的卵壳,胚膜的两极略隆起,生出 4～8 根细丝。

附:曼氏迭宫绦虫

1. 成虫大体标本(肉眼观察) 链体可长达 1 m 左右,节片均宽度大于长度,但远端节片长宽几乎相等,关节细小呈指状,背、腹面各有 1 条纵向的吸槽。

2. 头节染色玻片标本(低倍镜或放大镜观察) 睾丸为小泡状,有数百个,卵巢为左右对称的两叶,子宫位于节片中部呈螺旋状盘曲,紧密重叠。

3. 虫卵玻片标本(低倍镜观察) 近椭圆形,大小为(40～60) μm×(36～48) μm,两端稍尖,呈浅灰褐色,有卵盖,卵壳较薄,内含 1 个卵细胞和许多卵黄细胞。

4. 裂头蚴(肉眼观察) 长形,大小为 300 mm×(0.1～12) mm,体前端稍大,具有与成虫相似的头节,但具横皱纹状。常寄生在蛙的肌肉间隙内。

二、自己镜检

观察带绦虫卵、微小膜壳绦虫卵、猪带绦虫头节及孕节、牛带绦虫头节及孕节、原头蚴。

[实验报告]

绘制带绦虫卵及微小膜壳绦虫卵图并注明其构造。

[思考题]

(1)列表比较猪带绦虫与牛带绦虫的形态和生活史。为什么说猪带绦虫对人的危害比牛带绦虫大?

(2)为什么棘球蚴病多见于我国西北畜牧地区?

(3)如何解读猪囊尾蚴病的血清学诊断结果?

(田　芳　陆　凤)

实验十五　线　　虫

[实验目的]

(1)了解丝虫成虫、旋毛虫成虫及幼虫的形态特征。

(2)熟悉蛔虫、鞭虫、蛲虫及钩虫成虫的形态特征。

(3)掌握蛔虫卵、鞭虫卵、蛲虫卵、钩虫卵的形态特征。掌握两种微丝蚴的形态鉴别要点。

[实验材料]

示教标本(片)、显微镜、香柏油、二甲苯、擦镜纸、染色液等。

[实验内容]

一、示教内容

(一)似蚓蛔线虫(蛔虫)

1. 成虫大体标本(肉眼观察) 似蚓蛔线虫是寄生于人体的最大的线虫,形似蚯蚓,活时呈淡红色,死后呈黄白色。雌雄异体,雌虫比雄虫大,雌虫长 20～35 cm、宽 3～6 mm,尾端垂直;雄虫长 15～31 cm、宽 2～4 mm,尾部向腹面卷曲。体表为角皮层,有纤细环纹。左、右各有纵向侧线一条,背线、腹线不明显。

2. 成虫解剖标本(肉眼观察)

(1)消化器官:一纵行直管,开口于虫体顶端,下连短棒状食道,以下依次为中肠和直肠。雌虫直肠通后端肛门,雄虫直肠与射精管均通泄殖腔。

(2)生殖器官:雌虫的生殖器官为两组相同的管状构造。卵巢长如线,一端游离,另一端逐渐膨大形成输卵管、子宫,子宫为最粗部分,其内充满虫卵,两组子宫末端合并而成阴道,阴门开口于虫体腹面前 1/3 与中 1/3 交界处。雄虫的生殖器官为单组的管状构造,依次为睾丸、输精管、储精囊(最粗)、射精管,尾端有两根交合刺伸入泄殖腔而通至体外。

3. 蛔虫头部玻片标本(低倍镜观察) 唇瓣三个,一个在背面(称背唇),两个在腹面(称腹唇),呈"品"字形排列。

4. 蛔虫卵玻片标本(低倍镜及高倍镜观察) 蛔虫受精卵为短椭圆形,大小为(45～75) μm×(35～50) μm,呈黄褐色,卵壳厚,外有一层凹凸不平的蛋白质膜,内含一大而圆的卵细胞,卵细胞与卵壳两端有新月形空隙。蛔虫未受精卵大小为(80～94) μm×(39～44) μm,呈黄褐色,长椭圆形,蛋白质膜和卵壳均较薄,蛋白质膜分布不均匀,卵内含大小不等、反光性较强的卵黄颗粒。受精卵与未受精卵的蛋白质膜均可脱落,即脱蛋白质膜卵。此卵颜色变为无色,卵内结构不变。感染期虫卵(含蚴卵):外形与受精卵相同,但卵内是一卷曲的幼虫。

5. 病理标本(肉眼观察) 观察蛔虫寄生在胆道、肠道、阑尾及气管的大体病理标本。

(二)毛首鞭形线虫(鞭虫)

1. 成虫大体标本(肉眼观察) 灰白色,前 3/5 细长,后 2/5 粗短,形似马鞭,故得名鞭虫。雌虫较大,长 30～50 mm,尾部直而钝圆;雄虫较小,长 30～45 mm,尾部卷曲。

2. 雄虫染色玻片标本(低倍镜观察) 尾部有一根交合刺,交合刺外面有可伸缩的交合刺鞘。

3. 雌虫染色玻片标本(低倍镜观察) 阴门位于虫体中部以后、粗部前方的腹面,尾部末端钝圆。

4. 鞭虫卵染色玻片标本(低倍镜及高倍镜观察) 大小为(50～54) μm×(22～23) μm,黄褐色,橄榄形,卵壳厚,两端有透明栓,卵内含一长圆形卵细胞。

5. 病理标本(肉眼观察) 鞭虫寄生于肠壁,以其虫体前端的细长部侵入肠黏膜,而以粗短的虫体后部游离于肠腔中。

(三)蠕形住肠线虫(蛲虫)

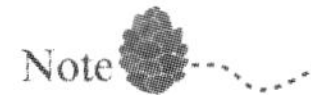

1. 成虫大体标本(肉眼观察) 虫体细小,乳白色,状似白棉线头。雌虫长 8～13 mm,尾尖部细长;雄虫长 2～5 mm,尾端向腹面卷曲。

2. 成虫染色玻片标本(低倍镜观察) 虫体前端有三个唇瓣,两侧角皮隆起形成头翼,食道末端呈球形隆起,称食管球。雄虫尾端有交合刺一根,雄虫阴门开口于虫体前 1/3 腹面正中线上。

3. 蛲虫卵染色玻片标本(低倍镜及高倍镜观察) 大小(50～60) μm×(20～30) μm,无色透明,柿核形,不对称,一侧隆起,一侧扁平,卵壳较厚,内含一接近成熟的幼虫。

(四)十二指肠钩口线虫和美洲板口线虫(钩虫)

1. 两种钩虫成虫大体标本(肉眼观察) 虫体呈细长圆柱形,长 1 cm 左右,乳白色,雌虫较雄虫略粗长,尾直,雄虫尾端膨大成伞状。十二指肠钩口线虫头部与身体弯曲方向一致,似"C"形;美洲板口线虫头部与身体弯曲方向相反,略似"S"形。

2. 成虫口囊玻片标本(低倍镜观察) 虫体前端为口囊,十二指肠钩口线虫口囊内有两对钩齿;美洲板口线虫口囊内仅一对板齿。

3. 成虫尾部玻片标本(低倍镜观察) 十二指肠钩口线虫雌虫尾部有透明的尾刺,雄虫交合伞撑开时呈圆形,交合刺一对,末端分开,背辐肋在末端 1/3 处分为 2 支,每一支再各分为 3 小支。美洲板口线虫雌虫无尾刺,雄虫交合伞撑开时呈扁圆形,交合刺一对,一刺末端呈钩状,包于另一刺的凹槽中,背辐肋在基部分为 2 支,每一支再各分为 2 小支。

4. 钩虫卵玻片标本(低倍镜及高倍镜观察) 大小(57～76) μm×(36～40) μm,卵壳薄,无色透明,椭圆形。随粪便排出时,卵内通常具有 2～8 个卵细胞,以 8 个卵细胞期为多见。如粪便放置较久,卵内细胞继续分裂,可呈桑椹形甚至发育为幼虫。

5. 杆状蚴玻片标本(高倍镜观察) 前端钝圆,后端尖细。食道前端粗大,中间狭小,后端略呈球形。食道长度等于体长的 1/4。

6. 丝状蚴玻片标本(高倍镜观察) 口腔封闭,食道前端细长,后端球状体不明显,尾端尖细。食道长度等于体长的 1/4。

7. 成虫寄生小肠的大体标本(肉眼观察) 观察成虫寄生小肠的大体标本。

(五)班氏吴策线虫和马来布鲁线虫(丝虫)

1. 丝虫成虫大体标本(肉眼观察) 虫体呈细长丝状,乳白色,体表光滑。雌虫较长,尾端不弯曲;雄虫较短,尾端向腹面卷曲 2～3 周。班氏吴策线虫雌虫长 58.5～105 mm、宽 0.2～0.3 mm,雄虫长 28.2～42 mm、宽 0.2～0.3 mm;马来布鲁线虫雌虫长 40～69 mm、宽 0.12～0.22 mm,雄虫长 13.5～28.1 mm、宽 0.07～11 mm。

2. 未染色微丝蚴玻片标本(低倍镜及高倍镜观察) 微丝蚴呈细长丝状,无色透明,反光性强,前端钝圆,后端尖细。

3. 两种微丝蚴染色玻片标本(高倍镜或油镜观察) 吉氏或苏木素染色,可见微丝蚴体外有鞘,体内有紫蓝色核点(表 2-15-1)。

4. 丝状蚴在蚊口器内玻片标本 观察丝状蚴在蚊口器内玻片标本。

5. 病理标本 观察阴囊象皮肿病理标本。

表 2-15-1 两种微丝蚴鉴别要点

鉴别要点	班氏微丝蚴	马来微丝蚴
大小/μm	(244～296)×(5.3～7)	(177～230)×(5～6)
体态	柔和,弯曲度较大而自然	僵直,大弯中有小弯
头间隙	较短,长宽相等或长度为宽度的 1/2	较长,长度约为宽度的 2 倍
体核	排列疏松,相互分开,清晰可数	排列紧密,常相互重叠,不易分清
尾核	无	有 2 个,前后排列,尾核处膨大

(六)旋毛虫

1. 成虫玻片标本(低倍镜观察) 虫体细小,前端较后端细,食道由长形单细胞组成,雌虫长3～4 mm,尾端钝圆;雄虫长1.4～1.5 mm,尾端有用于交配的附器。

2. 幼虫玻片标本(低倍镜观察) 虫体细长,卷曲成螺旋形,外有囊壁,形成椭圆形或棱形囊包,内含1～2条幼虫,囊包和横纹肌纤维平行排列。

二、自己镜检

观察蛔虫卵、鞭虫卵、蛲虫卵、钩虫卵玻片标本,以及未染色微丝蚴、两种微丝蚴染色玻片标本。

三、录像片

观看线虫录像片。

[实验报告]

绘制蛔虫受精卵和未受精卵、鞭虫卵、蛲虫卵、钩虫卵及班氏微丝蚴、马来微丝蚴图,并说明其结构名称。

[思考题]

(1)粪便检查未检获蛔虫卵能否排除蛔虫早期感染?
(2)经口食入蛔虫卵,是否能引起蛔虫感染?
(3)鞭虫生活史和蛔虫生活史有哪些异同点?
(4)简述十二指肠钩口线虫和美洲板口线虫主要鉴别点。
(5)输入含有微丝蚴的血液后能否引起丝虫病? 为什么?
(6)怎样诊断丝虫病? 为什么要这样做?
(7)怎样鉴别人体感染的丝虫虫体? 丝虫的种类鉴别有何临床价值?

(田　芳　陆　凤)

实验十六　常见蠕虫的检验方法

[实验目的]

(1)掌握粪便直接涂片法和饱和盐水浮聚法。
(2)熟悉透明胶纸法、钩蚴培养法、定量透明法(改良加藤氏法)、水洗沉淀法、毛蚴孵化法及环卵沉淀试验等技术。
(3)掌握粪便检查中可见的常见蠕虫卵的形态特征。

[实验内容]

一、粪便标本中蠕虫的检查方法

(一)粪便标本的收集

寄生于肠道的蠕虫和原虫,都是随粪便排出人体的。由于许多肠道寄生虫极易损坏,为保持

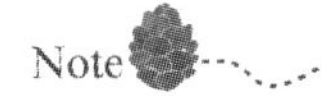

它们的原有形态以便准确鉴别,只有正确收集粪便才能做可靠的形态学诊断。

(1)给患者带盖的涂蜡纸盒或杯子(容器须洁净、干燥)以留取粪便,告诉患者直接将粪便排到容器内或一张纸上,然后用竹签转移粪便到容器内,防止污染。粪便不可混入尿液及其他体液等。

(2)粪便必须新鲜,送检时间一般不宜超过 24 h。

(3)在盛有标本的容器上清楚地标明下列内容:患者姓名、标本编号、标本收集日期、患者排便的时间。

(4)为了取得满意的检查结果,粪便标本一定要足量(鸽子蛋大小)。标本不能混有尿液等脏物。

(5)如不能立即检查标本,将装有标本的纸盒放在冰箱内,切忌将标本放在温暖的地方,也不要放在阳光下。

(二)常见蠕虫卵的检查

方法示教:透明胶纸法、钩蚴培养法、定量透明法(改良加藤氏法)、水洗沉淀法及毛蚴孵化法。

自己操作:粪便直接涂片法、饱和盐水浮聚法。

1. 粪便直接涂片法 粪便直接涂片法是检查粪便中蠕虫卵最常用的方法。为了不改变涂片的渗透压,一般用生理盐水作为粪便的稀释剂,使和粪便粘在一起的寄生虫和寄生虫卵,通过生理盐水的稀释作用,分散在涂片中,这样既不妨碍透光作用,又能暴露寄生虫及寄生虫卵的形态结构,便于在镜检中识别。此法是适用范围最广的一种方法。

实验材料:显微镜、载玻片、竹签或牙签、生理盐水等。

方法:在干净的载玻片上滴 3 大滴生理盐水,用竹签挑取火柴头大小的粪便,在生理盐水中调匀涂开,涂成长约 4 cm、宽约 1.8 cm 的椭圆形粪膜,置显微镜下观察。

注意事项:

(1)要求涂膜厚度适当,太厚则看不清虫卵易致漏检,太薄则涂材太少而影响虫卵检出率,涂片厚薄以能透过粪膜看清下面印刷的字为宜。

(2)粪便中如有脓血,应取此部分进行涂片。

(3)粪便涂片约占玻片大小的 2/3,粪便不要接近玻片边缘,涂片上的粗颗粒应除去,以免沾污载物台及手指。

(4)显微镜须平放,切忌倾斜。镜检时先用低倍镜观察,可疑时换用高倍镜。

(5)每份标本涂片 3 张,以提高检出率。

(6)注意防止涂片干燥,必要时滴加生理盐水。

2. 浮聚法 利用相对密度较大的液体,使蠕虫卵上浮,集中于液体表面进行检查。常用的方法有两种:饱和盐水浮聚法和硫酸锌离心浮聚法。

(1)饱和盐水浮聚法:利用饱和盐水这种相对密度较大的液体,使蠕虫卵上浮,集中于液体表面进行检查,主要用于钩虫卵的检查。

实验材料:漂浮杯(或用青霉素瓶、链霉素瓶代替)、竹签、载玻片、滴管、显微镜、饱和盐水(相对密度达 1.20)等。饱和盐水的配制:将食盐徐徐加入盛有沸水的容器内,不断搅动,至食盐不再溶解,容器底有食盐沉淀为止。

方法:用竹签取黄豆粒大小的粪便放入漂浮杯内,加入相当于漂浮杯 1/4 量的饱和盐水,调匀。再加入饱和盐水至漂浮杯的 3/4 量,混匀。将漂浮杯平置于搪瓷盘中,再轻轻加入饱和盐水使液面稍高出于杯口而不外溢,取一洁净(干燥无脂肪)的载玻片轻轻盖于杯口,静置 15～20 min,再将载玻片垂直提起并翻转,镜检。

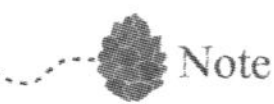

注意事项:①此法适用于相对密度较小的虫卵,检查钩虫卵效果最好,也可用于检查其他线虫卵和微小膜壳绦虫卵,但不适用于检查吸虫卵;②应挑去液面上漂浮的粗渣;③将载玻片盖于杯口时,避免留有气泡。④翻片速度不宜过快,防止粪液甩落于他处。

(2)硫酸锌离心浮聚法。

实验材料:离心管、离心机、33%硫酸锌溶液(相对密度为1.18)、吸管、40~60目金属筛等。

方法:取粪便约1 g,加10~15倍量的水,充分搅碎,用金属筛过滤。将过滤后的粪液倒入离心管中,1500~2000 r/min离心2 min,反复离心3~4次,至水清为止,最后倒去上清液,在沉渣中加入硫酸锌溶液,调匀后再加硫酸锌溶液至离管口1 cm,同法离心2 min。用金属环挑取表面的粪液置于载玻片上,镜检。

注意事项:①此法适用于检查原虫包囊、线虫卵和微小膜壳绦虫卵;②检查包囊时滴加碘液1滴,盖上盖玻片镜检;③挑取标本时,用金属环轻轻接触液面即可,切勿搅动;④离心后应立即取标本镜检,如果放置时间超过1 h,则会因包囊或虫卵变形而影响观察效果;⑤尚有硝酸钠漂浮法,即将硝酸钠溶于等量水中,煮沸后冷却(相对密度为1.40),以此代替硫酸锌溶液效果很好。

3.沉淀法 蠕虫卵相对密度大,可沉积于水底,有助于虫卵的浓聚,提高检出率。但相对密度较小的钩虫卵和某些原虫包囊用沉淀法则效果较差。

(1)水洗沉淀法:此法是传统的肠道寄生虫卵检查方法,适用于多种蠕虫卵的检查。

实验材料:500 ml或1000 ml三角量杯或搪瓷杯、40~60目金属筛、玻璃棒、吸管等。

方法:取粪便约30 g(鸡蛋大小),通过金属筛筛入盛满清水的三角量杯或搪瓷杯内,静置20~30 min,倒去上层粪水,留下沉淀物,然后加满清水,以后每隔20 min换水1次,直至水清(需3~5次)。最后倒去上层液,留取沉渣,以毛细管吸取底部沉渣涂片1~3张,镜检。

注意事项:①倾倒水时不能有间断,以免沉渣浮起而被倒掉;②操作过程应绝对防止相互污染,所用器材应反复清洗;③检查血吸虫卵时,沉淀时间不宜过长,尤其当室温高于15 ℃时,卵内毛蚴易孵化;④增加涂片数可提高检出率。

(2)离心沉淀法:将上述滤去粗渣的粪液以1500~2000 r/min离心1~2 min,倒去上层液,注入清水,再离心沉淀,如此反复沉淀3~4次,直至上层液澄清,最后倒去上层液,取沉渣镜检。本法省时、省力,适用于临床检验。

(3)汞碘醛离心(MIFC)沉淀法:本法既可浓集,又可固定和染色,适用于原虫包囊、滋养体及蠕虫卵和幼虫的检查。

试剂配方:①A液(汞碘醛液):1/1000硫柳汞酊200 ml、甲醛25 ml、甘油5 ml、蒸馏水200 ml。②B液(5%鲁氏碘液):碘5 g、碘化钾10 g、蒸馏水100 ml。检查时取A液2.35 ml、B液0.15 ml混合备用。

方法:取粪便约1 g,加上述混合液5 ml,调匀滤去粗渣,加入乙醚4 ml,充分振荡混匀,在离心管中静置2 min。1500~2000 r/min离心1~2 min,使分成乙醚、粪渣、汞碘醛液及沉淀物4层,倒去上3层,留沉淀涂片镜检。

注意事项:①本法不仅浓集效果好,而且不损伤包囊和虫卵的形态,易于观察和鉴定;②对于含脂肪较多的粪便,本法效果优于硫酸锌离心浮聚法。

4.定量透明法(改良加藤氏法) 粪便厚涂片经甘油透明后进行镜检,视野背景呈淡绿色。

实验材料:①100目金属筛、刮片、玻璃纸、聚苯乙烯定量板(大小为40 mm×30 mm×1.37 mm,模孔为一长圆孔或长条孔,所取的粪样平均为41.7 mg);②甘油-孔雀绿溶液:甘油100 ml、3%孔雀绿水溶液1 ml、蒸馏水100 ml;③将玻璃纸裁剪成24 mm×50 mm大小,浸泡于甘油-孔雀绿溶液中24 h,备用。

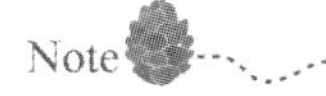

方法:置定量板于载玻片上,将金属筛覆盖在粪便标本上,自筛网上用刮片刮取粪便约50 mg,用一手的两指压住定量板的两端,将刮片上的粪便填满模孔,刮去多余粪便。掀去定量板,载

玻片上留下一个长形粪样，然后在粪条上覆盖含甘油-孔雀绿溶液的玻璃纸条，展平后加压，使玻璃纸下的粪便铺成长椭圆形。粪便经 1～2 h 透明后置镜下检查，可进行虫卵计数。

注意事项：

(1)本法适用于蠕虫卵检查，因粪便标本取材量大，故检出率高。

(2)必须掌握粪膜的合适厚度和透明的时间，如粪膜厚、透明时间短，则难以发现虫卵；如透明时间过长，则虫卵变形，卵壳破裂，也不易辨认。在检查钩虫卵时，透明时间为 30 min。

(3)模孔为两个长条孔的定量板更易压出厚度适宜的粪膜。

(4)每克粪便虫卵数(eggs per gram，EPG)＝每张片上虫卵数×24×粪便性状系数。粪便性状系数：成形粪便为 1，半成形粪便为 1.5，软湿粪便为 2，水泻粪便为 4。

5. 钩蚴培养法 本法是根据钩虫卵内幼虫在适宜的温度、湿度等条件下可在短时间内孵出的原理设计的。

实验材料：1.2 cm×12 cm 试管、滤纸条(滤纸剪成约 1.5 cm×10 cm T 形纸条)、恒温培养箱等。

方法：将滤纸条对折成一角度，取洁净试管，加入冷开水或蒸馏水 2～3 ml，使滤纸条插入试管后下端刚好能浸入水中。取粪便 0.2～0.4 g，均匀地涂在滤纸条中段，并将滤纸条插入试管，但不接触水底，同时注意勿使粪便混入水中，置 20～30 ℃环境中培养。3～5 d 后，肉眼观察或用放大镜检查管底部水中有无乳白色做蛇形运动的钩蚴。

注意事项：

(1)操作前用铅笔将受检者姓名或编号书写于滤纸条横边。

(2)培养期间每天沿管壁补充水分，以保持水面高度。

(3)在将滤纸条插入试管时，涂抹的粪便切勿接触水面。

(4)3 d 后如未发现钩蚴，应继续培养观察至第 5 天。

6. 毛蚴孵化法 本法是根据血吸虫卵内的毛蚴在适宜温度的清水中，短时间内可孵出的特性，结合水洗沉淀法而设计的方法，适用于早期血吸虫病患者的粪便检查。

实验材料：三角烧瓶、500 ml 或 1000 ml 锥形量杯、40～60 目金属筛、玻璃棒、吸管等。

方法：取粪便约 30 g(鸡蛋大小)，先经水洗沉淀法浓集处理，以毛细管吸取沉渣，涂片 3 张镜检虫卵。如未找到虫卵，则将全部沉渣倒入 500 ml 的三角烧瓶内，加清水至瓶口，在 20～30 ℃的条件下进行孵化。分别在 4 h、12 h、24 h 后用肉眼或放大镜观察结果。如见水面下有白色点状物做直线来往游动，即是毛蚴。

注意事项：

(1)粪便必须新鲜，不新鲜或粪量过少都会影响检出率。

(2)沉淀换水时必须使上层液澄清，否则影响观察结果。

(3)气温高时，毛蚴可在短时间内孵出，因此在夏季水洗粪便时要用 1.2%食盐水或冰水冲洗粪便，最后一次才改用室温清水。

(4)换水倾倒时不能有间断，以免沉渣浮起被倒掉。

(5)孵化用水必须是清水，适宜的 pH 为 7.2～7.6。含盐分或余氯过多或含 NH_2 均影响孵化。

(6)操作过程中应绝对防止相互污染。所用器材应反复清洗，并用沸水泡杀虫卵。

(7)观察结果时应仔细与水虫鉴别。毛蚴为针尖大小，长圆形，灰白色，折光，大小一致，常在离水面 1～4 cm 处做直线来往游动，碰壁才转向。必要时，将其吸至载玻片上，用显微镜观察。

7. 尼龙袋集卵法 主要用于血吸虫卵的浓集检查。

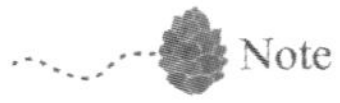

实验材料：60 目铜筛，120 目(内袋，袋深 10 cm，袋口直径 8 cm)、260 目(外袋，袋深 15 cm，袋口直径 9 cm)尼龙袋，三角量杯。将 120 目(孔径略大于血吸虫卵)尼龙袋套于 260 目(孔径略小

于血吸虫卵)尼龙袋内备用。

方法:先将粪便加水调匀,经60目铜筛滤去粗粪渣,将滤下的粪便淋入两只套在一起的尼龙袋中,移去铜筛,继续淋水冲洗袋内粪渣,并将袋轻轻振动,使之加速过滤,直至滤出液变澄清。然后收集260目尼龙袋内的粪渣做镜检或进行毛蚴孵化。

注意事项:本法与沉淀法比较,有费时短、虫卵丢失少、器材使用少、便于流动普查等优点,但尼龙袋必须严格清洗,防止交叉污染。

8. 绦虫检查法 为评价驱虫疗效,常需从粪便中淘取绦虫进行鉴定与计数。方法是取患者服药后24～72 h的全部粪便,加水搅拌,用40目筛或纱布滤出粪渣,经水反复冲洗后,倒在盛有清水的大玻璃皿内。在大玻璃皿下衬以黑纸检查虫体。

9. 带绦虫孕节检查法 在粪便内、衣裤、被褥上检得绦虫节片后,用清水洗净,置于两个玻片之间,轻轻压薄,对光观察内部结构,并根据子宫分支情况鉴定虫种,如一侧分支数<15,则为猪带绦虫,否则为牛带绦虫。若上法不能辨认,可用小注射器从孕节生殖孔徐徐注入碳素墨水或墨汁或卡红液(钾明矾饱和液100 ml、卡红3 g、冰醋酸10 ml,混合后置于37 ℃温箱内过夜,过滤后应用)于子宫内,待子宫分支显现后计数。检查完成后所用器皿均须消毒以杀死虫卵。

(三)蠕虫混合虫卵标本片镜检

用低倍镜寻找虫卵并确定是哪一种蠕虫卵。

线虫、吸虫和绦虫是医学上三类重要的蠕虫,常用的诊断方法是检查虫卵。用于鉴别各种虫卵的特征如下:①大小:虫卵长度和宽度可以测量,它们总是在一定范围内。②形状:每种虫卵均有其特殊的形状。③颜色:有些虫卵无色,有些为黄色或棕色。④卵壳的厚度:有些虫种卵壳厚,另一些卵壳薄。⑤具有特征性的结构,如卵盖、棘、塞或小钩等。⑥虫卵内容物:当虫卵随粪便被排出时,有些虫种的虫卵由单细胞组成,有些可能由多细胞组成;另有一些处于胚胎期(即含有1个幼虫);有时粪便标本已存放数小时或1～2 d之久,虫卵可发育到较晚期。由于发育期的变化,虫卵也会随之变化。蛔虫卵随粪便排出时通常仅有1个卵细胞,然而单细胞可能分裂,故陈旧的标本中可见到有2个或4个卵细胞的虫卵。在保存数小时的粪便标本内,钩虫卵内可含有16个、32个或更多个卵细胞,粪便排出后12～24 h,虫卵可能发育为胚胎,而后孵化出幼虫。因此诊断所用的理想标本应该是新鲜粪便。

二、肛门周围寄生虫的检查方法

透明胶纸法:主要适用于蛲虫卵、带绦虫卵的检查,蛲虫于肛周产卵,带绦虫卵常可黏附在肛门附近,利用透明胶纸的胶面粘贴后镜检。

实验材料:长约6 cm、宽约2 cm透明胶纸,二甲苯。

方法:用长约6 cm、宽约2 cm透明胶纸的胶面粘贴肛门周围的皮肤后,将胶面平贴在玻片上,镜检。

注意事项:

(1)检查时一端揭起,在玻片和透明胶纸之间滴加一滴二甲苯,再把胶纸粘回原处镜检。

(2)检查时间最好是清晨排便前。

(3)显微镜检查时注意区分虫卵与气泡。

三、血液标本中蠕虫的检查方法

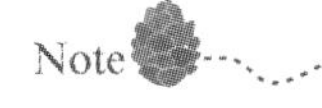

1. 血液标本中微丝蚴检查 在我国,寄生于人体的丝虫主要有班氏吴策线虫和马来布鲁线虫两种,它们的微丝蚴都是夜间出现在外周血液中。所以都必须在晚上9时以后取血检查。染色检查可以确定虫种。

(1)微丝蚴厚血膜检查法:取耳垂或指尖血3大滴(约60 μl)。滴于洁净干燥的载玻片中央,用另一张玻片的角将血滴涂成1 cm×2 cm的椭圆形厚血膜。血膜应厚薄均匀、边缘整齐,平放,自然晾干。用蒸馏水或冷开水滴在血膜上盖没血膜溶血,5～10 min后倒去血水,再加上清水重复溶血1次,至血膜无红色为止。血膜脱去血红蛋白变为灰白色后,镜检。厚血膜的制作、溶血、固定与吉姆萨染色同疟原虫检查法。用苏木素染色法染色效果更好。在10倍物镜下寻找微丝蚴。此时,微丝蚴容易查出。如果找到微丝蚴,换油镜鉴别虫种。观察完全片。

(2)苏木素染色法。

染液配制:取苏木素1 g溶于纯酒精或95%酒精10 ml中,加饱和硫酸铝铵(8%～10%)100 ml,倒入棕色瓶中,瓶口用两层纱布扎紧,在阳光下氧化2～4周,过滤,加甘油25 ml和甲醇25 ml。用时稀释10倍左右。

染色方法:将已溶血、固定的厚血膜在Delafield苏木素液内染10～15 min,在1%酸性酒精中分色1～2 min,蒸馏水洗涤1～5 min,至血膜呈蓝色,再用1%伊红染色0.5～1 min,以水洗涤2～5 min,晾干后镜检。

注意事项:①微丝蚴厚血膜检查法为最常用的丝虫病诊断方法,可用于普查,阳性者染色后可鉴别虫种;②由于血液量多,要待血膜干透再进行溶血,否则血膜在溶血过程中易脱落,一般在采血后第3天溶血最好,切勿加热或在太阳下晒干,以免红细胞变性而不能溶解;放置时间也不可太久,否则血膜难以溶血。

(3)活微丝蚴浓集法:在离心管内装半管蒸馏水,加血液10～12滴,再加生理盐水混匀,离心3 min,取沉渣检查。或取静脉血1 ml,置于盛有3.8%枸橼酸钠0.1 ml的试管中,摇匀,加水9 ml,待红细胞溶解后,3000 r/min离心2 min,倒去上层液,加水再离心,取沉渣镜检。

2. 环卵沉淀试验 环卵沉淀试验(circumoval precipitin test,COPT)是沉淀试验的一种特定类型,是以血吸虫卵为抗原的特异免疫血清学试验。由于虫卵内成熟毛蚴的分泌物、排泄物能透过卵壳上的微孔渗出,当与待检血清共同孵育一段时间后,在虫卵周围若出现泡状或指状沉淀物,即为阳性反应,若无沉淀物出现,即为阴性反应。

常规法用棉棒蘸液体石蜡在载玻片上画2条相距20 mm的粗蜡线,在蜡线间滴加受检血清2滴(相当于0.1 ml)。用针尖挑取血吸虫卵干粉少许(100～150只卵)于血清内混匀,覆盖24 mm×24 mm盖玻片,四周用石蜡密封,置37 ℃湿盒中48 h,低倍镜观察结果,必要时需观察72 h时的反应结果。典型的阳性反应为出现泡状、指状、片状或细长卷曲状的折光性沉淀物,边缘整齐,与卵壳牢固粘连。对阴性反应者必须观察全片。对阳性反应者观察100个成熟卵,计算环沉率及反应强度比例。环沉率是指100个成熟虫卵中出现沉淀物的虫卵数。凡环沉率≥5%者可报告为阳性,1%～4%者为弱阳性。

[思考题]

(1)吸虫纲与线虫纲在形态与生活史上有哪些主要区别?

(2)确诊钩虫感染有哪几种方法?比较这几种方法的优缺点。

(3)粪便检查法能不能用来诊断蛲虫感染?为什么?

(田　芳　陆　凤)

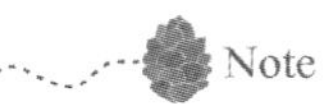

实验十七 阿 米 巴

[实验目的]

(1)掌握溶组织内阿米巴滋养体与包囊的形态特点及其与结肠内阿米巴的形态鉴别要点。
(2)了解微小内蜒阿米巴和布氏嗜碘阿米巴的滋养体和包囊的形态特点。

[实验材料]

示教标本(片)、显微镜、香柏油、二甲苯、擦镜纸等。

[实验内容]

一、示教标本

(一)溶组织内阿米巴(*Entamoeba histolytica*)

1. 溶组织内阿米巴滋养体铁苏木素染色标本(油镜观察) 虫体为蓝黑色,呈不规则形,直径25～60 μm,外质着色浅;内质颗粒状,着色深。内、外质界限清晰,外质常显示有舌状或指状的伪足;内质有1个圆弧形的细胞核,内含吞噬的红细胞,核泡状,核膜内缘有1圈大小均匀、排列整齐的染色质粒,核仁较小,多居中。核仁与核膜之间常可见网状的核纤维。

2. 溶组织内阿米巴包囊铁苏木素染色标本(油镜观察) 蓝黑色,圆球形,直径5～20 μm。囊壁薄,不着色,折光性强,其周围的空白圈为制作标本时包囊伸缩所致。囊内有1～4个细胞核,构造与滋养体相同。拟染色体为蓝黑色,棒状,有1个至数个。糖原在染色过程中溶解,故呈空泡状。在成熟包囊内,拟染色体和糖原泡一般均消失。

3. 溶组织内阿米巴包囊未染色标本(高倍镜观察) 在粪便生理盐水直接涂片标本中,其包囊呈圆球形,较小,细胞核不易看清,可见棒状、折光性强的拟染色体。

4. 溶组织内阿米巴包囊碘液染色标本(高倍镜观察) 囊壁薄,不着色,折光性强,囊内虫体呈黄色。细胞核1～4个,核仁小,不易见。在有1个或2个细胞核的包囊内,有棒状的拟染色体及棕黄色的糖原泡(在成熟包囊中多已消失)。

(二)结肠内阿米巴(*Entamoeba coli*)

1. 结肠内阿米巴滋养体铁苏木素染色标本(油镜观察) 通常略大于溶组织内阿米巴滋养体,外质较少,内质粗颗粒状,内、外质界限不清晰。内质食物泡内含有细菌、酵母及淀粉粒等,但不含红细胞。核膜内缘染色质粒大小均匀,排列不整齐,核仁稍大,多偏位。

2. 结肠内阿米巴包囊铁苏木素染色标本(油镜观察) 球形、较大,直径10～30 μm,细胞核1～8个,结构形态与滋养体相似。未成熟包囊内有糖原泡,拟染色体呈束状或碎片状,两端尖细、不齐。

3. 结肠内阿米巴包囊碘液染色标本(高倍镜观察) 圆球形,较大,囊壁稍厚,折光性强,囊内虫体呈淡黄色;细胞核1～8个,不着色,发亮;糖原泡为棕黄色,呈弥散状。

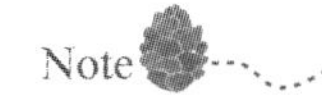

(三)微小内蜒阿米巴

1. 微小内蜒阿米巴滋养体铁苏木素染色标本(油镜观察) 虫体较小,直径3～12 μm。染色

后呈蓝黑色。伪足舌状,染色淡;内质食物泡内含有细菌。细胞核圆球形,核仁粗大而不规则,核囊着色浅,无核周染色质粒,核仁之间有核丝相连。

2. 微小内蜒阿米巴包囊铁苏木素染色标本(油镜观察) 类圆形或椭圆形,蓝黑色,大小(7～9) μm×(5～7) μm。细胞核 1～4 个;结构与滋养体相同;无拟染色体,成熟包囊有 4 个细胞核,糖原泡偶见。

(四)布氏嗜碘阿米巴

1. 布氏嗜碘阿米巴滋养体铁苏木素染色标本(油镜观察) 较微小内蜒阿米巴滋养体略大,虫体直径 6～20 μm,内、外质界限不明显,核单个,核膜内缘染色质粒小或缺如,核仁粗大,常被一层染色较浅的球状体所包绕。内质食物泡内含有细菌和其他有机物。

2. 布氏嗜碘阿米巴包囊铁苏木素染色标本(油镜观察) 椭圆形,直径 8～10 μm。细胞核 1 个,偶有 2 个。结构与滋养体相似,空泡状,常将细胞核推向一侧。

二、自己镜检

(1)观察溶组织内阿米巴包囊碘液染色标本。
(2)观察结肠内阿米巴包囊碘液染色标本。
(3)观察溶组织内阿米巴、结肠内阿米巴包囊铁苏木素染色标本。

三、录像片

观看阿米巴录像片。

[实验报告]

绘制碘液染色的溶组织内阿米巴和结肠内阿米巴滋养体及包囊的形态鉴别特征。

[思考题]

(1)说明组织内阿米巴与结肠内阿米巴的滋养体及包囊的形态鉴别特征。
(2)溶组织内阿米巴的生活史特点是什么?

(田　芳　陆　凤)

实验十八　孢　子　虫

[实验目的]

(1)掌握人体红细胞内间日疟原虫和恶性疟原虫各期的形态特征。
(2)初步掌握四种人体疟原虫的主要鉴别特征。
(3)了解疟原虫感染阶段及传播媒介。
(4)识别厚血膜中间日疟原虫和恶性疟原虫的基本形态特征。
(5)了解弓形虫滋养体的基本形态特征。

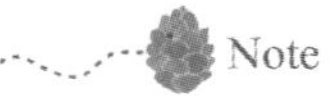

[实验材料]

示教标本(片)、显微镜、香柏油、二甲苯、擦镜纸等。

[实验内容]

一、示教标本

(一)间日疟原虫(*Plasmodium vivax*)薄血膜(油镜观察)

经吉氏或瑞氏染色后,细胞质呈淡蓝色,细胞核呈红色。自大滋养体阶段开始,被寄生的红细胞逐渐胀大,故着色浅,并有匀细的鲜红色薛氏小点。疟原虫细胞质内的疟色素呈棕黄色。

1. 小滋养体(环状体) 被寄生的红细胞大小正常。疟原虫细胞质少,环形,大小约为红细胞直径的 1/3。核点状,位于环的一端,中央为一空泡。整个虫体呈戒指状。

2. 大滋养体(阿米巴样体) 由小滋养体进一步发育长大而成。细胞质增多,并出现伪足,似阿米巴样,并有 1 个或多个空泡。虫体形状很不规则。核 1 个,较大,疟色素呈烟丝状。

3. 早期裂殖体(未成熟裂殖体) 大滋养体发育到一定阶段即停止活动,同时虫体变圆,细胞质内空泡逐渐消失,疟色素增多,核开始分裂(2 个以上)。

4. 裂殖体(成熟裂殖体) 核分裂为 12~24 个,细胞质亦随之分裂,每个核均被一部分细胞质所包裹,形成许多椭圆形的裂殖子。此时,疟色素集中成块,位于裂殖体中央或一边。

5. 雌配子体(大配子体) 虫体较大,圆形或椭圆形,常充满胀大的红细胞。细胞质呈蓝色;核 1 个,较小,核质致密,深红色,多位于虫体一侧。疟色素散在分布。

6. 雄配子体(小配子体) 虫体较雌配子体小,充满或略小于被寄生的红细胞。细胞质呈淡蓝色,有时略带红色;核 1 个,较大,核质疏松,淡红色,多位于虫体中央。疟色素均匀散在分布。

(二)间日疟原虫厚血膜

在厚血膜干燥过程中,原虫发生皱缩、断裂等;又因红细胞重叠或竖立或倾斜,原虫发生重叠、折叠及变形,故形态常不典型,可呈现飞鸟状、感叹号状或问号状等多种形态。同时,由于红细胞在溶血过程中被破坏,被疟原虫寄生的红细胞的某些特点也几乎消失殆尽。此外,经吉氏或瑞氏染色后,厚血膜上各种形态的其他物质亦较多,从而造成形态学诊断上的困难。因此,必须抓住疟原虫的细胞核、细胞质、疟色素、空泡四个要素反复观察和分析,并与薄血膜中疟原虫的形态特征进行对照,才能较快地掌握厚血膜的镜检技术,提高检验效率。

1. 小滋养体(环状体) 核点状,较小;细胞质少,形状不一,虫体可呈飞鸟状、感叹号状及问号状等。

2. 大滋养体(阿米巴样体) 虫体较大,形态多变,疟色素呈棕黄色,呈烟丝状。

3. 早期裂殖体(未成熟裂殖体) 形态变化大,虫体多断裂成块,核 2 个以上,疟色素呈棕黄色。

4. 裂殖体(成熟裂殖体) 虫体较大,裂殖子 12~24 个,似一串葡萄状,疟色素集中成块,呈棕黄色。

5. 配子体 圆形或椭圆形,虫体和细胞核均较大。细胞质常断裂,有时出现腐蚀现象,甚至完全消失。雌、雄配子体区别常不明显,应与大滋养体鉴别。

(三)恶性疟原虫(*Plasmodium falciparum*)薄血膜(油镜观察)

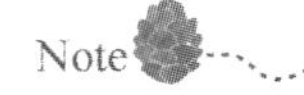

在以末梢血涂制的玻片标本上,通常只能见到环状体和成熟配子体,被疟原虫寄生的红细胞大小正常或略缩小。在吉氏或瑞氏染色的标本中,虫体的情况与间日疟原虫相似,疟色素呈深褐

色或黄棕色。红细胞边缘常皱缩，有时可见几颗粗大呈紫褐色的茂氏小点。恶性疟原虫的大滋养体和裂殖体通常不能在外周血中查见。

1. 小滋养体(环状体) 细胞质少，呈环状，较纤细，直径约为红细胞的 1/5；核 1～2 个，细小，点状。在 1 个红细胞内常同时寄生多个环状体，环状体有时可位于红细胞边缘。

2. 配子体 被寄生的红细胞随虫体伸长受牵拉而不见，或仅能见到一小部分，附于配子体凹面的一侧。

(1)雌配子体：两端较尖，呈新月状，细胞质蓝色；核小而致密，深红色，位于虫体中央。疟色素呈短杆状，核周较多。

(2)雄配子体：两端钝圆，呈腊肠状，细胞质淡蓝色，略带红色；核大而疏松，淡红色，位于虫体中央。疟色素呈棕黄色，短杆状，核周较多。

(四)疟原虫在蚊体内的发育时期(油镜观察)

1. 囊合子(卵囊) 在按蚊胃壁的弹性纤维下发育成熟；呈圆形，边缘规则，内含 1000～10000 个子孢子。

2. 子孢子 虫体呈梭状或新月状，大小约 8 μm×1 μm。经吉氏或瑞氏染色后，细胞质淡蓝色；核 1 个，红色，点状，位于虫体中央。

(五)弓形虫滋养体染色标本(油镜观察)

经吉氏或瑞氏染色后，虫体呈香蕉状或半月状，一端较尖，另一端钝圆；一侧扁平，另一侧略弯曲。大小为(4～7) μm×(2～4) μm，细胞核红色，位于虫体中央，虫体一端常见一较小的红色副核。铁苏木素染色后，尚可见核膜及核仁。

二、自己镜检

(1)观察间日疟原虫薄血膜吉氏或瑞氏染色标本。

(2)观察恶性疟原虫薄血膜吉氏或瑞氏染色标本。

镜检时，注意将有血膜的一面朝上，先在低倍镜下观察，找红细胞分布比较均匀、染色较好的部位，然后加香柏油滴，用油镜按顺序仔细观察。切勿将所见到的红点或蓝斑误认作疟原虫。观察时，可一边调节细螺旋，一边辨认疟原虫，并判别其发育阶段。

三、疟原虫厚、薄血膜检查法示教

厚、薄血膜同片制作法是检查疟原虫较准确的方法。薄血膜中疟原虫数量少，不易检获，但因疟原虫结构完整，且发现被疟原虫寄生的红细胞亦可能有助于诊断的确立，鉴别虫种虫期较容易。厚血膜血量较多而疟原虫集中，形态虽常不典型，但因疟原虫密度高而易于发现。

(一)器材和试剂

一次性刺血针、标记笔、载玻片、滴管(带橡皮胶头)、染色架、水槽、推片(凹玻片)，pH 7.0～7.2 磷酸盐缓冲液、吉氏染色液或瑞氏染色液等。

(二)方法

1. 取血与涂片

(1)将用于涂制血膜的载玻片自右向左分为 6 等份(6 格)，第 1、2 格贴标签备用。

(2)以 75%酒精棉球消毒受检者耳垂或无名指尖，用左手拇指与食指使受检者局部皮肤绷紧，右手用一次性刺血针刺破皮肤(深 1～2 mm)，挤出血滴，再以推片一端中部蘸取一小滴血。

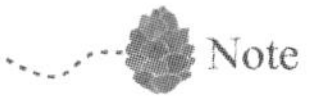

(3)左手拇指、食指及中指夹持载玻片两端，将推片蘸取的血滴置于第 4 格起始部。当血液沿推片边缘和载玻片之间扩展至 2 cm 宽时，使两片之间的角度为 30°～45°，然后将推片自右向左

匀速推进，制作成长约 3 cm 的舌状或长方形薄血膜。

(4)以推片的一角刮取一小滴血，置上述载玻片的第 3 格中央，自内向外做螺旋形(只能向一个方向)涂布，制作成直径 1.2 cm 的圆形厚血膜。

(5)将涂制了血膜的载玻片贴好标签，平置阴凉处，待其自然晾干。

2. 固定与染色

(1)用玻璃蜡笔在厚、薄血膜之间及载玻片两端各画一条直线，便于染色及溶血或固定血膜。

(2)以滴管将蒸馏水加于厚血膜上(切勿累及薄血膜)，溶血 15 min 左右，当厚血膜呈灰白色时，倾去载玻片上含血色素的蒸馏水，然后晾干。

(3)染色：可用瑞氏染色或吉氏染色。

瑞氏染色：滴加 1 ml 瑞氏染色液覆盖血膜，固定半分钟左右，然后加入等量蒸馏水或 pH 7.0～7.2 磷酸盐缓冲液，混匀，染色 5～10 min。

吉氏染色：先用甲醇固定薄血膜半分钟，然后加入用 pH 7.0～7.2 磷酸盐缓冲液稀释的吉氏染色液染色 30 min。此时不必先对厚血膜溶血，因溶血在染色过程中已同时完成。

(4)用水冲洗后晾干或以滤纸吸干，进行镜检。

镜检厚血膜可出现下列特征：背景清洁，无杂质，由于红细胞溶解而呈斑驳的淡灰色。白细胞核被染成深紫色。疟原虫染色质呈深红色，细胞质呈蓝紫色。在间日疟原虫感染者中，可在标本片边缘的红细胞影迹中见到薛氏小点。至少要观察 100 个视野。

镜检薄血膜可出现下列特征：背景清洁，无杂质，红细胞被染成淡灰红色。中性粒细胞有被染成深紫色的核，以及明显的粉红色颗粒。疟原虫的染色质呈深紫红色，而细胞质呈鲜明的蓝色。在含有间日疟原虫和卵形疟原虫的红细胞中，薛氏小点清晰可见，而在被恶性疟原虫大环状体寄生的红细胞中，可见茂氏小点。

3. 注意事项

(1)理想的薄血膜血细胞分布均匀，细胞间没有较大空隙，但也不相互重叠。理想的厚血膜厚薄均匀，没有气泡，边缘光滑；在油镜下，每个视野内可见 10～15 个白细胞。

(2)瑞氏染色法操作简便，适用于临床诊断，但甲醇蒸发很快，掌握不当时易在标本片上发生染料沉淀，并较易褪色，保存时间不长。多用于临时性检验。

(3)水洗时标本片应平放，待染料浮起顺水漂去后再倾斜标本片，否则染料易沉淀在标本片上。

(4)所用载玻片应清洁、不油腻、光滑、无刻痕。

[实验报告]

(1)绘制红细胞内间日疟原虫各期形态图。

(2)绘制薄血膜(吉氏或瑞氏染色)中恶性疟原虫环状体和雌、雄配子体图，并说明各部结构名称。

[思考题]

(1)如何在薄血膜上鉴别间日疟原虫和恶性疟原虫？

(2)试述间日疟原虫生活史与发作、再燃、复发的关系。

(3)试述弓形虫的形态特征及其对人体的危害。

(田　芳　陆　凤)

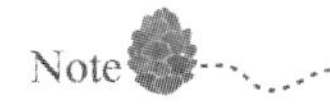

实验十九　鞭　毛　虫

[实验目的]

(1)掌握杜氏利什曼原虫和阴道毛滴虫的形态特征。

(2)熟悉蓝氏贾第鞭毛虫的形态特征和检查方法。

(3)了解人毛滴虫的形态特点。

[实验材料]

示教标本(片)、显微镜、香柏油、二甲苯、擦镜纸等。

[实验内容]

一、示教标本

(一)杜氏利什曼原虫

1. 杜氏利什曼原虫无鞭毛体吉氏或瑞氏染色标本(油镜观察)　虫体圆形或椭圆形,在巨噬细胞内或散在于细胞外,大小为 2.8～4.4 μm。细胞质呈淡蓝色或淡白色;细胞核呈紫红色,大而圆,常靠近细胞膜。动基体细小,呈杆状,着色较深,前方有点状的基体,向前发出一根丝体。

2. 杜氏利什曼原虫前鞭毛体吉氏或瑞氏染色标本(油镜观察)　生长于白蛉消化道或 NNN 培养基内。虫体呈梭形或纺锤形,细胞核呈圆形、紫红色,位于虫体中部。动基体杆状,紫红色,在虫体前端有一点状的基体,由此发出一根鞭毛,向前游离,长度与体长相当。有时,多个前鞭毛聚集在一起,呈菊花状排列,或相互交织成网状。

(二)阴道毛滴虫

1. 阴道毛滴虫吉氏或瑞氏染色标本(油镜观察)　虫体呈蓝紫色,梨形或圆形,体长 7～23 μm。细胞核 1 个,呈长椭圆形,位于虫体前 1/3 处的中央;细胞核前缘有 5 颗基体,排列成环形。从基体发出 4 根前鞭毛和 1 根后鞭毛。前鞭毛等长,向前游离,后鞭毛与波动膜外缘相连,末端不游离。波动膜较短,在一侧通常不超过虫体长度的 1/2,轴柱纵贯虫体中央,并从末端伸出。轴柱和鞭毛以及细胞核均被染成紫红色。此外,在轴柱对侧,有 1 根副基纤维,波动膜内缘尚有 1 根基染色杆,均被染成紫红色。细胞质内有很多着色较深的染色质粒,在轴柱和基染色杆附近较为密集。

2. 阴道毛滴虫活体标本(高倍镜观察)　在适宜温度(25～30 ℃)下,可见虫体随前鞭毛的摆动而前进,并以波动膜的颤动做螺旋式运动。虫体伸缩力强,常可改变体形来通过障碍物。如虫体运动剧烈,不便于观察,可加入 1∶10 血清 1 滴。

(三)蓝氏贾第鞭毛虫

1. 蓝氏贾第鞭毛虫滋养体铁苏木素染色标本(油镜观察)　虫体呈瓢状或呈倒置梨形,长 9～21 μm、宽 5～15 μm、厚 2～4 μm,两侧对称,前端宽圆,后端渐细,背面隆起,腹面前部凹陷,形成吸器。细胞核 1 对,泡状,左右并列,核仁显著,位于核中央。1 对轴柱纵贯虫体,其中部有 1 对半月形的中央小体,4 对鞭毛自两细胞核之间的基体复合体发出,从前向后依次为前鞭毛、中鞭毛、腹鞭毛及后鞭毛各 1 对。

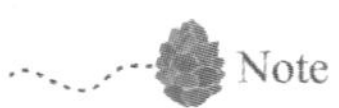

2. 蓝氏贾第鞭毛虫包囊铁苏木素染色标本(油镜观察) 虫体呈长圆形或卵圆形，大小为(8～14) μm×(7～10) μm，囊壁厚，不着色。虫体与囊壁之间间隙明显，不对称。具 2 个或 4 个细胞核，以 4 个细胞核为多见，常偏于一侧。轴柱居中央，并可见中央小体及鞭毛轴丝。

3. 蓝氏贾第鞭毛虫包囊碘液染色标本(高倍镜观察) 黄绿色，囊壁不着色，具折光性，囊内细胞核、中央小体及鞭毛轴丝等不着色、折光性强。

附：人毛滴虫

人毛滴虫铁苏木素染色标本(油镜观察) 人毛滴虫只有滋养体期。虫体呈梨形或椭圆形，前鞭毛 3～5 根，后鞭毛 1 根，轴柱纵贯虫体，末端游离。波动膜和染色基杆与虫体等长，后鞭毛附着于波动膜外缘，末端游离。细胞核呈椭圆形，位于虫体前端，细胞质内有多个食物泡，常含有细菌。

二、自己镜检

(1)观察杜氏利什曼原虫无鞭毛体吉氏或瑞氏染色标本。

(2)阴道毛滴虫活体标本检查及染色标本观察：取滴虫性阴道炎患者的阴道分泌物或人工培养物，制成悬滴标本或涂片标本。加盖玻片，先在低倍镜下找到滴虫，然后转换成高倍镜，仔细观察其形态及运动特点。

(3)蓝氏贾第鞭毛虫包囊碘液染色标本检查：取蓝氏贾第鞭毛虫包囊悬液(摇匀后吸取)1 小滴于载玻片上，并覆以盖玻片。然后，从盖玻片的一侧加 1 滴碘液，使之逐渐向对侧渗透。用低倍镜寻找包囊，再在高倍镜下仔细观察其结构形态。

[实验报告]

(1)绘制杜氏利什曼原虫无鞭毛体及阴道毛滴虫图，并注明各部结构名称。

(2)绘制碘液染色的蓝氏贾第鞭毛虫包囊图，并注明各部结构名称。

[思考题]

(1)寄生于人体的鞭毛虫主要有哪些种类?

(2)试述常见人体鞭毛虫的形态特征。

(3)为什么滴虫性阴道炎容易发生流行? 如何防治?

(田 芳 陆 凤)

实验二十 纤 毛 虫

[实验目的]

了解结肠小袋纤毛虫的基本形态特征。

[实验材料]

示教标本(片)、显微镜、香柏油、二甲苯、擦镜纸等。

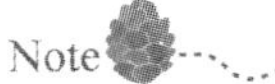

[实验内容]

示教标本:结肠小袋纤毛虫铁苏木素染色标本(油镜观察)。

1. 滋养体 近似椭圆形,大小平均为 60 μm×45 μm,前端有胞口、胞咽,后端有胞肛。周身有纤毛,内含一肾形的大核,其凹入面一侧的附近有一圆形的小核,细胞质内尚有伸缩泡和食物泡等结构。

2. 包囊 圆形或卵圆形,直径为 40～60 μm,囊壁厚而透明,内含虫体,小核已消失,食物泡亦已排空。随着包囊的成熟,虫体上的纤毛逐渐消失。

[思考题]

试述结肠小袋纤毛虫的形态特征及对人体的危害。

(田　芳　陆　凤)

实验二十一　原虫检查方法

[实验目的]

(1)掌握粪便直接涂片碘液染色法。
(2)初步掌握厚、薄血膜涂片制作及染色技术。
(3)掌握阴道分泌物直接涂片法检查阴道毛滴虫。

[实验材料]

阴道毛滴虫活体标本、显微镜、香柏油、二甲苯、擦镜纸、盖玻片、载玻片等。

[实验内容]

一、粪内原虫检查

直接涂片法对检查粪便中的原虫滋养体和包囊是必不可少的。原虫滋养体用生理盐水涂片法可以观察它的动态,如伪足、鞭毛、波动膜、纤毛等的运动情况。而对包囊来讲,有些构造只有在新鲜涂片中才能看清楚,如溶组织内阿米巴包囊的拟染色体、布氏嗜碘阿米巴包囊的糖原块等。所以检查原虫时首先应做直接涂片。做直接涂片时应注意涂片要薄而均匀,若涂片厚了,则原虫细小、看不清楚而容易漏检。

原虫中的鞭毛虫、纤毛虫由于活动较快,在视野中容易被发现;而阿米巴伪足伸缩活动不明显,故难以观察,故需转换为高倍镜细心观察才能判断是否为阿米巴。但除了溶组织内阿米巴滋养体通过伪足伸缩快、做定向运动、体内有红细胞可以确定外,其他的许多种阿米巴在生理盐水涂片中是较难确定的,因此,需要经铁苏木素染色才能加以鉴别。

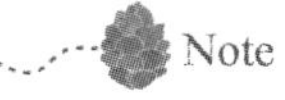

检查原虫的包囊时,首先在低倍镜中看清它的大小、形状、折光强度,是否有明显的囊壁构造,要与其他结构如白细胞、人酵母、脂肪球,以至小气泡相鉴别。当转换成高倍镜观察时,首先

看包囊的囊壁是否完整，然后观察包囊内的折光强度有什么不同，如溶组织内阿米巴包囊的拟染色体呈短棒状，它的折光强度比包囊的细胞质强，再如布氏嗜碘阿米巴包囊糖原块的折光强度也较强，通过这些特点可以初步鉴别它们。而要确定是哪一种原虫，则还需要用碘液染色，以便进一步看清它的核、糖原块的特点来做出判断，如果尚不能看清它们的构造特点，最后就需要用铁苏木素染色法来确定。

(一)原虫包囊碘液染色法

1. 器材和药品 碘液(将碘化钾 4 g 溶于 100 ml 蒸馏水中，再加入碘 2 g，待溶解后即可使用)等。

2. 方法 以 1～2 滴碘液代替生理盐水做直接涂片，在涂抹的标本上盖上盖玻片即可镜检。若同时需检查活滋养体，可在生理盐水直接涂片的一侧滴 1 滴碘液，再盖上盖玻片。片中滴碘液的一侧查包囊；另一侧查活滋养体。

3. 注意事项

(1)碘液染色后包囊的细胞质被染成黄色或浅褐色，而细胞核被染成深褐色，核周染色小体被染成浅黄色，但可能不是很清晰；包囊内含有的糖原被碘液染为深褐色。在被碘液染色的鞭毛虫包囊中可见丝状物。

(2)采集标本的用具要干净，不能被污水、药物或水生原虫等污染。

(3)粪便等留检标本应留在便盆、痰盂内，而不要在潮湿的地面上或公共厕所中挑取材料，以防止污染标本。

(4)原虫标本应用新鲜材料立刻检查，不要放置过久，原虫死亡后难以鉴别。

(5)涂片取材时应注意挑选粪便中的异常部分，如含血液、脓液、黏液等的部分。

(二)原虫滋养体和包囊的铁苏木素(iron-hematoxylin)染色法

铁苏木素染色法是观察原虫滋养体或胞囊的最佳染色方法，并且是长久保存标本的理想方法。

1. 器材和药品 22 mm×22 mm 盖玻片、染色皿、盖玻镊、毛笔等。

肖定氏(Schaudinns)固定液：饱和氯化汞水溶液 2 份＋95％酒精 1 份，每 100 ml 中加冰醋酸 5 ml。

碘酒精：碘 1 g 溶于 100 ml 的 70％酒精中。

4％(2％)硫酸铁铵(铁明矾)水溶液：硫酸铁铵 4 g(2 g)溶于蒸馏水 100 ml。

苏木素原液：苏木素 1 g 溶于 10 ml 无水酒精中。使用时取 0.5 ml 加于 100 ml 蒸馏水中。

各级酒精：30％酒精、50％酒精、70％酒精、80％酒精、90％酒精、95％酒精、无水酒精。

透明剂：二甲苯或冬青油。

封片剂：中性树胶或加拿大树胶。

2. 方法

(1)用盖玻片或毛笔将粪便薄而均匀地涂刮在盖玻片上，迅速投入已温热至 40 ℃的固定液中，滋养体固定 10 min，包囊固定 20～30 min。

(2)倒出固定液，加入碘酒精作用 30 min。

(3)倒出碘酒精，加入 70％酒精漂洗 2～3 次，直至碘色褪尽。

(4)置于流水中轻轻冲洗 10 min。

(5)加入 4％硫酸铁铵水溶液，滋养体作用 15 min，包囊作用 30 min。

(6)倒出硫酸铁铵水溶液，用自来水过 3 次(即加满后倾倒，重复 3 次)。

(7)加入苏木素原液，染色 5～10 min 或稍久，时间根据染液性能而定。

(8)倒去染液，用自来水洗数次。

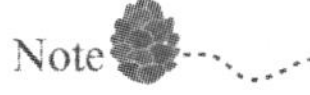

(9)加入2%硫酸铁铵水溶液使褪色,褪色时间视颜色深浅而定。

(10)倒出硫酸铁铵水溶液,在流水中轻轻冲洗20 min。

(11)依次用30%酒精、50%酒精、70%酒精、80%酒精、90%酒精、95%酒精、无水酒精1、无水酒精2脱水,每种酒精脱水2~5 min。

(12)放入二甲苯-无水酒精(1∶1)混合液或冬青油纯酒精混合液中10 min。

(13)放入二甲苯或冬青油中5 min。

(14)用中性树胶或加拿大树胶封片。

虫体染色后呈蓝黑色,在光学显微镜下细胞结构清晰。

3. 注意事项

(1)涂抹粪便时宜薄而不宜厚。

(2)染色时间根据铁苏木素染色液着色力而定。染色液配制后宜放置一段时间再使用。

(3)脱水过程不宜过急,在透明时如发现标本片出现乳白色雾状,应立即更换新的二甲苯。

(4)固定液、碘酒精、硫酸铁铵水溶液均可重复使用。

(三)溶组织内阿米巴培养方法

(1)营养琼脂双相培养基组成如下。

液体部分:NaCl 8 g、KCl 0.2 g、$CaCl_2$ 0.2 g、$MgCl_2$ 0.01 g、Na_2HPO_4 2 g、KH_2PO_4 0.3 g、水1000 ml。

固体部分:牛肉浸膏3 g、蛋白胨5 g、琼脂15 g。

(2)消毒米粉:将大米粉分装至小管,放180 ℃烤箱中消毒3次。

(3)配制方法:先配液体部分2000 ml,$CaCl_2$、$MgCl_2$另装小瓶,高压灭菌(54.89 kPa,20 min)后冷却,混合。取1000 ml配好的固体部分,经沸水浴2~3 h,使完全溶解。若有残渣,可用4层纱布过滤,趁热将滤液分装至试管,每管5 ml,高压灭菌,放成斜面冷却,置冰箱中备用。

接种前,每管加液体部分4.5 ml和无菌小牛血清0.5 ml,并用铂金环加消毒米粉约20 mg。

目前,BIS-33培养基具有较广的使用范围,已在多种寄生虫的体外无菌培养中应用。

二、阴道分泌物检查

阴道内常见的寄生虫是阴道毛滴虫,此外尚有偶尔误入阴道的蠕虫,如蛲虫以及其他的线虫,留取标本检查的容器一定要干净,以避免外界虫体污染而误认为阴道内寄生虫。

(一)阴道分泌物直接涂片检查

用消毒的棉签在受检者阴道后穹隆、子宫颈及阴道壁上拭取分泌物,然后放入有生理盐水的瓶或管内,天气较冷时,要注意标本保温。检查时可用棉签做直接涂片检查。活动的阴道毛滴虫滋养体比较容易识别,滋养体不活动时就较难区别,因此还可以做涂片进行染色后再鉴别。直接涂片如虫体少不易发现,可将瓶内盐水在1000 r/min离心3 min,吸取沉淀镜检。

(二)阴道毛滴虫染色检查法

阴道毛滴虫不活动时难以鉴别,需要用染色方法使其构造显示而识别。常用的有瑞氏染色法或吉氏染色法,即将分泌物涂片后让其干燥,然后染色,方法同血片染色。也可用铁苏木素染色后进行检查。

(三)阴道毛滴虫培养检查法

因阴道内原虫太少,直接取分泌液不容易查出,可以采用培养基增殖培养,使原虫数目增多而容易检出。做培养检查时取材方法同上,但要求在无菌条件下取材并接种于培养基中。

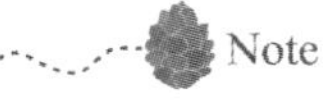

阴道毛滴虫培养基种类较多,一般认为比较好的是肝浸汤培养基。

1. 肝浸汤培养基 牛肝或兔肝 15 g、蛋白胨 2 g、NaCl 0.5 g、半胱氨酸盐酸盐 0.2 g、麦芽糖 1 g、水 100 ml。配制方法：先将肝研碎，浸入 100 ml 水中混匀，置冰箱冷藏过夜，次日加热煮沸半小时，用四层纱布过滤，并补足蒸发掉的水量到 100 ml。然后加入上述成分，加热使其充分溶解，再用滤纸过滤，调节 pH 至 5.5～6.0，每管 8 ml 分装于 15 mm×150 mm 的试管中，用硅胶塞封口，于 54.89 kPa 灭菌 20 min。待冷却后取出，并取两管放入 37 ℃温箱中 24～48 h，证明无菌，其余放冰箱保存备用。

培养方法：培养基使用前每管加灭活无菌的小牛血清 2 ml，以铂金环挑取青霉素、链霉素粉少许(200～400 U/ml)，用消毒棉签从受检者阴道后穹隆、子宫颈及阴道壁上拭取分泌物接种到培养基中。置 37 ℃温箱中 24～48 h，吸取悬液于显微镜下观察结果。

2. 1640 蛋白胨培养基 RPMI1640 1.02 g、蛋白胨 0.8 g、NaCl 0.5 g、半胱氨酸盐酸盐 0.2 g、麦芽糖 0.4 g、水 100 ml。配制方法：加热使上述成分充分溶解，用不锈钢滤菌器过滤后，分装于已灭菌的试管中，每管 5 ml。无菌试验方法同上。

培养方法：培养基使用前每管加灭活无菌的小牛血清 0.5 ml，其他操作同上。

应用 1640 蛋白胨培养基替代肝浸汤培养基，可使试剂成品化，培养基配制方便、经济。

三、厚、薄血膜涂片制作及染色

见本书第二篇实验十八。

[思考题]

阴道分泌物直接涂片检查阴道毛滴虫要注意哪些事项？

(田 芳 陆 凤)

实验二十二 医学节肢动物

[实验目的]

(1)掌握蚊、蝇生活史各期的一般形态特征。
(2)初步掌握三属蚊及常见蚊、蝇重要虫种的鉴别特点。
(3)了解白蛉生活史各期的一般形态特征。
(4)认识蚤、虱、臭虫、蜱、螨类的一般形态特征。

[实验材料]

示教标本(片)、显微镜、香柏油、二甲苯、擦镜纸等。

[实验内容]

一、示教标本

(一)蚊

1. 成蚊针插标本(肉眼及放大镜观察) 体长 1.6～12.6 mm，体呈灰褐色、棕黄色或黑色等，

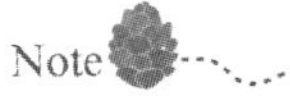

由头、胸、腹三个部分组成。

头部:似球形,有复眼、触角及触须各 1 对,喙细长,自唇基向前下方伸出。雄蚊的触角轮毛长而密,雌蚊的触角轮毛短而稀,库蚊和伊蚊的雄、雌蚊触须短,约为喙长的 1/4。按蚊的雌、雄蚊触须与喙几乎等长。

胸部:分为前、中、后胸 3 节,每节各生有足 1 对。中胸发达,有翅 1 对,后胸有 1 对平衡棒。

腹部:分 10 节,仅前 8 节明显可见,第 9、10 节衍化为外生殖器。腹节背板上有时可见由鳞片组成的淡色横带,其有无及形状和位置的变化,均为鉴定虫体的重要依据。

(1)中华按蚊:中等大小,体色灰暗。触须上有 4 个白环,以顶白环为最宽。翅前缘脉上有 2 个大白斑,第六纵脉上有 2 个暗斑。后足末节白环较窄。

(2)白纹伊蚊:体形小至中等,黑色。中胸背板前半部正中有 1 条银白色纵纹,后足末节全白。

(3)淡色库蚊:中等大小,淡褐色,但中胸背板呈红褐色。第 2~6 腹节背板基部有淡色横带,横带的后缘直或凹入,或有一部分后缘凸而圆,背板两侧无分离的淡色侧斑,足黑色,无白环。

2. 雌蚊口器玻片标本(低倍镜观察) 刺吸式,有上唇。舌 1 个及上、下颚各 1 对。上、下颚末端呈尖刀状,并有锯齿样构造。雌蚊口器由 6 根口针构成,这 6 根针样结构,在不吸血时,均藏于鞘状结构的下唇内,下唇末端有 2 个小的唇瓣。

3. 蚊翅玻片标本(放大镜观察) 狭长、膜状,脉序从前向后依次为前缘脉、亚前缘脉、第 1 纵脉、第 2 纵脉(末端分 2 支)、第 3 纵脉、第 4 纵脉(末端分 2 支)、第 5 纵脉(末端分 2 支)及第 6 纵脉,因此,蚊翅的脉序可记作 1、2.1、2.2、3、4.1、4.2、5.1、5.2、6。该脉序是蚊科动物最重要的特征。翅上有很多鳞片,色泽因种属而异:在翅后缘的长鳞片称为缘缨,由鳞片组成的色斑的数目及位置是分类上的重要依据之一。

4. 蚊卵玻片标本(低倍镜观察) 蚊卵甚小,最长不超过 1 mm,通常为 0.5 mm×0.2 mm。

(1)按蚊卵:船形,两侧各有 1 个浮囊,故能单个浮于水面。

(2)伊蚊卵:纺锤形,表面有条纹,无浮囊,因单个地产出,故沉于水底。

(3)库蚊卵:长圆形,钝端向下,无浮囊,因数十个甚至几百个卵顺纵轴聚集成卵块,故形成筏状,浮于水面。

5. 幼虫(孑孓)玻片标本(放大镜观察) 虫体分头、胸、腹三个部分。头部有单眼、复眼及触角各 1 对。口器咀嚼式,有口刷 1 对。胸部背、腹面有毛,其长短、分支及排列情况,在按蚊分类上有重要意义,腹部分 9 节,前 7 节形状相似,第 7、9 节变化很大。

(1)按蚊幼虫:腹部第 1~7 节背面有成对的掌状毛。末端有呼吸孔 1 对,在水面静止时,虫体与水面平行。

(2)库蚊幼虫:腹部背面无掌状毛。末端有呼吸管 1 根。呼吸管细而长。

(3)伊蚊幼虫:与库蚊幼虫类似,但呼吸管较粗短。在水面静止时,库蚊和伊蚊的幼虫以呼吸管口接触水面,所以体与水面成一角度。

6. 蛹(放大镜观察) 逗点状,体分头胸部与腹部两个部分。头胸部膨大,背面有 1 对呼吸管。在水面静止时,呼吸管口接触水面。

(1)按蚊蛹:呼吸管粗短,口宽呈漏斗形,前方有一裂隙。

(2)库蚊蛹:呼吸管细长,口窄。

(3)伊蚊蛹:呼吸管短而宽,口呈三角形。

(二)蝇

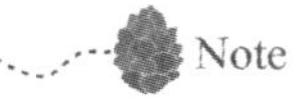

1. 成蝇针插标本(肉眼及放大镜观察) 体长 4~14 mm,大小较悬殊,分头、胸、腹三个部分,全身密生鬃毛。不同种类的成蝇的体形及色泽亦不一样。

头部:通常呈半球形。有复眼 1 对,单眼 3 个,除麻蝇外,雌蝇二复眼间距较宽,雄蝇二复眼间距较近。有触角 1 对,分 3 节,在第 3 节近基部外前方有一触角芒,其形式多样,是分类的依据之一。口器多为舐吸式,但也有的蝇具刺吸式口器。

胸部:分为前胸、中胸和后胸三个部分。中胸发达,生有 1 对透明的膜质翅。纵脉包括前缘脉、亚前缘脉及第 1～6 纵脉。第 4 纵脉末段的弯曲情况在分类上有重要意义。有 3 对足,足分节,多毛。

腹部:圆钝,筒状,分 10 节,但外观上仅有 5 节明显可见,其余腹节为外生殖器,不用时,缩入腹内。

(1)舍蝇:亦称南方家蝇、饭蝇等。体长 5～8 mm,中等大小,灰褐色。中胸背板上有 4 条黑色纵纹。触角芒呈羽状,翅第 4 纵脉末段向上弯曲,末端几乎与第 3 纵脉接触。

(2)夏厕蝇:体长 5～7 mm,灰色。翅第 4 纵脉挺直,第 3、第 4 纵脉的梢端有相当的距离。

(3)厩腐蝇:体长 6～9 mm,深灰色,胸背板上有 4 条黑色纵纹,中间 2 条较明显,翅第 4 纵脉末端呈弧形。

(4)厩螫蝇:体长 5～8 mm,暗灰色,形似舍蝇。喙细长,口器为刺吸式,胸背部有不清晰的 4 条纵纹。腹部第 2、3 节各有 3 个黑点。

(5)丝光绿蝇:体长 5～10 mm,中等大小,体色为略带黄绿色的金属光泽,触角芒短,羽状。复眼暗紫色,颊部银白色。

(6)大头金蝇:体长 8～11 mm,躯体肥大。体色带有蓝绿色的金属光泽。头大而红,俗称“红头蝇”。颊部呈杏黄色或橙色。

(7)巨尾阿丽蝇:体长约 10 mm,中胸背板前缘中央有 3 条短黑色纵纹,中间的一条最宽,腹部背面有深蓝色金属光泽。

(8)黑尾黑麻蝇:体长 6～12 mm,暗灰色。触角芒栉状,呈羽状分支,中胸背板上有 3 条黑色纵纹。胸部背面具有闪光的、黑白相间的棋盘状斑,第 4 纵脉呈深弯曲状。

2. 蝇头部玻片标本(体视显微镜观察) 仔细观察舐吸式口器的构造。口器末端有 1 对膨大的唇瓣,上有很多凹沟式的小管道,与食道相通,用于舔食,此称假气管。

3. 蝇足玻片标本(体视显微镜观察) 足分 5 节,即基节、转节、股节、胫节及跗节。跗节又分为 5 节。末端有爪及垫各 1 对,爪间突 1 个。爪垫上密布细毛,并能分泌黏液。足部生有很多鬃,鬃的数量及分布位置均有分类学意义。

4. 蝇卵玻片标本(低倍镜观察) 乳白色,香蕉状或椭圆形,长约 1 mm,常堆积成卵块。

5. 幼虫(蛆)玻片标本(低倍镜观察) 多为乳白色。包括头部在内,由 14 节组成,仅 11 节明显可见。虫体圆柱形,前端较尖细,后端粗而钝,呈截断状。有前、后气门各 1 对,后气门由气门环、气门裂和钮孔组成,其形状、构造有重要分类学意义。

6. 蛹瓶装标本(肉眼观察) 棕褐色至黑色,长椭圆形,长 5～8 mm。不食不动,外有蛹壳。

(三)白蛉

1. 成虫玻片标本或针插标本(放大镜观察) 体长 1.5～4 mm,呈黄色或淡黄色,虫体分头、胸、腹三个部分。头部有 1 对大而黑的复眼。口器刺吸式,胸部向背面隆起,呈驼背状。翅 1 对,末端尖,较狭长,翅脉特殊。足 3 对,细长分节。腹部由 10 节组成,最后 2 节特化为外生殖器。雌蛉腹部末端钝圆,雄蛉外生殖器构造复杂。

2. 卵玻片标本(低倍镜观察) 长椭圆形,长约 0.4 mm,深棕色或黑色(初产出时呈灰白色),壳表面有纹迹。

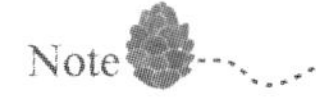

3. 幼虫玻片标本(低倍镜观察) 除头部外,虫体分为 13 节,淡褐色或白色,第 1 龄幼虫末端有 1 根粗长的尾鬃,第 2～6 龄幼虫尾鬃均为 2 对。

（四）蚤

1. 成蚤玻片标本(低倍镜及放大镜观察) 虫体左、右侧扁，长约 3 mm。棕黄色至深棕色，体表有很多向后突出的鬃，虫体分头、胸、腹三个部分。

头部：小，呈三角形，口器刺吸式，触角 1 对，位于触角窝内，由 3 节构成，窝前可有单眼 1 对，黑色，有的种类缺如。眼鬃位置、颊栉的有无、栉的刺数均为分类的依据。

胸部：分前、中、后 3 节，前胸背板后缘可有向后生长的前胸栉，栉的有无及其刺数和侧板杆的有无，均为分类的重要依据。足 3 对，后足特别发达，适于跳跃。

腹部：由 11 节组成，前 7 节为正常腹节，其余腹节为生殖节和肛节，雌蚤腹部末端钝圆，在透明的标本第 7、8 腹板的部位可见有角质性的受精囊，雄蚤末端尖，外生殖器的构造复杂，为重要的分类依据。

(1)致痒蚤：又称人蚤。眼发达，眼鬃位于眼下方。无颊栉和前胸栉，中胸侧板亦无垂直的侧板杆。

(2)印鼠客蚤：眼发达，眼鬃位于眼前方，无颊栉和前胸栉，中胸侧板有垂直的侧板杆。

(3)猫栉头蚤：头长而尖削。眼发达，眼鬃位于眼前方，有颊栉和前胸栉。

2. 卵玻片标本(低倍镜观察) 近似椭圆形，直径为 0.4～2 mm，白色或淡黄色。

3. 幼虫玻片标本(低倍镜观察) 体形似蛆而小，白色，长约 6 mm，口器咀嚼式，触角 1 对，腹部末端有 1 对指状突起。

4. 蛹玻片标本(低倍镜观察) 具有成蚤的雏形，淡黄色至淡棕色，外包有茧。茧由成熟幼虫唾腺分泌的丝，与尘埃和其他物质的碎屑黏合而成(制作标本时，通常已去除)。

（五）虱

1. 成虱玻片标本(低倍镜及放大镜观察) 人虱：灰色或灰白色，无翅，头小，呈菱形。口器刺吸式，位于头内，触角 1 对，分 5 节，约与头等长，位于头部两侧。眼 1 对，位于触角之后，胸部 3 节融合，有 3 对足，胫节末端内方生一指状胫突，跗节端部生一弯曲的爪，与胫突相对，形成抱握器，用于抓握毛发或衣服纤维。通常雌虱较大，体长 2.5～4.2 mm，末端分 2 叶，呈“W”形；雄虱稍小，末端钝圆，呈“V”形，近尾端部有一交尾刺。人体虱一般较人头虱大(表 2-22-1)。

2. 虱卵玻片标本(低倍镜观察) 俗称虮子，呈长圆形，长约 0.8 mm，白色或黄白色，卵壳透明，表面具有胶质，一端有小盖，常黏附在毛发或衣服纤维上。

3. 若虱玻片标本(低倍镜观察) 形似成虱但较小，腹部甚小且短，生殖器官尚未发育成熟。

表 2-22-1 三种成虱的区别(含亚种)

区别点	人体虱	人头虱	耻阴虱
体形	狭长	狭长	短宽似蟹状
体色	色淡	色深	色淡
腹侧突起	无	无	有 4 对
触角	较细长，第 3 节呈长方形	较粗短，第 3 节呈方形	无特殊

（六）臭虫

1. 成虫玻片标本(放大镜观察) 体长 4～6 mm，卵圆形，红褐色，背腹扁平，虫体分头、胸、腹三个部分。

头部：两侧有突出的复眼 1 对，无单眼。触角 1 对，由 4 节组成。口器刺吸式，不吸血时向右弯折在头及胸部的腹面沟内。

胸部：前胸大而明显，其前缘不同程度地凹入。中胸背面有翅基 1 对，足 3 对，在第 2、3 足基

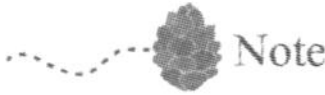
Note

之间有 1 对臭腺孔开口。

腹部：10 节，但仅有 8 节明显可见。雄虫腹部末端狭而尖，有一镰刀状交尾器，雌虫腹部末端钝圆，在第 5 腹节后缘右侧有一三角形凹陷，称柏氏器，为交配器官。

温带臭虫：前胸较宽，其前缘凹入较深，两侧缘略呈翼状向外延伸。

2. 卵玻片标本(低倍镜观察) 长 0.8～1.3 mm，长圆形，黄白色。卵壳表面有网纹，前端有一卵盖，略偏于一侧。

3. 若虫玻片标本(低倍镜观察) 外形似成虫，但体形较小，体色较浅，无翅基，生殖器官未发育成熟。

(七)蜱

成蜱玻片标本(放大镜及低倍镜观察)：蜱有硬蜱与软蜱之分(表 2-22-2)，未吸血时虫体为卵圆形，背腹扁平，体长 2～13 mm。前端为颚体(假头)，后部为躯体，由胸、腹部愈合而成。口器由口下板、螯肢及须肢三个部分组成。成虫与若虫有 4 对足，幼虫仅有 3 对足。

表 2-22-2 硬蜱与软蜱成虫的主要区别

区别点	硬蜱	软蜱
大小	较小	较大
假头	较大，突出于前端，从背面可见	较小，隐藏于前端，从背面不可见
盾板	有	无
雌雄区别	雌：盾板小；雄：盾板大	雌雄区别不明显

1. 全沟硬蜱 盾板褐色，触须为细长圆筒状，无眼和缘垛。肛沟在肛门前方呈倒“U”形，雄虫躯体背面几乎完全为盾板覆盖，雌虫的盾板小，仅见于背面前部。

2. 波斯锐缘蜱 躯体长圆形，体缘扁而锐，有缝线，体缘表面结构为方格形。无盾板，雌雄不易区别。

(八)螨

1. 革螨 成虫玻片标本(低倍镜观察)：外形似蜱，但较小，虫体一般长 0.2～0.5 mm，大的可达 3 mm，呈卵圆形，黄褐色，背腹扁平，分颚体与躯体两个部分。在腹面，近体前缘的正中，有一叉形的胸叉。雌虫躯体腹面有胸板、生殖板、腹板、肛板及其他背板，生殖板与腹板合成生殖腹板。雄虫躯体腹面的骨板常愈合为全腹板。雌虫生殖孔呈横裂隙状，位于胸板之后，雄虫生殖孔位于胸板前缘，呈漏斗状。有气门 1 对，气门沟长度因虫种而异，气门和气门沟外围以气门板。足 4 对，腿分为 6 节，末端有爪及爪垫。

2. 恙螨 成虫躯体呈“8”字形，全身密被绒毛，有 4 对足，第 1 对足特别长，其幼虫寄生在人体或脊椎动物的体表，与医学的关系密切。

恙螨幼虫玻片标本(低倍镜观察)：椭圆形，呈红色、橙色、淡黄色或乳白色，体长 0.2～0.5 mm，分为颚体及躯体两个部分，颚体包括螯肢和触须各 1 对，触须在外，分为 5 节，螯肢在内，基节呈三角形。躯体背面前部有盾板，生有 5 根毛，并有感器 1 对，盾板后方有背毛，盾板的形状及背毛排列的行、数目和形状等，均因虫种而异。有足 3 对，分为 6～7 节，末端有爪 1 对和爪间突 1 个。

3. 疥螨 寄生于人体的疥螨的生活史分为卵、幼虫、两期若虫和成虫 5 个时期。

成虫玻片标本(低倍镜观察)：类圆形或椭圆形，背面隆起，乳白色，大小为 0.2～0.4 mm。颚体短小，螯肢呈钳状，触须 3 对。躯体背面有波状横纹：后部有长刚毛。腹面光滑，有 4 对足，足粗短，呈圆锥形，前、后 2 对相距较远。前 2 对足末端均有一带细长柄的吸垫。雄虫第 4 对足末端也具有吸垫。而雌虫第 3、4 对足末端均为长刚毛。

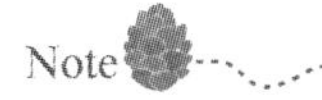

附:皮肤中寄生昆虫的检查

1. 疥螨的检查 从疥螨寄生的"隧道"盲端用利刀刮取病变部位,做涂片检查,寻找疥螨成虫或虫卵。

2. 蠕形螨检查 寄生于人体面部毛囊内,严重时引起酒渣鼻。常用检查方法有两种。

(1)挤压涂片法:用小镊子挤压毛囊四周,使蠕形螨从毛囊内挤出,置载玻片上加甘油一滴镜检。

(2)透明胶纸粘贴法:用透明胶纸在晚上睡觉前粘贴于待检查部位,次日取下贴于载玻片上镜检。

3. 蝇蛆病检查 皮下蝇的幼虫可寄生在皮下组织形成蝇蛆病,被寄生部位可形成疖肿,幼虫亦可在皮下组织移行,定居形成疖肿后中间有一小孔为幼虫呼吸开口处,可在疖肿四周挤压,将幼虫挤出进行检查。

二、自己观察

观察并比较三属蚊生活史各期的形态特征。

三、录像片

观看蚊和寄生虫病原学检查录像片。

[思考题]

(1)试述我国常见蚊、蝇的种类及其主要鉴别特征。

(2)蚊、蝇与医学的关系如何?怎样防治?

(田 芳 陆 凤)

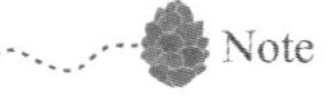

第三篇　综合性实验

实验一　多克隆抗体的制备及效价测定

［实验目的］

（1）掌握颗粒性抗原多克隆抗体制备的原理，加深对影响抗原免疫原性因素的理解。

（2）掌握颗粒性抗原多克隆抗体制备及效价测定的流程。

［实验材料］

（1）免疫原：商品化诊断菌液伤寒沙门菌 H901 和伤寒沙门菌 O901。

（2）体重 2.5 kg 左右的健康家兔，两耳光滑，可见明显耳静、动脉。

（3）无菌磷酸盐缓冲液（PBS）。

（4）兔头固定器、离心机、水浴锅、超净台、1 ml/10 ml 一次性注射器、1.5 ml/15 ml 离心管等。

［实验内容］

1. 免疫原的处理

（1）原理：商品化诊断菌液中含有防腐剂甲醛，不适合直接免疫，需要用 PBS 清洗除去甲醛。

（2）方法。

①伤寒沙门菌 H901 和伤寒沙门菌 O901 诊断菌液的含菌量皆为 7×10^{9}/ml，计算免疫所需的菌量。

②充分摇匀诊断菌液，在超净台上转移所需量的菌液至 1.5 ml 离心管，于 10000 r/min 离心 1 min，弃去上清。

③用 1 ml 无菌 PBS 充分吹打洗涤沉淀，于 10000 r/min 离心 1 min，弃去上清，如是操作 2 次。

④将细菌重悬于 0.2～0.5 ml 无菌 PBS 中。

2. 免疫动物

（1）原理：决定多克隆抗体最终滴度的因素很多，包括抗原本身的理化性质、实验动物的遗传和生理状况、免疫程序以及是否使用佐剂等。

①相比于可溶性抗原而言，颗粒性抗原的免疫原性一般较强，比较容易诱导出高滴度的抗体，可以不用佐剂。

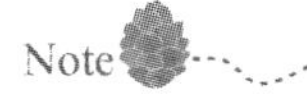

②实验动物的选择方面,最重要的一点是要与抗原来源物种之间有较远的亲缘关系,再根据所需的多克隆抗体的量来选择,其他还要考虑动物的遗传背景、性别、年龄、健康状况等。

③免疫程序对多克隆抗体的产量影响很大,需要充分考虑免疫原剂量、接种途径、免疫次数与间隔时间等多种因素。

a. 免疫原剂量太大或者太小,都会诱导免疫耐受而不是免疫应答,导致抗体制备的失败。

b. 同剂量接种时,一般抗体产量是皮内注射>皮下注射>静脉注射≈腹腔注射≈肌内注射>口服,滴鼻则主要用于诱导黏膜免疫。但不同免疫途径可以接种的免疫原剂量是有差异的,皮内注射最少,腹腔注射最多。

c. 根据抗体生产的一般规律,相比于初次应答,再次应答可以诱导更高水平和亲和力更强的抗体,所以制备抗体时经常需要多次免疫,免疫次数及间隔时间往往需要通过预实验来确定。我们实验中比较腹腔大剂量短间隔接种与耳缘静脉小剂量长间隔接种的结果,来说明不同免疫程序对抗体产量的影响。

(2)方法。

①接种动物前须收集一些正常血清,以备检测抗体效价时作为阴性对照。待家兔在新环境中稳定数天至 1 周,即可进行耳动脉取血,一般取 5 ml 即可。

②所有同学分为 4 个实验组,每个实验组分为 3 个小组,作为重复实验。

a. 实验组一为伤寒沙门菌 H901 耳缘静脉小剂量长间隔接种组。

b. 实验组二为伤寒沙门菌 O901 耳缘静脉小剂量长间隔接种组。

c. 实验组三为伤寒沙门菌 H901 腹腔大剂量短间隔接种组。

d. 实验组四为伤寒沙门菌 O901 腹腔大剂量短间隔接种组。

③实验组一/二于第 1、6、11、16 天接种 4 次,菌量分别为 0.2×10^9、0.5×10^9、1×10^9、1.5×10^9;实验组三/四每隔 2 天接种 1 次,至第 19 天共接种 10 次,菌量皆为 7×10^9。

3. 取血 第 21 天时,通过耳动脉取血检测抗体效价。

(1)用 15 ml 离心管收集血样,于 37 ℃水浴孵育 30 min。

(2)于 2500 r/min 离心 10 min。

(3)吸取血清至一新的 15 ml 离心管中,加入 NaN_3 至终浓度为 0.02%(*W/V*)进行防腐,分装后于−20 ℃保存。

4. 效价测定

(1)方法采用肥达试验,同本书第二篇实验五。

(2)凝集效价达到或超过 1∶2560 说明实验成功。

5. 注意事项 实验过程中要充分保证动物福利。

[实验报告]

报告抗血清的凝集效价,和其他小组比较,并分析产生差异的原因。

[思考题]

思考各种因素对多克隆抗体制备的影响,给出你对免疫程序优化的建议。

Note

(潘兴元　孔桂美)

实验二　流式细胞术检测小鼠脾脏T、B细胞的比例

［实验目的］

(1)掌握小鼠脾脏单细胞悬液的制备方法。

(2)掌握流式细胞术的基本操作及数据分析。

(3)了解小鼠脾脏中T、B细胞的比例。

［实验材料］

(1)C57BL/6小鼠,6周龄,雌雄不限。

(2)75%酒精、红细胞裂解液、pH 7.2～7.4无菌PBS等。

(3)制冰机、离心机、剪刀、镊子、培养皿、不锈钢网、玻璃注射器、超净台、细胞计数板、1.5 ml/15 ml离心管、流式细胞仪等。

［实验内容］

1. 小鼠脾脏单细胞悬液的制备

(1)小鼠颈椎脱臼处死,75%酒精浸泡3 min,取出脾脏,放入盛有5 ml PBS的培养皿中。

(2)将脾脏放置在不锈钢网(100或200目)上,用注射器针芯轻轻研压脾脏,经过过滤获得单细胞悬液。

(3)裂解红细胞,进行细胞计数,调整到1×10^6/ml。

2. 荧光抗体标记细胞

(1)准备4个1.5 ml离心管,每管中加入100 μl细胞悬液(1×10^6/ml)。

(2)1号离心管为未标记空白管,不加任何抗体;2号离心管为CD3-FITC单标管,加入0.5 μl mCD3-FITC荧光抗体;3号离心管为CD19-APC单标管,加入0.5 μl mCD19-APC荧光抗体;4号离心管为双标管,两种荧光抗体各加入0.5 μl。

(3)冰上避光孵育20 min。

(4)400 μl PBS洗涤1次。

(5)于6000 r/min离心5 min,弃上清,用200 μl PBS重悬细胞。

3. 流式细胞检测

(1)打开专用分析软件,通过FSC-SSC散点图(图3-2-1),设门圈定淋巴细胞进行分析。通过调整电压、阈值等参数使细胞处于合适位置,并排除碎片干扰。

(2)分别开启含有目的抗体检测通道的散点图,并限定其获取的细胞为上一步设门圈定的淋巴细胞。

(3)用空白对照调节电压,使未染色细胞的自发荧光完全处于阴性区域,所使用的通道内荧光直方图的淋巴细胞阳性率<2%,双荧光散点图内的未染色细胞位于散点图的左下象限内。

(4)用抗体单标对照调节荧光补偿(图3-2-2)。

(5)上样测试,获取数据。

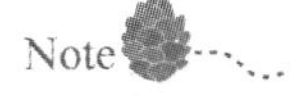

4. 注意事项

(1)红细胞裂解必须充分,否则会对结果分析产生干扰。

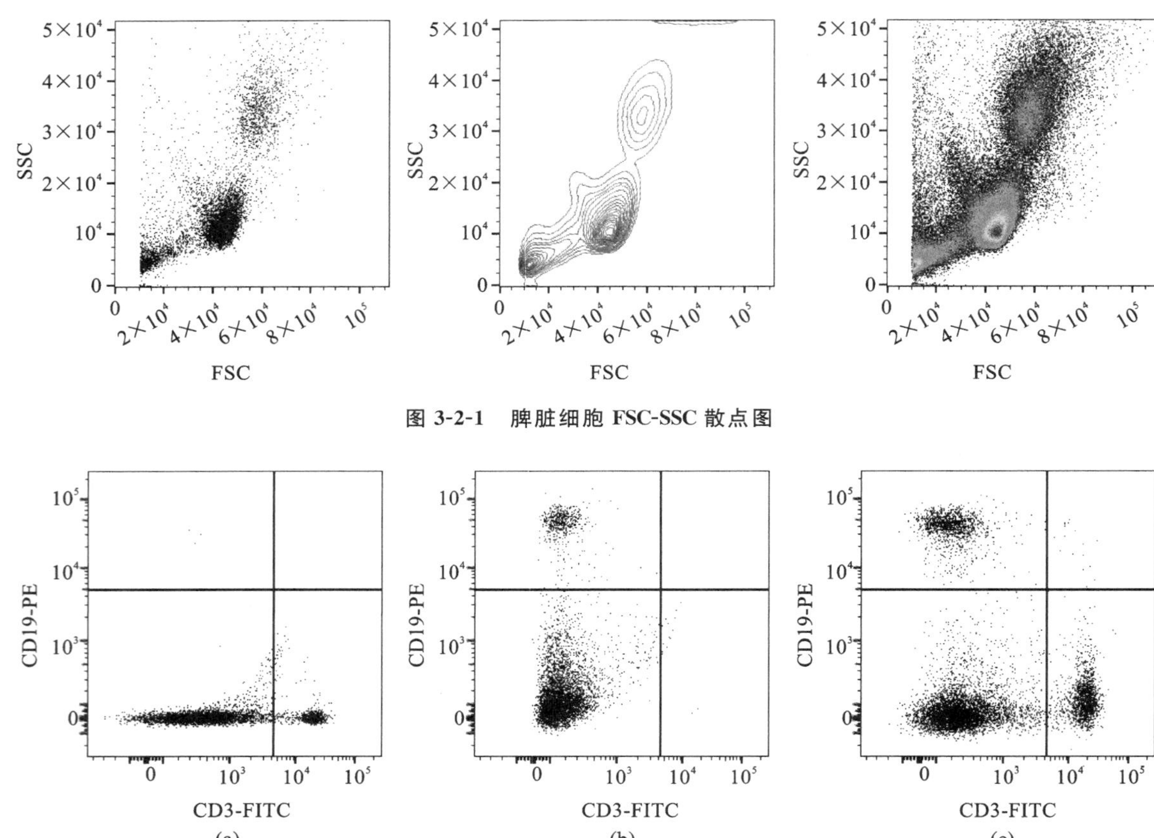

图 3-2-1　脾脏细胞 FSC-SSC 散点图

图 3-2-2　脾脏细胞 CD3-CD19 染色

(a)CD3 单标记;(b)CD19 单标记;(c)CD3-CD19 双标记

(2)流式细胞仪是贵重仪器,用完后需要按照使用规范进行维护,并做好记录。

[实验报告]

(1)说明 4 个离心管的作用。

(2)报告流式图,分析小鼠脾脏中 T、B 细胞的比例。

[思考题]

不同免疫器官和组织中 T、B 细胞的比例分别是什么样的?

(蔺志杰　潘兴元)

实验三　呼吸道感染常见病原微生物的实验室检查

[实验目的]

(1)掌握呼吸道标本的细菌学检验方法。

(2)了解呼吸道标本中的其他微生物。

[实验材料]

(1)标本:模拟痰液、支气管冲洗液、鼻咽拭子,或疑似呼吸道感染者的痰液、支气管冲洗液、鼻咽拭子。

(2)培养基:血琼脂平板、巧克力琼脂平板、麦康凯琼脂平板、科玛嘉念珠菌显色培养基和常用生化鉴定管。

(3)试剂:革兰染液、过氧化氢酶试剂、氧化酶试剂、各种生化反应相关试剂等。

(4)其他:一次性无菌注射器、75%酒精棉球、记号笔、擦镜纸、香柏油、载玻片。

(5)仪器:光学显微镜、恒温培养箱、二氧化碳(CO_2)培养箱。

[实验内容]

一、上呼吸道标本

上呼吸道标本主要包括鼻、鼻咽、口咽拭子及提取物,多有口咽正常菌群存在。

1. 直接检查

(1)疑为白喉棒状杆菌感染的标本:用棉拭子标本制作两张涂片,一张做革兰染色,另一张做美蓝或异染颗粒染色。若发现排列不规则的革兰阳性棒状杆菌,并且有明显的位于菌体一端或两端的蓝黑色异染颗粒,可初步报告“有异染颗粒的革兰阳性棒状杆菌”。

(2)疑为奋森疏螺旋体和梭形杆菌感染的标本:将棉拭子轻轻涂在载玻片上制片,进行革兰染色,注意复染时间加长至 2 min。若见淡红色、细长的疏螺旋体及微弯弧形细长、两头尖的革兰阳性或阴性杆菌,报告“咽拭子涂片找到形似奋森疏螺旋体及梭形杆菌”。

(3)疑为念珠菌感染的标本:将棉拭子涂于干净的载玻片上,加一滴生理盐水后混匀,高倍镜下观察。如发现有酵母样细胞及菌丝,报告“找到酵母样真菌,形似念珠菌”。亦可做涂片,革兰染色镜检。若发现革兰阳性菌,散在或丛生聚集的卵圆形芽生的酵母样真菌,可报告“找到酵母样真菌,形似念珠菌”。

2. 分离培养

(1)普通细菌培养:一般情况下将标本接种于血琼脂平板、巧克力琼脂平板、麦康凯琼脂平板,置于 CO_2 培养箱中,于 37 ℃培养 24～48 h,挑取可疑菌落进行涂片染色、生化反应、血清学试验及动物实验等鉴定,根据结果做出报告。同时做药敏试验。

(2)特殊细菌培养。

①疑为白喉棒状杆菌感染时,将标本接种于吕氏血清斜面或鸡蛋培养基上,35 ℃培养 12 h 后观察菌苔生长情况。如出现灰白色、有光泽的菌苔,或呈圆形、灰白色或淡黄色的菌落,涂片做革兰染色,镜检发现菌体形态和异染颗粒等典型特征者,再结合临床症状发布初步报告,并将菌落划线接种到亚碲酸钾血琼脂平板上,35 ℃纯培养 48 h 并做生化鉴定和毒力试验,报告结果。

②疑为百日咳鲍特菌感染时,将鼻咽拭子接种于鲍-金(Bordet-Gengou)平板中,将平板置于盛有少许水的有盖玻璃缸内培养。35 ℃培养 48～72 h,如有细小、隆起、灰白色、不透明、周围有狭小溶血环的水银滴样菌落,涂片染色观察,如为革兰阴性成双或单个的卵圆形小杆菌,结合菌落特征可初步诊断。进一步做生化反应、血清凝集试验和营养需求等鉴别试验。若培养 7 d 仍无细菌生长,做阴性报告。

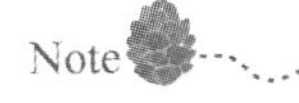

③疑为溶血性链球菌感染时,将标本接种于血琼脂平板,置于 5%～10% CO_2 培养箱,35 ℃

培养 18～24 h,取 β 溶血的小菌落进行染色、生化鉴定和血清学分群,报告鉴定结果。

④疑为流感嗜血杆菌时,将标本接种于血琼脂平板和巧克力琼脂平板,并在血琼脂平板中央划直线接种金黄色葡萄球菌,置于 5%～10% CO_2 培养箱,35 ℃孵育 24～48 h。如有卫星现象出现并发现水滴样小菌落,革兰染色为阴性小杆菌,可进一步鉴定,具体内容参见相关章节。

⑤疑为奈瑟菌感染时,将标本接种于已预温的血琼脂平板(或卵黄双抗琼脂平板)及巧克力琼脂平板,置于 5%～10% CO_2 培养箱,35 ℃培养 24～48 h,挑选可疑菌落涂片染色和做氧化酶试验,若为氧化酶阳性的革兰阴性双球菌,继续做生化反应和血清学鉴定,报告结果。

二、下呼吸道标本

下呼吸道标本包括各种痰液和支气管镜下采集的支气管刷、冲洗液等。痰液可有少量口咽等正常菌群,支气管镜下采集的标本正常菌群较少或无。

1. 标本观察 肉眼观察标本,包括颜色、黏度、有无血丝或脓等性状并记录。将标本做直接涂片镜检,低倍镜下观察白细胞和上皮细胞数目,评定标本是否适合做细菌培养,并初步判断是否有病原菌存在。痰标本镜下分类见表 3-3-1。

表 3-3-1 痰标本镜下分类

分级	白细胞/个	上皮细胞/个	结果
A	>25	<10	合格
B	>25	<25	合格
C	<10	>25	不合格

注:A、B 级两种情况为合格的痰标本,适合做培养;C 级为不合格标本,应要求重新留标本。

对于确定来自下呼吸道的标本,根据镜下观察到的细菌的染色及形态特征做出初步病原学诊断。

2. 直接检查

(1)挑取标本中脓性或带血部分涂片,革兰染色镜检,发布初步报告。

(2)对于疑为白喉棒状杆菌感染的标本,取标本做两张涂片,分别进行革兰染色和 Albert 异染颗粒染色,根据结果发布初步报告。

(3)对于疑为结核分枝杆菌感染或需要排除结核分枝杆菌感染的标本,取干酪样或脓性标本直接做厚涂片或通过离心收集细菌后做厚涂片,抗酸染色,油镜下观察红色的抗酸杆菌,根据结果发布初步报告。

3. 分离培养

(1)痰标本前处理:痰标本接种前应进行前处理。

①洗涤:将标本加入有 10～20 ml 无菌生理盐水的试管中,剧烈振荡 5～10 s,然后用接种环将粘于管底的浓痰挑出,再放入另一试管内,以同样方法反复洗涤 2 次,最后将剩余的浓痰取出接种,也可用无菌培养皿代替试管。

②均质化:向痰(洗涤后)标本中加入等量的 pH=7.6 的 1%胰酶,35 ℃孵育 90 min。

(2)普通细菌培养:将前处理后的痰液或无菌采集的标本(支气管刷或冲洗液等)接种于血琼脂平板、巧克力琼脂平板、麦康凯琼脂平板,置于 5%～10% CO_2 培养箱,35 ℃培养 18～24 h。如发现疑似病原菌菌落(表 3-3-2),做涂片染色镜检,根据菌落和镜下特点选择相应的生化试验及血清学试验进行鉴定,同时做药敏试验。如未长出菌落,继续孵育至 48 h,观察平板、记录并报告。

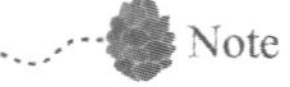
Note

表 3-3-2 呼吸道标本中常见正常菌群及病原菌

种类	革兰阳性细菌及真菌	革兰阴性细菌
正常菌群	甲型溶血性链球菌、微球菌、表皮葡萄球菌、四联球菌、白喉棒状杆菌以外的棒状杆菌、乳杆菌	除脑膜炎奈瑟菌和淋病奈瑟菌外的其他奈瑟菌
上呼吸道常见病原菌	B群链球菌、肺炎链球菌、金黄色葡萄球菌、厌氧菌、白念珠菌、米勒链球菌属、曲霉菌	流感嗜血杆菌、铜绿假单胞菌、肠杆菌科细菌、嗜麦芽窄食单胞菌
上呼吸道偶见病原菌	白喉棒状杆菌、百日咳棒状杆菌、副百日咳棒状杆菌	脑膜炎奈瑟菌
下呼吸道常见病原菌	肺炎链球菌、金黄色葡萄球菌、乙型溶血性链球菌、白念珠菌、曲霉菌	流感嗜血杆菌、卡他莫拉菌、非发酵菌、肠杆菌科细菌、巴斯德菌、嗜血杆菌、脑膜炎奈瑟菌

常见革兰阴性杆菌鉴定：取菌进行氧化酶试验、过氧化氢酶试验、硝酸盐还原试验，如氧化酶试验阴性、过氧化氢酶试验阳性和硝酸盐还原试验阳性，可判断为肠杆菌科细菌，接种 KIA、MIU、IMViC 及肠杆菌科系统生化鉴定管，鉴定至属或者种。如生物学特性符合沙门菌或者志贺菌，用诊断血清进行凝集试验确定种或型。如氧化酶试验阳性或阴性，不发酵葡萄糖或不利用葡萄糖者，可判断为非发酵菌。

常见革兰阳性球菌鉴定：取菌进行过氧化氢酶试验，阳性者为微球菌科细菌，通过 O-F 试验鉴别葡萄球菌属（F 型）和微球菌属（O 型）。过氧化氢酶试验阴性者，常为链球菌或肠球菌。

（3）常规真菌培养：疑为真菌感染时，可将标本接种于沙氏培养基于 35 ℃培养，如未生长，则孵育至第 5 天，记录并报告。怀疑念珠菌感染的可直接接种至科玛嘉念珠菌显色培养基。

（4）厌氧菌培养：无菌操作取气管或环甲膜穿刺液接种于已预还原的厌氧血琼脂平板或巧克力琼脂平板，厌氧培养 24～48 h，观察并记录。

（5）特殊细菌培养：对于怀疑有特殊细菌感染的标本，进行特殊病原菌的分离培养。①结核分枝杆菌：具体内容参见相关章节。②嗜肺军团菌：取器官分泌物接种于活性炭-酵母浸出液（buffered charcoal yeast extract，BCYE）琼脂，35 ℃、2.5% CO_2 培养箱培养 14 d，每天观察结果。③诺卡菌：在镜下观察到革兰阳性或丝状分支可怀疑其存在。④支原体、衣原体等：分离培养及鉴定参见相关章节。

4. 药敏试验 具体内容参见相关章节。

[结果报告]

1. 直接检查

（1）上呼吸道标本：根据形态染色结果，对具有特殊形态或染色性的细菌，发布相应报告。如“咽拭子涂片找到形态似奋森疏螺旋体及梭形杆菌”“找到酵母样真菌，形似念珠菌”。

（2）下呼吸道标本：根据染色后白细胞和鳞状上皮细胞计数、细菌形态和染色性，发布初步报告。如“找到革兰阳性球菌，形似葡萄球菌”“找到革兰阴性球菌，疑似脑膜炎奈瑟菌”。

2. 培养

（1）阳性：查见病原菌，报告菌名和药敏试验结果。

（2）阴性：①上呼吸道标本如无可疑病原菌生长，有咽部正常菌群生长，报告“未检出病原菌”，或报告“甲型溶血性链球菌（正常菌群）生长”“奈瑟菌（正常菌群）生长”“培养基无真菌生长”“培养基无嗜血杆菌生长”。注意在血琼脂平板上未检出特定病原菌，而某种常居菌生长茂盛或接近乃至呈纯培养时，应考虑这种菌可能与疾病有关，应鉴定后报告“××菌生长茂盛”。②下呼

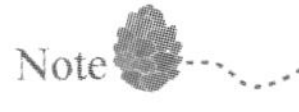

吸道标本痰液如无可疑病原菌生长,报告"未检出病原菌"。支气管刷或冲洗液等深部无菌部位来源标本可报告无细菌生长。

[思考题]

(1)如何判断痰标本是否来自深部?

(2)如何进行下呼吸道标本的细菌学检验?

(3)呼吸道标本检查中可能存在哪些生物安全问题?如何避免这些问题以确保生物安全?

(阴银燕　刘翠翠)

实验四　肠道杆菌的分离和鉴定

[实验目的]

掌握粪便标本细菌学检验方法。

[实验材料]

(1)粪便标本或肛拭子。

(2)培养基:SS 琼脂平板、麦康凯琼脂平板、CAMPY 血平板、中国蓝平板、伊红美蓝(EMB)平板、KIA 培养基、MIU 培养基、GN 增菌液、碱性蛋白胨水、TCBS 琼脂平板及副溶血性弧菌选择平板、CCFA 琼脂平板等。

(3)试剂:靛基质试剂、志贺菌属诊断血清、沙门菌属诊断血清、霍乱弧菌诊断血清、肠致病性大肠埃希菌(EPEC)及肠侵袭性大肠埃希菌(EIEC)诊断血清等。

(4)其他:显微镜、生理盐水、玻片等。

[实验内容]

1. 显微镜直接观察

(1)粪便标本直接涂片镜检:对于炎症性腹泻患者,可取粪便(肛拭子)标本直接涂片、干燥、固定后,进行革兰染色,在显微镜下直接观察。对于沙门菌、志贺菌、耶尔森菌、弯曲菌、EIEC 以及一些弧菌属细菌引起的腹泻,常在粪便标本涂片中观察到白细胞存在,对于有肠壁出血的患者,还可以观察到红细胞存在;如果观察到有"革兰阴性、弯曲的、伴有海鸥展翅形杆菌"存在,患者可能被弯曲菌或弧菌属细菌感染。

(2)观察细菌动力:将粪便标本制成湿片或使用悬滴法观察细菌动力,如果是弯曲菌或弧菌属细菌感染,可见其特征性的"投标样"运动。

2. 细菌分离培养　鉴别选择培养基常用于粪便中病原菌的分离培养,这些培养基通常含有抗菌药物或化学抑制剂,可抑制肠道正常菌群的生长,有利于肠道病原菌生长。

(1)麦康凯琼脂平板:用于发现肠杆菌科细菌和其他非苛养革兰阴性杆菌,抑制革兰阳性菌和某些苛养革兰阴性杆菌。在此培养基上,致病性沙门菌、志贺菌(极少数除外)、爱德华菌为透明、无色或淡黄色菌落;肠道正常菌群,发酵乳糖的细菌如埃希菌属、克雷伯菌属、肠杆菌属和某些枸橼酸杆菌属的细菌为深粉红色到微红色菌落;迟缓发酵乳糖的细菌如某些枸橼酸杆菌属、沙

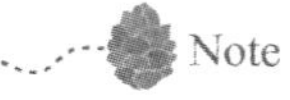
Note

雷菌属，培养 24 h 是无色菌落，而培养 24～48 h 是轻微的粉红色菌落；不发酵乳糖的细菌如变形杆菌属、某些枸橼酸杆菌属、普鲁威登菌属和摩根菌属细菌为透明、无色菌落。

(2)SS 琼脂平板：用于发现沙门菌属和志贺菌属细菌，抑制革兰阳性菌和常见肠道正常菌群的生长，加入指示剂可检测 H_2S 的产生。在此培养基上，沙门菌属和志贺菌属为透明或半透明、无色或淡黄色菌落，肠道正常菌群的生长与麦康凯琼脂平板上生长状况一致。

(3)CAMPY 血平板：用于从粪便中初步分离弯曲菌的选择培养基。在此培养基上，空肠弯曲菌在 42 ℃孵育后为粉红灰色、湿润、流动样菌落。

(4)TCBS 琼脂平板：用于从粪便标本中发现弧菌属细菌的强选择性培养基。因为此培养基 pH 高、胆盐水平高，所以可抑制绝大多数肠道菌群的生长。气单胞菌属也可以在此培养基上被检出，因含蔗糖，所以发酵蔗糖的弧菌属细菌如霍乱弧菌、溶藻弧菌为黄色菌落，而不发酵蔗糖的副溶血性弧菌、创伤弧菌是蓝绿色菌落，除了偶尔可见的假单胞菌呈现蓝绿色菌落外，绝大部分肠道菌群被抑制。

(5)CCFA 琼脂平板：从可疑抗菌药物相关性腹泻或假膜性肠炎患者粪便中初步分离艰难梭菌的选择性培养基。艰难梭菌因可发酵果糖表现为黄色菌落，此培养基可抑制包括革兰阳性球菌和革兰阴性杆菌在内的绝大多数肠道菌群。

3. 粪便标本常见的病原菌

革兰阳性菌：葡萄球菌属、白念珠菌、艰难梭菌、结核分枝杆菌、蜡样芽孢杆菌。

革兰阴性菌：志贺菌属、沙门菌属、肠致病性大肠埃希菌、霍乱弧菌、副溶血性弧菌、亲水气单胞菌、类志贺邻单胞菌、空肠弯曲菌、小肠结肠炎耶尔森菌。

(1)志贺菌属和沙门菌属。

细菌培养：急性腹泻患者的粪便标本分别划线接种至 SS(或 HE，或 XLD)琼脂平板和麦康凯琼脂平板，37 ℃培养箱培养 18～24 h；对慢性腹泻怀疑感染志贺菌属的患者或携带者，应将标本接种至 GN 增菌液，对于怀疑沙门菌属感染的患者或携带者，应将标本接种至亚硒酸盐增菌液，放于 37 ℃培养箱培养 6 h 后，再转接种至 SS 琼脂平板和麦康凯琼脂平板，放于 37 ℃培养箱培养 18～24 h。观察 SS 琼脂平板中有无微小、透明或半透明、无色或浅黄色的可疑菌落生长；有时 SS 琼脂平板上可见中心黑色菌落(产生 H_2S)；在麦康凯琼脂平板上，沙门菌属、志贺菌属(极少数除外)为透明、无色或淡黄色菌落。

挑取三个可疑菌落，分别接种三支 KIA 和 MIU 培养基(做动力、吲哚及脲酶(MIU)复合试验)，37 ℃培养箱中培养 18～24 h，观察反应结果。可同时挑取可疑菌落进行涂片、革兰染色，观察细菌形态与排列等。

如果 KIA 和 MIU 培养基上的生化反应结果与表 3-4-1 中志贺菌属细菌生化反应结果相符，则初步认定该菌株属于志贺菌属；随后用志贺菌属诊断血清对 KIA 管生长的细菌进行血清学分型鉴定。

表 3-4-1 志贺菌属和沙门菌属的初步生化反应

细菌	KIA			MIU				硝酸盐还原试验	过氧化氢酶试验
	斜面	底层	H_2S	产气	动力	吲哚	脲酶		
志贺菌属	K	A	−	−/+	−	+/−	−	+	+
甲型副伤寒沙门菌	K	A	−/+	+	+	−	−	+	+
乙型副伤寒沙门菌	K	A	+	+	+	−	−	+	+
伤寒沙门菌	K	A	+/−	−	+	−	−	+	+
鼠伤寒沙门菌	K	A	+	+	+	−	−	+	+

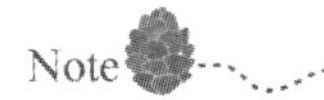

如果 KIA 和 MIU 培养基上的结果符合表 3-4-1 中的沙门菌属的生化反应结果,则初步认定该菌株属于沙门菌属,需进一步与肠杆菌科的其他属细菌进行鉴别(表 3-4-2)。确定为沙门菌属细菌后,用沙门菌属诊断血清对 KIA 管生长的细菌进行血清学分型鉴定。

表 3-4-2　沙门菌属与肠杆菌科其他细菌的鉴别

试验	沙门菌属	枸橼酸杆菌属	亚利桑那菌	爱德华菌属
赖氨酸脱羧酶试验	+	−	+	+
KCN 生长试验	−	+	−	−
丙二酸盐利用试验	−	+/−	+	+
靛基质试验	−	−/+	−	+

(2)肠致病性大肠埃希菌(EPEC)。

细菌培养:取可疑粪便接种于麦康凯琼脂平板(或中国蓝平板或 EMB 平板),放于 37 ℃培养箱中培养 18～24 h;挑取红色的乳糖发酵菌落(中国蓝平板上为蓝色菌落,EMB 平板上则为紫红色菌落),移种于 KIA 和 MIU 培养基管,放于 37 ℃培养箱培养过夜后观察结果,选择符合大肠埃希菌培养结果的可疑细菌,根据 EPEC、EIEC 等细菌的血清学、生化特性进行进一步鉴定。

(3)霍乱弧菌。

①直接镜检:取可疑患者的水样便或米泔水样便制成涂片 2 张,干燥后用酒精或甲醇固定,分别进行革兰染色和苯酚复红染色(1∶10 稀释),油镜下观察有无革兰阴性、呈鱼群样排列的弧菌。

另取可疑标本制成悬滴片或压滴片,向其中一份加入一滴不含防腐剂的霍乱弧菌多价诊断血清,显微镜下观察:如发现不加抗血清的标本有“投标样”运动的细菌,加入抗血清的标本中细菌停止运动并凝集成块为制动试验阳性,则可报告“霍乱弧菌抗血清制动试验阳性”,具有诊断意义。

②细菌培养:疑为霍乱的患者的粪便标本应接种于碱性蛋白胨水,放于 37 ℃培养箱培养 4～6 h,取菌膜或培养液进行革兰染色和制动试验;并取菌膜或培养液接种于 TCBS 琼脂平板(或碱性琼脂平板,或庆大霉素-亚碲酸钾平板),37 ℃培养箱培养 18～24 h,观察 TCBS 琼脂平板上有无黄色菌落;用霍乱弧菌的多价抗血清进行凝集试验(须用生理盐水作阴性对照观察有无自凝现象),若可疑菌抗血清凝集试验阳性,而生理盐水无凝集,结合菌落、菌体形态、氧化酶试验等,可初步判定为霍乱弧菌。

(4)副溶血性弧菌。

细菌培养:将可疑标本接种于副溶血性弧菌选择平板或 TCBS 琼脂平板,放于 37 ℃培养箱中培养 18～24 h,观察菌落形态。副溶血性弧菌在副溶血性弧菌选择平板上形成圆形、边缘整齐、隆起、混浊、绿色、湿润的菌落,在 TCBS 琼脂平板上为绿色或蓝绿色的菌落。将可疑菌落接种于含 3.5%NaCl 的 KIA 和 MIU 培养基中进行耐盐生长试验(表 3-4-3),可以进一步鉴定。

表 3-4-3　副溶血性弧菌的初步生化反应

实验	KIA 培养基(加 3.5% NaCl)				MIU 培养基(加 3.5% NaCl)			蛋白胨水		
	斜面	底层	气体	H_2S	动力	吲哚	脲酶	0%NaCl	7%NaCl	10%NaCl
结果	−	+	−	−	+	+	−	−	+	−

(5)小肠结肠炎耶尔森菌。

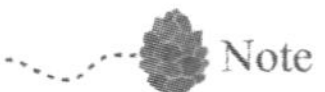

细菌培养:将标本划线接种于耶尔森菌专用(CIN)培养基和麦康凯琼脂平板上,放于 37 ℃培养箱孵育。带菌者的粪便和肛拭子可在 pH 7.4～7.8 的 PBS 中经 4 ℃增菌 21 d,然后于第 7、14

及 21 天各取 0.1 ml 菌液移种于选择培养基上培养 48 h。小肠结肠炎耶尔森菌在麦康凯琼脂平板上呈乳糖不发酵菌落，透明或半透明、较小、扁平、无色、稍隆起；在 CIN 培养基上呈红色菌落，菌落周围偶尔有一圈胆盐沉淀。将疑似菌落移种于 KIA、MIU 及其他生化反应培养基做进一步鉴定。

(6)空肠弯曲菌。

细菌培养：取液状或带血粪便接种于弯曲菌选择性培养基（CAMPY-BA、Skirrow 血琼脂或 Butzler 血琼脂培养基），或接种于 CEM 增菌液（经 42 ℃微需氧培养 18～48 h，再移种于上述选择培养基上做划线分离），在 42 ℃微需氧（可用烛缸法，最好采用混合气体（85% N_2、10% CO_2和 5% O_2））培养条件下孵育 24～48 h，观察细菌生长情况及菌落特点。弯曲菌形成直径 1～2 mm、凸起、湿润、略带红色、有光泽的半透明菌落；若培养基表面较湿润，空肠弯曲菌和大肠弯曲菌可扩散生长，形成扁平的大菌落；各型菌落均不溶血，取此类菌落用悬滴法或压滴法观察动力时，可见呈摆动的"投标样"运动；革兰染色为阴性、细长、两端稍尖的弧形细菌，亦有 S 形、螺旋形或纺锤形者。弯曲菌的鉴定必须结合多种试验加以确定。

(7)葡萄球菌属。

细菌培养：取绿色、海水样或糊状粪便划线接种于高盐甘露醇平板或血平板上，放于 37 ℃培养箱孵育过夜后观察菌落；挑取高盐甘露醇平板上的黄色菌落，进行涂片、革兰染色、镜检。如见革兰阳性、呈葡萄串状排列的球菌，则需做凝固酶、DNA 酶及甘露醇发酵等试验加以确定。

(8)艰难梭菌。

细菌培养：取黄色带有假膜的新鲜粪便，立即接种于环丝氨酸-头孢西丁-果糖琼脂（CCFA）平板上（10～20 min 完成接种）；将接种的平板放于 35 ℃含 80% N_2、10% CO_2及 10% H_2的厌氧环境中培养 48 h 后，选择粗糙的黄色菌落做悬滴动力检查和革兰染色镜检。如显微镜下观察到卵圆形或长方形芽孢位于近端的革兰阳性杆菌（在厌氧琼脂平板上更易产生芽孢），则可做进一步鉴定。

(9)真菌。

真菌培养：真菌性腹泻多继发于抗菌药物治疗后，常见病原菌有白念珠菌和光滑念珠菌。将标本接种于含氯霉素的沙氏培养基及血琼脂培养基上，分别置于 25～30 ℃的空气环境和 37 ℃培养箱孵育 24～48 h，根据菌落形态及涂片革兰染色结果，决定后续鉴定方法。

[实验报告]

(1)描述粪便标本分离的肠杆菌科细菌形态。

(2)分离肠杆菌科细菌过程中需注意的问题有哪些？

[思考题]

(1)不同肠道杆菌在鉴别培养基上的菌落形态有何区别？

(2)大肠埃希菌和志贺菌的生化反应有何不同？

(3)肠道标本检查中可能存在哪些生物安全问题？如何避免以确保生物安全？

（孔桂美　高成凤）

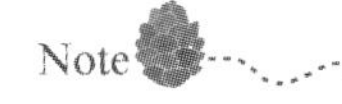

实验五　泌尿生殖道感染常见病原微生物的实验室检查

[实验目的]

掌握泌尿生殖道标本的细菌学检验方法和注意事项。

[实验材料]

(1)标本:尿道或宫颈拭子。

(2)培养基:血平板、巧克力琼脂平板、解脲支原体及人型支原体培养基等。

[实验内容]

1. 涂片检查　分泌物涂片经革兰染色后于油镜下观察,若发现中性粒细胞内(外)有典型的革兰阴性肾形双球菌,可报告"查见细胞内(外)革兰阴性双球菌,疑似淋病奈瑟球菌"。若发现形态细小的革兰阴性杆菌,有时两极浓染,散在或成丛,可报告"查见革兰阴性杆菌,形似杜克雷嗜血杆菌"。梅毒螺旋体可用暗视野显微镜或镀银染色法检查,沙眼衣原体的包涵体可用吉姆萨染色法检查(见相关章节)。念珠菌涂片可用生理盐水制成湿片,加盖玻片,直接镜检或革兰染色后镜检。

(1)淋病奈瑟球菌(*Neisseria gonorrhoeae*):标本经革兰染色后于油镜下观察。注意其形态为肾形,成对排列,革兰染色呈阴性。若用感染性分泌物涂片,可见细菌被中性粒细胞吞噬在细胞质内。

(2)白念珠菌(*Candida albicans*):标本经革兰染色或乳酸酚棉蓝染色后,显微镜下观察显示孢子呈椭圆形,革兰染色呈阳性。注意观察是否存在出芽形成的假菌丝。

(3)衣原体(chlamydia):将感染衣原体的上皮细胞经吉姆萨染色后于油镜下观察。细胞质呈淡红色,细胞核呈紫色,细胞质内的嗜碱性包涵体呈深紫色,且结构致密。

(4)支原体(mycoplasma):支原体菌落经吉姆萨染色,在低倍镜下可呈典型的"油煎蛋"状,边缘整齐透明,颜色较浅;菌落中心致密,呈蓝紫色。

2. 常见细菌的培养和鉴定　将标本接种于血平板上,根据菌落特征和细菌形态进行初步鉴定。

3. 淋病奈瑟球菌的分离、培养和鉴定　将标本接种于淋病奈瑟球菌培养基或巧克力琼脂平板上,置于 35 ℃、5%～10% CO_2 培养箱中培养 24～48 h 后,可观察到圆形、凸起、灰白色、直径 0.5～1 mm 的光滑型菌落。淋病奈瑟球菌在生长过程中可产生大量氧化酶,能将无色的氧化酶试剂(5%～10%盐酸四甲基对苯二胺溶液)氧化成红色的醌类化合物,淋病奈瑟球菌菌落的颜色可变成紫红色或黑色。取可疑菌落涂片,革兰染色镜检,并做氧化酶试验和糖(葡萄糖、麦芽糖、蔗糖、果糖、乳糖)发酵试验进行鉴定。

淋病奈瑟球菌氧化酶试验:在混有杂菌的淋病奈瑟球菌平板上进行试验,用 0.5 ml 吸管滴加 2～3 滴氧化酶试剂于可疑灰白色小菌落上,菌落变为红色即为氧化酶阳性菌,报告"检出淋病奈瑟球菌"或"未检出淋病奈瑟球菌"。淋病奈瑟球菌氧化酶试验对快速诊断早期淋病具有一定意义。

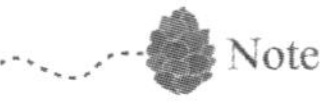

4. 解脲支原体的分离、培养和鉴定　将标本接种于解脲支原体培养基中,置于 35 ℃培养箱中孵育 24～48 h,若培养基由清亮变为紫红色,可按以下方法进行实验。

(1)取此培养基 0.1 ml 接种于解脲支原体固体培养基上，置于 35 ℃、5% CO_2 培养箱中孵育 24～48 h，于低倍镜下观察，如发现“油煎蛋”或“颗粒样”菌落，参照相关章节进行解脲支原体的鉴定。

(2)将上述液体培养物接种于 A7B 鉴定培养基中，置于 5% CO_2 培养箱中孵育 24～48 h 后，解脲支原体产生较小的深棕色或黄色菌落，而其他支原体产生比解脲支原体菌落大的微琥珀色菌落。

根据以上阳性结果，报告“检出解脲支原体”；若孵育 72 h 仍无菌落生长，报告“未检出解脲支原体”，必要时可用 PCR 方法或代谢抑制试验(metabolic inhibition test，MIT)鉴定型别。

5. 衣原体的分离、培养和鉴定

(1)标本处理：将标本拭子放入试管内，猛烈振荡使其洗脱于运送培养基中，使感染细胞破碎，释放出衣原体。立即接种或置于－70 ℃冰箱保存(接种前于 37 ℃水浴中迅速熔化)。

(2)制备单层小鼠成纤维细胞(McCoy 细胞)：McCoy 细胞在细胞瓶中形成致密单层，用 0.25%胰酶消化后，调整细胞浓度为 1×10^5/ml，将细胞爬片置于 24 孔细胞培养板中，加入 1 ml 细胞悬液，置于 35 ℃、5% CO_2 培养箱中孵育 24～48 h。

(3)接种标本：每孔加入 0.2 ml 标本，2000 r/min 离心 1 h。置于 5% CO_2 培养箱中继续孵育 24～72 h。

(4)弃上清，PBS 清洗 2～3 次后用甲醇固定。使用吉姆萨染色法、碘染色法(包涵体呈褐色)、免疫荧光法检测包涵体，结果观察方法同前所述。

6. 念珠菌的培养和鉴定 将念珠菌接种于 2 个沙氏培养基管，分别置于室温(18～25 ℃)和 35 ℃孵育，鉴定方法参考相关章节。

[注意事项]

(1)淋病奈瑟球菌抵抗力差，可以分泌自溶酶，因此标本采集后应尽快接种和进行涂片检查。尽量在床旁接种，如需运送，应将标本置于 35 ℃选择性培养基中，并预热接种的平板。

(2)阴道中存在大量正常菌群，需正确评价正常菌群的致病性。

(3)沙眼衣原体是胞内寄生微生物，在处理标本时，需使上皮细胞破碎从而释放出细胞内的衣原体。

(4)泌尿生殖道感染常见病原微生物的鉴定如图 3-5-1 所示。

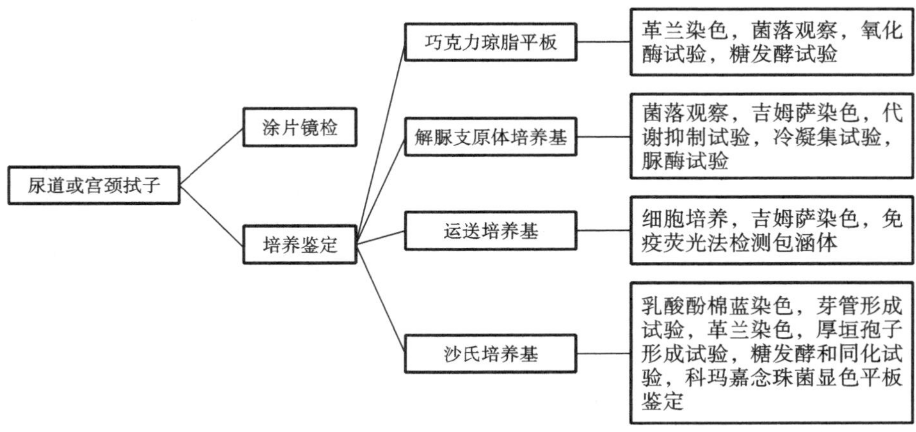

图 3-5-1 泌尿生殖道感染常见病原微生物的鉴定

[思考题]

(1)引起性传播疾病的病原微生物有哪些？

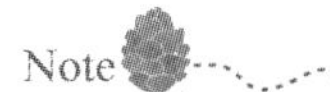

(2)与其他化脓性球菌相比,淋病奈瑟球菌有何特点?

(3)泌尿生殖道标本检查中可能存在哪些生物安全问题?如何避免这些问题以确保生物安全?

(阴银燕　刘翠翠)

实验六　皮肤创伤感染常见细菌的实验室检查

[实验目的]

掌握脓液标本的细菌学检查方法。

[实验材料]

(1)标本:穿刺液、脓液或创面分泌物,或模拟标本等。

(2)血平板、厌氧培养瓶,以及 O-F 试验管、克氏双糖铁琼脂(KIA)管、硝酸盐生化鉴定管、枸橼酸盐生化鉴定管等常用生化鉴定管。

(3)革兰染色液、3%过氧化氢溶液、1%盐酸四甲基对苯二胺溶液、吲哚试剂、新鲜人或兔血浆等。

(4)载玻片、显微镜等。

[实验内容]

脓液及创面分泌物是感染过程中较常检测的标本,检验人员与临床医生应密切配合,以确保正确采集和快速送检此类标本。从脓液及创面分泌物中能够检测出多种细菌,主要的致病菌为金黄色葡萄球菌、化脓性链球菌,其次为铜绿假单胞菌、肠杆菌科细菌等。

1. 肉眼观察　观察标本的性状、颜色及有无硫黄样颗粒。若标本呈绿色,则可能为铜绿假单胞菌感染;若标本有恶臭,则可能为厌氧菌或变形杆菌感染;若脓液中有硫黄样颗粒,则提示放线菌感染。

2. 涂片检查

(1)一般细菌涂片检查:待检标本固定后进行革兰染色镜检,根据镜下所见细菌的形态和染色特点,可做出初步报告。对疑有结核分枝杆菌感染的标本,可做抗酸染色检查。

(2)以色列放线菌和星形诺卡菌涂片检查:用肉眼或放大镜检查脓液、创面分泌物或者敷料内有无直径 1 mm 以下的灰白色或硫黄样颗粒。用接种环挑取含有硫黄样颗粒的标本置于洁净的载玻片上,覆以盖玻片,轻轻挤压;若颗粒结构不明显,可滴加 2～3 滴 50～100 g/L 的氢氧化钾溶液,消化后于低倍镜及高倍镜下仔细观察。或将标本直接涂片,革兰染色后镜检(必要时进行抗酸染色),根据镜下细菌的形态和染色特点,可报告“直接涂片找到革兰阴/阳性菌”。如存在以色列放线菌颗粒,可见中央为交织的菌丝,菌丝的末端稍膨大、似棒状排列并呈放射状,有时可见嵌于类似明胶的鞘膜内。星形诺卡菌与以色列放线菌形态基本相同,但分枝菌丝末端一般不膨大成棒状,革兰染色呈阳性,抗酸染色呈阳性;而以色列放线菌革兰染色呈阳性,抗酸染色呈阴性。如查见中间部分菌丝革兰染色呈阳性,向四周放射的末端菌丝革兰染色呈阴性,抗酸染色呈阴性者,可报告“找到以色列放线菌”;若查见革兰染色反应与以色列放线菌相同,而抗酸染色呈

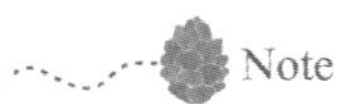

阳性者，可报告“找到星形诺卡菌”；如查见革兰染色呈阴性，抗酸染色呈阴性者，可报告“未找到以色列放线菌及星形诺卡菌”。

3. 培养检查

（1）一般细菌：取脓液棉拭子或用接种环将脓液接种于血平板上进行划线分离，置于 37 ℃培养箱中培养 18～24 h，观察培养结果；如有细菌生长，可按菌落特征挑取各种单一菌落，分别涂片进行革兰染色镜检，初步判断细菌的种类，再按各类细菌的鉴定要点进行鉴定。

①乙型溶血性链球菌：若菌落小如针尖，周围伴有大而透明的溶血环，则可能为溶血性链球菌，结合镜检有助于鉴别。必要时用血清肉汤培养，若出现沉淀且涂片染色后呈长链状排列，则疑为乙型溶血性链球菌。

②金黄色葡萄球菌：金黄色葡萄球菌在血平板上为中等大小、凸起、湿润的金黄色或白色圆形菌落，有 β-溶血环；涂片染色镜检为革兰阳性、葡萄状或簇状排列的球菌；过氧化氢酶试验、甘露醇发酵试验、血浆凝固酶试验均呈阳性，对新霉素敏感，耐热核酸酶试验呈阳性。如果在血平板上见中等大小的脂溶性金黄色色素或无特殊色素，有透明溶血环，涂片染色镜检为呈葡萄串状排列的革兰阳性球菌，可通过甘露醇发酵试验、血浆凝固酶试验等进一步鉴定。

③肺炎链球菌：菌落小，周围有草绿色溶血环，涂片染色镜检为革兰阳性，呈短链状排列者多为甲型溶血性链球菌，呈双排列者多为肺炎链球菌，做进一步鉴定和鉴别试验可确诊。

④普通变形杆菌：血平板上，菌落扁平，呈迁徙性弥漫生长，湿润，灰白色。由于细菌蛋白酶的作用，可见类似溶血的现象，并伴有恶臭。革兰阴性杆菌呈多形性，氧化酶试验阴性、过氧化氢酶试验阳性、苯丙氨酸脱氨酶试验阳性。KIA：K/A、H_2S（＋）、产气。MIU：动力（＋）、靛基质（＋）、脲酶（＋）。

⑤铜绿假单胞菌：血平板上，菌落扁平、边缘不规则，湿润，向四周扩散，培养基上常有水溶性的蓝绿色色素，有 β-溶血环和特殊气味。革兰染色呈阴性的直杆菌，两端钝圆；氧化酶试验阳性；能氧化分解葡萄糖和木糖，产酸不产气；能将硝酸盐还原为亚硝酸盐并产生氮气；可利用枸橼酸盐；精氨酸双水解酶试验阳性；42 ℃可生长。

（2）炭疽杆菌：疑为炭疽杆菌感染时，可取患者脓液接种于血平板上；对于污染严重的标本，可首先在肉汤培养基内增菌过夜，然后在 80 ℃加热 20 min 以杀灭非芽孢细菌，再移种于血平板进行分离培养。经 37 ℃培养 18～24 h，如在血平板上看到大而扁平、毛绒状、灰白色、边缘不整齐，形似卷发状（低倍镜下观察更为清楚）的不溶血菌落，则挑取菌落进行涂片、染色、镜检；如为革兰阳性、竹节状大杆菌，呈链状排列，悬滴检查无动力，则动物接种、串珠试验和噬菌体裂解试验可用于鉴别诊断。

（3）厌氧菌：疑为厌氧菌感染的标本应接种于牛心、牛脑浸出液或布氏肉汤培养基中，亦可直接接种于 KVA 血平板（或 LKV 平板），置于厌氧环境中培养。分离厌氧芽孢杆菌如破伤风芽孢梭菌时，应将已接种标本的液体培养基先置于 80 ℃水浴中加热 20 min 以杀灭非芽孢细菌，然后经 37 ℃培养 24～48 h，根据细菌生长情况及涂片染色镜检结果，按该厌氧菌的生物学特性（生化反应和动物实验）进行鉴定。

（4）以色列放线菌及星形诺卡菌。

①以色列放线菌：疑有杂菌污染的瘘管引流液，应首先将标本倒入无菌培养皿内，以无菌蒸馏水洗涤溶解血细胞后，再挑选典型或可疑的硫黄样颗粒，将其压碎，然后分别接种于两份葡萄糖肉汤琼脂平板上并置于 37 ℃进行需氧及厌氧培养。同时接种至沙氏葡萄糖琼脂斜面（或平板）上，置于 22～28 ℃培养，如无硫黄样颗粒，可取标本直接接种于上述培养基。

对于未被细菌或真菌污染的标本，可直接采集硫黄样颗粒或脓液接种于硫乙醇酸钠肉汤或深层葡萄糖肉汤琼脂平板，置于 37 ℃进行厌氧培养，同时接种至沙氏葡萄糖琼脂斜面，置于 22～28 ℃培养。培养 4 d 后，若在厌氧培养的葡萄糖肉汤琼脂平板上见有白色、粗糙或结节状菌落，

Note

且黏附于培养基上不易用接种环取下,也不易在生理盐水中乳化,而在需氧培养的平板上无类似菌落生长,则可疑为以色列放线菌。

将疑为以色列放线菌的菌落移种于硫乙醇酸钠肉汤管的底部,置于 37 ℃培养 4～6 d,可见有白色绒毛样菌团长出,摇动后破碎,上部培养液仍保持澄清;将其移种于葡萄糖肉汤琼脂进行深层培养,经 37 ℃培养 4～6 d,可在深层培养管表面下层发现分叶状的菌落,取菌落涂片镜检,可见有交织成团或小碎片状菌丝,抗酸染色呈阴性。

②星形诺卡菌:在沙氏培养基上需氧培养后出现光滑、不规则折叠或颗粒状的黄色至橙黄色菌落,可取菌落做湿片镜检,如发现精细分枝状,革兰染色呈阳性,抗酸染色呈红色的菌丝,即判定为阳性。

[实验报告]

(1)简述葡萄球菌的革兰染色和培养特性。
(2)简述铜绿假单胞菌的培养特性。

[思考题]

(1)简述硫黄样颗粒在细菌鉴定中的意义。
(2)如何处理被杂菌污染的样本?
(3)在检查脓液或脓性分泌物标本时可能存在哪些生物安全问题? 如何避免这些问题以确保生物安全?

(孔桂美　高成凤)

实验七　日本血吸虫感染小鼠致病及免疫学诊断

[实验目的]

(1)掌握日本血吸虫的感染途径、寄生部位及成虫形态特征。
(2)掌握日本血吸虫病的免疫学诊断方法。
(3)了解日本血吸虫卵引起的病理变化。

[实验内容]

(一)日本血吸虫感染小鼠模型的建立

(1)实验动物:6～8 周龄的昆明小鼠 20 只。

(2)将感染日本血吸虫的阳性钉螺置于装有清洁除氯水的小烧杯中,20～25 ℃、光照条件下日本血吸虫尾蚴从钉螺中逸出。用接种环挑取水面的尾蚴,移至盖玻片上,在解剖镜下计数,共收集(30±5)条。小鼠麻醉后,腹部朝上固定于鼠板上,拔除小鼠腹部毛发,用除氯水湿润小鼠腹部皮肤,将盖玻片直接贴附于小鼠腹部皮肤上,保留 20 min 后取下盖玻片。小鼠饲养到 6 周。

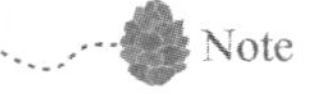

(二)日本血吸虫感染小鼠致病结果观察

1. 日本血吸虫成虫计数　采用生理盐水心脏灌注法。将小鼠颈椎脱臼处死后,剥离皮肤,打开腹腔、胸腔，用注射器吸取生理盐水经左心室进针灌注，待门静脉充盈后，切开一侧，继续灌注生理盐水冲出虫体。灌洗后，将整个肠及系膜组织取出，压于两块厚玻璃板间，计数肠系膜静脉中残留未冲出的虫体。每只小鼠最终所得虫数为灌洗所得虫数加上压板所得虫数。

2. 日本血吸虫虫卵计数 取小鼠肝脏左前叶于10%甲醛溶液中固定，剩余肝脏称量后置10 ml 5% KOH溶液中于37 ℃消化过夜。将消化液混匀后取1 ml至1.5 ml EP管，再从中取10 μl滴加到载玻片上，盖上盖玻片后于100倍光镜下计数虫卵，公式如下：

每克肝脏中的虫卵数=(光镜下计数虫卵数/消化肝脏质量)×1000

3. 肝脏病理学观察 将肝脏病变严重部分浸泡于10%甲醛溶液中，固定12 h以上，制作病理切片并进行苏木精-伊红染色，显微镜下观察，并拍照记录。主要观察虫卵肉芽肿分布情况。

(三)ELISA法辅助诊断日本血吸虫病

1. 实验原理 酶联免疫吸附试验(enzyme linked immunosorbent assay，ELISA)是常用于诊断日本血吸虫病的免疫学方法。将日本血吸虫的可溶性抗原包被在特制的聚苯乙烯反应孔内，将待测血清加到反应孔内，如血清中含有相应的特异性抗体，则可形成抗原-抗体复合物，若在反应孔内加入相应的辣根过氧化物酶(HRP)标记二抗，则可通过底物的显色反应来判断试验结果。

2. 试剂 PBS(10 mmol/L，pH 7.4)、PBST(含0.05% Tween-20的PBS)、包被液(pH 9.6，0.05 mol/L碳酸盐缓冲液)、底物显色液。封闭液：3%脱脂奶(3 g脱脂奶粉/100 ml PBS)。

鼠抗血清(血吸虫感染动物实验获得，−20 ℃冻存备用)、羊抗鼠IgG-HRP、日本血吸虫成虫抗原等。

3. 主要步骤

(1)包被：用包被液稀释上述抗原至5 μg/ml，每孔加入100 μl，置于4 ℃湿盒中孵育过夜。

(2)洗涤：以PBST洗涤5次。

(3)封闭：以3%脱脂奶封闭，每孔加入300 μl，室温下放置1 h。

(4)与抗血清反应：加入鼠抗血清(1∶100)，每孔加入100 μl，室温下放置1 h。

(5)同上述方法洗涤6次。

(6)与酶标二抗反应：加入羊抗鼠IgG-HRP(1∶5000)，每孔加入100 μl，室温下放置1 h。

(7)同上述方法洗涤6次。

(8)显色：加入底物显色液，每孔加入200 μl，室温下放置0.5 h，注意避光。

(9)终止：以50 μl 1 mol/L H_2SO_4终止反应。

4. 实验结果观察和分析 于490 nm波长处读取结果(阳性反应呈棕色或棕黄色)。

5. 注意事项

(1)严格遵守实验操作规程，严防孔间交叉污染。

(2)实验应设置无抗原的空白对照、阳性对照和阴性对照。

[思考题]

请根据实验结果分析日本血吸虫病抗体检测结果的意义。

(田　芳)

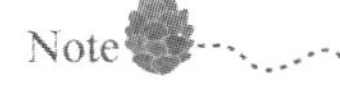

Chapter 1 Basic Experiments of Immunology

Experiment 1 Measure of the 50% Haemolytic Complement (CH_{50}) Activity of Serum

[Experimental Objective]

To master the principle and method of measuring the overall activity of the complement system, especially evaluate the classic complement activation pathway.

[Experimental Materials and Equipment]

(1) NaCl, $MgCl_2$, $CaCl_2$, 1 mol/L HCl solution, barbitone, sodium barbitone, distilled water, 2% sheep red blood cell (SRBC) suspension, hemolysin, human serum from healthy volunteers, etc.

(2) Ice machine, water bath, centrifuge, spectrophotometer, volumetric flasks, 15 ml centrifuge tubes, pipette, mark pens, etc.

[Experimental Contents]

Normal Results: The total blood complement level is 50-100 hemolytic units/ml.

1. Principle

The complement system is a group of proteins that will lead to target cell lysis and facilitate phagocytosis through opsonization when activated. Individual complement component can be quantified; however, this does not provide any information as to the activity of the pathway. The CH_{50} assay is a screening assay for the activation of the classical complement pathway, and it is sensitive to the reduction, absence and/or inactivity of any component of the pathway. The test is named CH_{50} assay for the reason that it is most sensitive around 50% lysis.

The CH_{50} assay tests the functional capability of serum complement components of the classical pathway to lyse SRBC pre-coated with rabbit anti-sheep red blood cell antibody (hemolysin). When antibody-coated SRBC are incubated with test serum, the classical pathway of complement is activated. If a complement component is absent, the CH_{50} level will be zero; if one or more components of the classical pathway are decreased, the CH_{50} will be decreased. A fixed volume of optimally sensitized SRBC is added to each serum dilution. After incubation, the mixture is centrifuged, and the degree of hemolysis is quantified by measuring the absorbance of

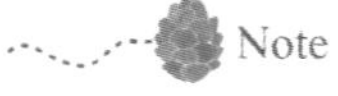

the hemoglobin released into the supernatant at 540 nm. The amount of complement activity is determined by examining the capacity of various dilutions of test serum to lyse antibody-coated SRBC.

A CH_{50} assay is often ordered to evaluate complement component deficiency and evaluate complement activity in cases of immune complex disease, glomerulonephritis (inflammation of the kidneys' filters), rheumatoid arthritis (RA) and cryoglobulinemia (abnormal proteins in the blood that thicken in cold temperature). It can also be used to evaluate a patient's response to systemic lupus erythematosus (SLE) therapy and predict disease flares.

This test is usually ordered for people with a family history of complement deficiency and those who have symptoms of RA, kidney disease, SLE, myasthenia gravis, infectious diseases such as meningitis and cryoglobulinemia.

Increased levels of complement may indicate acute-phase immune response, cancer, ulcerative colitis, heart attack (acute myocardial infarction) and sarcoidosis. Decreased levels of complement may indicate acquired deficiency, RA, vasculitis, severe trauma, SLE, membranous glomerulonephritis, cryoglobulinemia, liver disease or cirrhosis.

The CH_{50} assay is subject to many interferences. Some SRBCs are more fragile than others, resulting in spontaneous hemolysis that is unrelated to complement activity. The affinity of the rabbit antibody varies from lot to lot and from one manufacturer to another; this affects the amount of antibody that binds to the SRBC. Also, the process of sensitizing SRBC with antibodies results in cells with differing amounts of antibody coating the SRBC. Specimen collection and storage are an important potential source of error. Complement components, e.g. C1q, C3, C4 and C5 are extremely labile, so proper sample handling is critical. Prolonged exposure to heat will decrease complement activity and will produce inactive fragments of complement components. To detect as many sources of error as possible, it is critical to test a control serum with a known CH_{50} value every time the assay is performed and to reproduce the accepted value of the known serum control. One way to determine if there are any differences between different batches of SRBC and hemolysin is to test new test materials against a standard sample of serum several times and then determine if there are any changes in the basal level of hemolysis or in the CH_{50} value for the control serum.

2. Method

(1) Sensitisation of SRBCs with hemolysin.

① Prepare the hemolysin by diluting it with 2000 times PBS (final concentration: 2 U/ml).

② Incubate 2 U/ml hemolysin at 56 ℃ for 30-35 min in a water bath to inactivate contaminating complement compounds in hemolysin. Gently mix every 10 min.

③ Centrifuge 2% SRBC suspension at 2000 r/min for 10 min. Discard the supernatant and wash the cells for 2-3 times. After the final wash, centrifuge the cells at 2000 r/min for 10 min to pack the cells. Discard the supernatant and resuspend the cells in sufficient PBS to prepare a 2% solution.

④ Transfer 6 ml 2% SRBC to a small beaker. Dropwise add an equal volume of 2 U/ml hemolysin to the beaker while swirling continuously. Incubate at 37 ℃ for 15 min in a water bath. Gently mix the beaker every 5 min.

⑤ Store sensitized SRBC on ice.

(2) Preparation of 50% lysis tube.

① Add 0.5 ml of 2% SRBC suspension and 2 ml distilled water into a 15 ml centrifuge

tube.

②Add 2 ml 1.8% NaCl solution to make the isotonic solution.

③Add 0.5 ml of 2% SRBC suspension. Gently mix and label it as 50% hemolytic standard solution.

(3) The CH_{50} assay.

①Label a series of tubes. Prepare all tubes on ice according to the Tab. 1-1-1.

Tab. 1-1-1 CH_{50} assay method

Tube number	1	2	3	4	5	6	7	8	9	10	11
Test serum volume/ml	0.1	0.15	0.2	0.25	0.3	0.35	0.4	0.45	0.5	0	50% hemolytic standard solution 2.5 ml
PBS volume/ml	1.4	1.35	1.3	1.25	1.2	1.15	1.1	1.05	1	1.5	
Sensitized SRBC suspension volume/ml	1										
CH_{50}/(U/ml)	200	133	100	80	66.6	57.1	50	44.4	10	—	—

②Gently mix all tubes. Incubate at 37 ℃ for 30 min in a water bath, mixing after 15 min.

③Centrifuge the samples at 2000 r/min for 3 min to precipitate the SRBCs.

④Compare the color of the supernatant with the 50% lysis tube. The amount of the serum in the nearest tubes will be used to calculate CH_{50} activity as the formula below.

$$CH_{50}=\frac{1}{\text{the amount of serum causing 50\% hemolysis(ml)}}\times \text{dilution ratio}$$

[Notes]

(1) Complement is sensitive to heat, so all operations should be performed on ice to maintain complement activity.

(2) Sensitized SRBC suspension and other reagents should be freshly prepared. If contaminated by bacteria, it may lead to hemolysis.

(3) Glassware must be clean. Acid and alkali can affect the accuracy of the experiment.

(4) The hemolytic activity of complement is related to the pH, ionic strength, calcium and magnesium ions content, SRBC, total volume and temperature of the reaction. Therefore, the reaction should be strictly controlled to ensure the accuracy and repeatability of the experiment.

[Experimental Report]

(1) Describe the principle and procedure of the CH_{50} assay.

(2) Calculate CH_{50} activity and give your tentative diagnosis.

[Questions]

(1) What kind of patients need to be tested for CH_{50}?

(2) What other methods are available for the detection of complement activity? Try to compare the advantages and disadvantages of various methods.

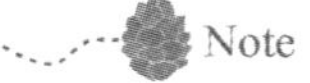

Note

(Xingyuan Pan, Liangliang Cai)

Experiment 2 Isolation of Human Peripheral Blood Mononuclear Cells

[Experimental Objective]

To master the principle and method of isolating human peripheral blood mononuclear cells (PBMCs) with Ficoll-Paque solution.

[Experimental Materials and Equipment]

(1) Human venous blood (anticoagulated by heparin or EDTA).

(2) Ficoll-Paque solution, pH 7.2-7.4 PBS, etc.

(3) Centrifuge, 15 ml centrifuge tubes, pipettes, etc.

[Experimental Contents]

1. Principle

The density of all kinds of blood cells in peripheral blood is not the same; the density gradient centrifugation with Ficoll-Paque solution is used to make a certain proportion of cells distribute according to the density gradient, and all kinds of blood cells can be separated. Human PBMCs include lymphocytes and monocytes, and their density ranges from 1.075 to 1.090 g/ml. While the densities of platelets, granulocytes and erythrocytes are 1.030-1.035 g/ml, 1.092 g/ml, and 1.093 g/ml, respectively.

Anticoagulant-treated blood is layered on the Ficoll-Paque solution (has a density of (1.077 $\pm$0.001) g/ml at 20 ℃) and centrifuged for a short period of time. Differential migration during centrifugation results in the formation of layers containing different cell types. The bottom layer contains erythrocytes, which have been aggregated by the Ficoll-Paque solution, therefore, sediment completely through the Ficoll-Paque solution. The layer immediately above the erythrocyte layer contains mostly granulocytes, which, at the osmotic pressure of the Ficoll-Paque solution, attain a great enough density to migrate through the Ficoll-Paque layer. Because of their lower density, the lymphocytes are found at the interface between the plasma and the Ficoll-Paque layer with other slowly sedimenting particles (platelets and monocytes). The lymphocytes are then recovered from the interface and subjected to short washing steps with a balanced salt solution to remove any platelets, Ficoll-Paque solution and plasma.

2. Method

(1) Take a 15 ml centrifuge tube and add 2 ml of Ficoll-Paque solution (pre-balanced to room temperature). Insert a pipette directly into the bottom of the tube to prevent the solution from touching the tube wall.

(2) Pour 2 ml intravenous anticoagulation into another 15 ml centrifuge tube and add 2 ml PBS to dilute the blood. When mixing, blow slowly along the tube wall to avoid forming bubbles.

(3) Carefully layer the diluted blood on the Ficoll-Paque solution along the tube wall, ensuring a clear interface between them.

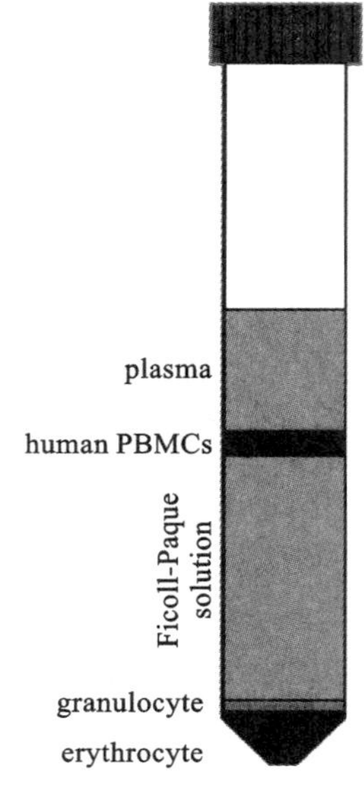

Fig. 1-2-1 Separated human peripheral blood

(4) Centrifuge at 1500-2000 r/min for 20 min at room temperature. Remember to set "No break" to avoid re-mixing the already layered cells after centrifugation because of rapid deceleration.

(5) Using a clean dropper to transfer the lymphocyte layer (i. e. human PBMCs) (Fig. 1-2-1) to a clean centrifuge tube. It is critical to remove all of the interface but a minimum amount of Ficoll-Paque solution and supernatant. Removing excess Ficoll-Paque solution causes granulocyte contamination; removing excess supernatant results in unnecessary contamination by platelets and plasma proteins.

(6) Add at least 5 times the volume of PBS to the human PBMCs. Gently draw the cells in and out of a dropper to suspend them. Centrifuge at 1500 r/min for 10 min at room temperature.

(7) Remove the supernatant. Gently draw the lymphocytes in and out of the dropper to suspend them in 1 ml PBS. The cell concentration is $(1\text{-}2)\times 10^6$/ml. The cell counting plate can be used to count accurately when needed. Stained with 7-ADD or PI fluorescent dyes, the percentage of the living cells detected by flow cytometry in the human PBMCs should be greater than 95%.

[Notes]

(1) Ficoll-Paque solution should be adequate, and peripheral blood should be fully diluted.

(2) Temperature directly affects the density and separation effect of Ficoll-Paque solution.

(3) Lymphocytes of different species have different densities, so different Ficolls-Paque solution for different species should not be exchanged.

[Experimental Report]

Describe the principle, method and matters needing attention of the separation of human PBMCs with Ficoll-Paque solution.

[Questions]

What impurities are theoretically present in the separated product? Under what circumstances do we need to continue separation and purification? What methods can be used?

(Xingyuan Pan, Zhijie Lin)

Experiment 3 E-rosette Forming Test

[Experimental Objectives]

(1) To master the principle, method, and application of E-rosette forming test.

(2)To be familiar with the morphology and counting method of E-rosette under the light microscope.

[Experimental Materials and Equipment]

(1)Isolated human PBMCs (prepared from Chapter 1 Experiment 2).

(2)pH 6.4-6.8 PBS,pH 7.2-7.4 PBS,1% SRBC suspension,0.8% glutaraldehyde,Wright-Giemsa stain solution,etc.

(3) Ice machine, centrifuge, water bath, microscope, 15 ml centrifuge tubes, pipettes, slides,etc.

[Experimental Contents]

1. Principle

The receptor on the surface of T cells that can bind with LFA-3 on the surface of SRBCs is called an E-receptor (CD2 molecule),which has been proven to be a specific surface marker of human T cells. SRBCs can stick to the surface of T cells through these E-receptors to form rosettes (Fig. 1-3-1).

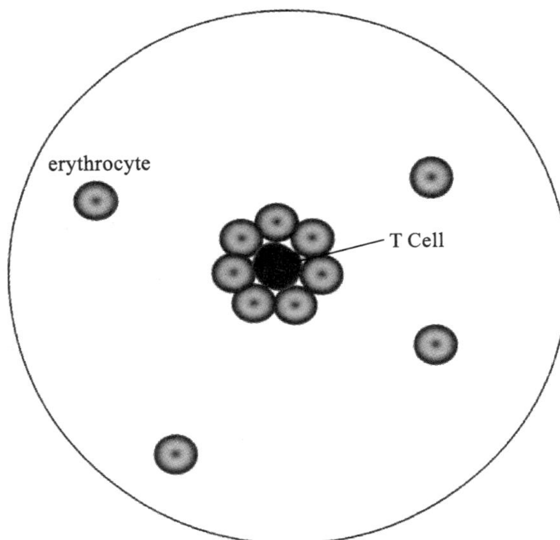

Fig. 1-3-1 E-rosette

The E-rosette forming test is a method of checking T cells by E-rosette formation. According to the number of E-rosettes,the number of T cells can be measured,thus indirectly reflecting the body's cellular immune function. This test is widely used in the study of tumor immunity,transplantation immunity and immune diseases. It provides important references for the immunological diagnosis, immunological prevention, immunological treatment of some diseases,prognosis judgment,and evaluation of drug efficacy,etc.

T cells are highly heterogeneous,with different expression levels of CD2 molecule on the surface,thus showing different affinity to SRBCs and different E-rosette forming abilities. The majority of T cells are at rest,and the expression level of CD2 molecules are low,so they need to react with SRBCs at 4 ℃ for more than 2 h (usually overnight) to form E-rosettes. This

Note

experiment was called the total E-rosette test, representing the total number of T cells in the specimen examined. Some T cells express high levels of CD2 molecules due to antigen stimulation and thus can form E-rosettes with SRBCs only for a short period of incubation. This active E-rosette test, which reflects the number of activated T cells, can better reflect the cellular immune function and dynamic changes in the body.

2. Method

(1) Active E-rosette test.

①Add 0.1 ml PBMCs suspension (about 10^6/ml) into equal volume 1% SRBC suspension (the ratio of lymphocyte to SRBC is about 1 : 20), and mix gently.

②Incubate at 37 ℃ for 5 min, gently rock it 2-3 times during incubation. Note: the combination between T cells and SRBCs is not strong, so it is needed to try to avoid severe shaking during subsequent operations.

③Centrifuge at 500 r/min for 5 min at 4 ℃. Incubate on ice for 20 min.

④Remove most of the supernatant and resuspend the cells gently in the remaining solution. Add 1-2 drops of 0.8% glutaraldehyde (prepared freshly, use within 15 min) to fix E-rosettes, mix gently and incubate on ice for 15 min.

⑤Gently rotate the centrifuge tube to resuspend the precipitated cells. Take 1 drop of the cell suspension and drop it on the slide pre-soaked in the pre-cooled distilled water. Let the cells spread out naturally and evenly. Blow it to dry with a hair dryer (cold wind).

⑥Add a few drops of Wright-Giemsa stain solution to completely cover the specimen and stain for 2 min. Add the same number of drops of pH 6.4-6.8 PBS, gently shake the slide to mix the stain solution well, stain for 5 min.

⑦Rinse with pH 7.2-7.4 PBS (do not tilt the slide to rinse; it should be rinsed horizontally), dry, and observe under high-power microscope.

(2) Total E-rosette test.

①Add 0.1 ml PBMCs suspension (about 10^6/ml) into 0.5 ml 1% SRBC suspension (the ratio of lymphocyte to SRBC is about 1 : 100), and mix gently.

②Incubate at 37 ℃ for 10 min, gently rock it 2-3 times during incubation.

③Centrifuge at 500 r/min for 5 min at 4 ℃. Incubate on ice for 2 h or overnight at 4 ℃.

④～⑦The same as active E-rosette test.

3. Result

Blue lymphocytes and monocytes can be seen under high-power microscope. The smaller lymphocytes are easily distinguished from the larger monocytes. SRBCs are red and form a rosette around the lymphocyte. Cells attached with 3 or more SRBCs are E-rosette forming cells (T cells). Count 200 lymphocytes and calculate the percentage of E-rosette formation, which is the percentage of T cells.

4. The normal value

The total E-rosette test positive lymphocytes ratio is 60%-80%, and the active E-rosette test positive lymphocytes ratio is 10%-40%.

[Notes]

(1) NK cells also express CD2 molecule and can form E-rosettes, but they are few in number

and larger than T cells thus they can be easily distinguished. Monocytes do not express CD2 molecule and can not form E-rosettes.

(2) The isolated PBMCs should not be placed for more than 4 h. Otherwise, the CD2 molecule will fall off from the cell membrane. At the same time, the percentage of the living cells in PBMCs should not be less than 95%.

(3) The freshness of SRBCs also plays an important role in this experiment. It is generally not recommended to keep it for more than 2 weeks; otherwise, its ability to bind with the lymphocyte decreases.

(4) The ratio of lymphocyte to SRBC is different for the active E-rosette test and total E-rosette test.

(5) Temperature greatly influences the experimental results. The samples should be counted immediately after being removed from 4 ℃ or ice.

(6) Before counting, the cells should be resuspended, but the tube should only be rotated gently, so that the cell mass can be loosened. Don't blow too hard or strong, otherwise, the E-rosettes will disappear or reduce.

[Experimental Report]

(1) Describe the principle and method of the E-rosette forming test.

(2) Discuss your results.

[Questions]

(1) When do we need to test T cell function?

(2) What other methods can be used to determine T cell function?

(Xingyuan Pan, Zhijie Lin)

Experiment 4 Neutrophil Phagocytosis Test

[Experimental Objectives]

(1) To master the principle and method of neutrophil phagocytosis test.

(2) To deepen the understanding of the body's innate immune mechanism through this experiment.

[Experimental Materials and Equipment]

(1) Human venous blood (anticoagulated by sodium citrate) and *Staphylococcus albus*.

(2) Broth medium, alkaline methylene blue solution, methanol, pH 7.2-7.4 PBS, etc.

(3) Centrifuge, 15 ml centrifuge tubes, droppers, etc.

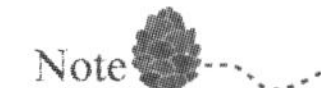

[Experimental Contents]

1. Principle

Neutrophils are the most abundant immune cells in the peripheral blood and immune system. Due to their functions of amoeboid movement and phagocytosis, they play important roles in resisting diseases and protecting the body. Neutrophils can adhere to the surface of endothelial in the large veins, can be quickly mobilized during infection and stress, and have many biological functions, such as chemotaxis, phagocytosis and antimicrobial activity. Neutrophils are very important weapons of our innate immune system. The phagocytic function of neutrophils can be judged by measuring the phagocytic percentage and phagocytic index of neutrophils.

2. Method

(1) Preparation of bacterial solution: inoculate *Staphylococcus albus* in broth medium and incubate at 37 ℃ for 12 h. Kill the bacteria by heating them in a water bath at 100 ℃ for 10 min, then diluted them with PBS to 6×10^{8}/ml.

(2) Mix 50 μl anticoagulant blood with 50 μl diluted bacterial solution, incubate at 37 ℃ water bath for 30 min, and shake one time during the incubation.

(3) Blow the mixed blood gently, take one drop onto the slide and push it into a smear.

(4) After air-drying, fix with methanol for 4-5 min, stain with alkaline methylene blue solution for 2-3 min, and observe under an oil immersion lens.

(5) Count 100 neutrophils randomly and record the number of phagocytic and non-phagocytic neutrophils. For phagocytic neutrophils, the number of phagocytic bacteria should also be recorded.

3. Results

(1) The phagocytic percentage is the percentage of neutrophils that phagocytic neutrophils. The normal percentage is 60%-70%.

(2) Phagocytic index: the total number of bacteria phagocytized by 100 neutrophils devided by 100 to get the average number of phagocytic bacteria per neutrophil.

[Notes]

(1) EDTA affects phagocytic function, and heparin may affect the effect of certain staining methods, such as Wright's staining, so sodium citrate anticoagulants may be appropriate.

(2) Blood smears should not be too thick otherwise it is not easy to observe the results.

(3) Because of the age and health conditions of different specimens are different, their phagocytic capacity is different.

(4) The phagocytic percentage and phagocytic index of the same person to different pathogens are different.

[Experimental Report]

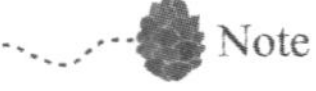

(1) Describe the principle and method of the neutrophil phagocytosis test.

(2) Report and discuss the patient's health status as reflected in the results of the experiment.

[Questions]

The neutrophil is the largest number of white blood cells, so why is the body designed this way?

(Xingyuan Pan, Liangliang Cai)

Experiment 5 Double Immunodiffusion Test

[Experimental Objectives]

(1) To master the principle and method of the double immunodiffusion test.

(2) Through this classic serological experiment, to deepen the understanding of the principles and characteristics of antigen-antibody binding.

[Experimental Materials and Equipment]

(1) Serum of healthy volunteers, pH 7.2-7.4 PBS, rabbit anti-human IgG antiserum, etc.

(2) Incubator, microwave oven, Pasteur pipettes, conical flasks, wet boxes, slides, etc.

[Experimental Contents]

1. Principle

The double immunodiffusion test uses agar gel as the medium. In this reaction, the antigen and the corresponding antibody meet in two places to form antigen-antibody complex. The precipitation line will occur when the ratio is appropriate.

According to the presence, shape and position of the precipitation line, we can analyze the presence or absence of antigen or antibody, the relative concentration and relative molecular weight of antigen and antibody, the nature of the antigen, the purity of the antigen or antibody, etc. This test also allows for a rough semi-quantification of antibody titers.

2. Method

(1) Prepare 1%-1.5% agar solution with PBS in a conical flask and heat in a microwave oven to promote dissolution. When the agar solution is cooled to 50-60 ℃, it is absorbed by a Pasteur pipette and dropped in the middle of the slide until the gel thickness reaches about 2 mm, allowing the sample volume of antigen/antibody to reach 10 μl.

(2) Let it cool at room temperature for a few minutes. When fully solidified, use a dropper to drill plum blossom holes 5-8 mm apart (Fig. 1-5-1). After drilling, the slide is fired several times on the alcohol lamp to seal the hole bottom and prevent the added antigen/antibody solution from leaking and affecting the experimental results.

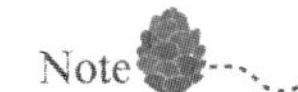

(3) Add 10 μl rabbit anti-human IgG antiserum (antibody) to the center hole and 10 μl diluted serum (antigen) of healthy volunteers to the surrounding five holes, leaving one hole

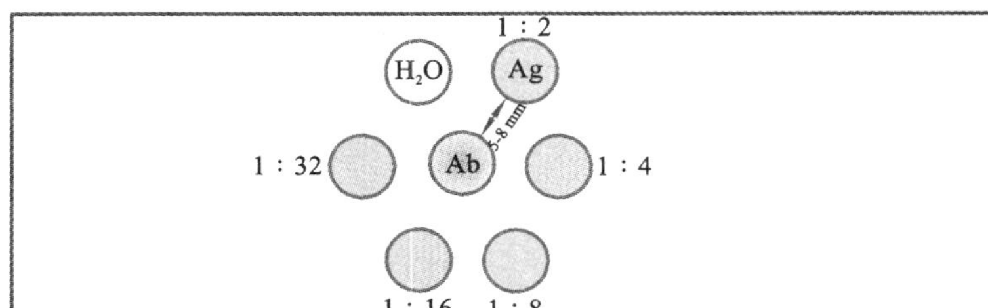

Fig. 1-5-1 Plum blossom holes of the double immunodiffusion test

with water as a negative control.

(4)Place the slide in a wet box lined with moisture-absorbing paper and incubate overnight at 37 ℃ in the incubator. You'll see the results the next day.

[Notes]

(1)Pour the agar solution fast to ensure that the agar gel is well-distributed.

(2)Don't overheat, otherwise the agar gel will melt.

[Experimental Report]

(1)Describe the principle and method of the double immunodiffusion test.

(2)Draw your results, including the position, shape and thickness of the precipitation line.

(3) Estimate the relative concentration and relative molecular weights of antigens and antibodies.

[Questions]

(1) What are the advantages of a double immunodiffusion test over a single immunodiffusion test?

(2)How to speed up the double immunodiffusion test?

(Xingyuan Pan, Zhijie Lin)

Experiment 6 Detect the HLA-A* 02 Gene by PCR-SSP

[Experimental Objectives]

(1)To master the principle and method of detecting the HLA-A* 02 gene by PCR-SSP.

(2)To deepen the understanding of HLA polymorphism through experiment results.

[Experimental Materials and Equipment]

Note

(1)Primers (Tab. 1-6-1).

Tab. 1-6-1 The primer sequences and product length

Primers	Sequences	Product length
HLA-A* 02 5′-primer	5′-TCCTCGTCCCCAGGCTCT-3′	813 bp
HLA-A* 02 3′-primer	5′-GTGGCCCCTGGTACCCGT-3′	
Control 5′-primer	5′-ATGATGTTGACCTTTCCAGGG-3′	256 bp
Control 3′-primer	5′-ATTCTGTAACTTTTCATCAGTTGC-3′	

(2) Peripheral blood of healthy volunteer, blood advanced direct PCR kit, TAE buffer, GoldView Ⅱ nuclear staining dye (Solarbio), DNA molecular weight marker, etc.

(3) PCR amplifier, centrifuge, JY-SPDT horizontal eletrophoresis tank, pipettes, disposable PE gloves, etc.

[Experimental Contents]

1. Principle

The HLA system is the most polymorphic system in the human body, which influences the susceptibility to human disease and the result of organ transplantation. With the development of technology, more and more HLA types have been identified, and the traditional serological detection technology can not meet clinical needs. At present, PCR is mainly used in HLA typing.

HLA-A* 02 is one of the hotspots in cancer research and organ transplantation because of its high proportion in the Han population. This experiment aims to detect the proportion of HLA-A* 02 alleles in the population by the basic low-resolution PCR-SSP typing technique. More precise PCR typing is often required in clinical and scientific research.

2. Method

(1) PCR reaction system (25 μl): as shown in Tab. 1-6-2.

Tab. 1-6-2 PCR reaction system

Components	Volume/μl
Blood sample (peripheral blood)	3
5′-primer (10 μmol/L)	1
3′-primer (10 μmol/L)	1
2×PCR buffer	12.5
DNA polymerase	0.5
Water	7

(2) PCR conditions: 95 ℃ pre-denature for 5 min, followed by 95 ℃ denature for 30 s, 60 ℃ anneal for 30 s, and 72 ℃ extension for 90 s, 30 cycles.

(3) Detection of PCR products: prepare a 2% agarose gel containing 0.02% GoldView Ⅱ nuclear staining dye with 1×TAE buffer. Centrifuge the PCR products at 1000*g* for 2 min to precipitate blood cell fragments. 15 μl of the supernatant was spotted and electrophoresed at 5 V/cm for 25 min.

[Notes]

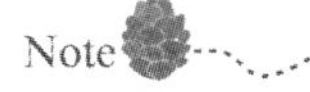

(1) Avoid taking blood clots when taking blood samples.

(2)This experiment involves human blood components, so we need to follow the pollutant treatment procedures strictly.

[Experimental Report]

(1)Describe the principle and method of detecting the HLA-A* 02 gene by PCR-SSP.

(2)Post your electrophoretogram to see if the volunteer is HLA-A* 02 gene positive.

[Questions]

(1)What does HLA data mean for national security?

(2)Is there any possibility of a false negative in this test? Each group is required to find a suitable positive control.

(3)Calculate the proportion of HLA-A* 02 alleles in the population of the YangZhou area according to the data of your class.

(Xingyuan Pan, Liangliang Cai)

Experiment 7 Purify IgG Antibody by SPA Affinity Chromatography

[Experimental Objectives]

(1)To master the principle and method of SPA affinity chromatography.

(2)To purify high-purity IgG antibodies from human serum.

[Experimental Materials and Equipment]

(1)SPA-sepharose 4B, serum of healthy volunteer, physiological saline, pH 3.2 glycine-HCl buffer, 0.1 mol/L $NaHCO_3$ solution, 7 mol/L urea solution, PBS, etc.

(2) 2 cm × 10 cm chromatographic column, 751 spectrophotometer, peristaltic pump, universal power supply, Mini-PROTEAN® tetra cell, etc.

[Experimental Contents]

1. Principle

Affinity chromatography is a kind of chromatography system that is based on the principle of reversible binding between biopolymers and ligands. Immunoaffinity chromatography is a method that utilizes the high specific affinity between antigens and antibodies for separation; it often requires only one step to separate a target protein from a complex protein mixture, and the product is often highly pure.

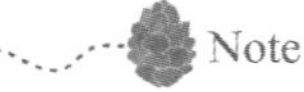
Note

Sepharose 4B is an agarose gel filter media often used in affinity chromatography. Its separation range is 60000-2000000 Da, and the working pH is 4-9. Sepharose 4B is suitable for the separation and purification of many kinds of biomacromolecules. SPA is a cell wall protein isolated from *Staphylococcus aureus*. It binds to mammalian IgG mainly through Fc fragments. It does not affect the binding of Fab fragments and antigens and shows different binding abilities with different IgG subclasses. Different IgG subclasses bound to the column can be eluted by changing pH and ionic strength. Sepharose 4B conjugated with SPA can directly purify IgG antibodies in human serum or mouse ascites and obtain IgG with high purity.

2. Method

(1) Column loading: pour full-swelled SPA-sepharose 4B into a 2 cm × 10 cm chromatographic column. After settling naturally, it is fully balanced with more than 10 times the column volume of physiological saline.

(2) Sample adding: dilute the serum 5 times with physiological saline, and then add the diluted serum to a column at a ratio of 25-30 mg IgG/g wet gel. After 15 min incubation at room temperature, elute the column with physiological saline at a flow rate of 20 ml/h. IgG was adsorbed by SPA on the chromatographic column, and other proteins flowed out with the eluent until the OD_{280} of the eluent was less than 0.02.

(3) Elution: elute the column with pH 3.2 glycine-HCl buffer. Quickly neutralize the eluted protein solution to pH 7 by 0.1 mol/l $NaHCO_3$ solution, the protein is the purified IgG.

(4) Purity identification: subject 10 μl purified IgG for SDS-PAGE electrophoresis, using the diluted serum as a control to check the purification.

(5) Regeneration: wash the used chromatographic column with 10 times column volume of 7 mol/L urea solution, then wash with 10 times column volume of physiological saline, and finally equilibrated with PBS.

[Notes]

(1) SPA-sepharose 4B is expensive. If necessary, the serum sample may be centrifuged to remove impurities and then filtered with a 0.22 μm filter to protect the chromatographic column.

(2) The gel should be fully suspended before column loading, and column loading should be done at one time so as to avoid the formation of abruption, which will affect the purification effect.

(3) After regeneration, add NaN_3 solution (with a final concentration of 0.02%) to the gel. Store the gel at 4 ℃, so that it can be repeatedly used 10-20 times.

(4) This experiment involves human blood components, so we need to follow the pollutant treatment procedures strictly.

[Experimental Report]

(1) Describe the principle and method of SPA affinity chromatography.

(2) Post your electrophoretogram to check how well your purification works.

[Questions]

What is the role of SPA affinity chromatography in the development of vaccines?

(Xingyuan Pan, Liangliang Cai)

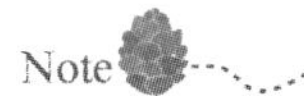

Experiment 8　Detection of Total IgE in Human Serum

[Experimental Objectives]

To master the principle and method of quantitative detection of total IgE in serum by ELISA.

[Experimental Materials and Equipment]

(1) Negative and positive control, sample diluent, enzyme conjugate, standards (10 IU/ml、50 IU/ml, 100 IU/ml, 200 IU/ml, 400 IU/ml), 30 × wash solution, color-substrate solution (A/B), stop solution (2 mol/L H_2SO_4 solution), etc.

(2) Pre-coated reaction plate, microplate reader, shaker, absorbent paper, etc.

[Experimental Contents]

1. Principle

The concentration of IgE in serum is extremely low, accounting for about 0.02% of immunoglobulin. IgE mainly exists in the skin and mucosa. It is generally believed that IgE is produced by plasma cells at the base of the nasopharynx, tonsil, bronchus and gastrointestinal mucosa and can bind to mast cells and basophilic granulocytes in the blood. When the allergen interacts with IgE bound to the cell, it causes the cell to degranulate and release histamine, which causes allergic reactions, such as serum sickness and seasonal allergic rhinitis. Increased IgE is commonly seen in allergic asthma, parasitic infections, drug allergy, IgE myeloma, liver disease, systemic lupus erythematosus, rheumatoid arthritis and other diseases. The decrease is commonly seen in ataxia telangiectasia, agammaglobulinemia, non-IgE myeloma, chronic lymphatic leukemia, immune deficiency, etc.

Double-antibody sandwich ELISA method is used in this experiment. The biotinylated anti-human IgE monoclonal antibody A is pre-coated on the reaction plate by reacting with avidin to maximize the immunological activity of antibody A. The total IgE level in human serum can be quantitatively detected by HRP-labeled anti-human IgE monoclonal antibody B. After adding substrate TMB for color development, the OD_{450} values of each hole are proportional to IgE content.

2. Method

(1) Sample adding: add 80 μl sample diluent into each reaction well, then add 20 μl standard products with different concentrations or samples to be tested. Set one well negative control (100 μl, not diluted), one well positive control (100 μl, not diluted), and one well blank control (100 μl sample diluent).

(2) Incubate at 37 ℃ for 60 min. Remove the liquid, wash the plate with the wash solution for 3 times, and pat it to dry on the absorbent paper.

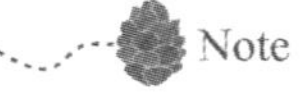
Note

(3) Enzyme conjugate adding: 2 drops (or 100 μl) per well, mix and incubate at 37 ℃ for 30

min. Wash 3 times as in step (2)and pat it to dry on the absorbent paper.

(4)Color development: add 1 drop (or 50 μl) of color-substrate solution A and B to each well, mix with a shaker and incubate at 37 ℃ for 10 min.

(5)Absorbance measurement: add 1 drop (or 50 μl) of stop solution to each well, mix and measure the OD value of each well at 450 nm.

(6)The OD value of 5 standard products is taken as the vertical coordinate, and the concentration (10 IU/ml, 50 IU/ml, 100 IU/ml, 200 IU/ml, 400 IU/ml) is taken as the horizontal coordinate to draw the standard curve. The concentration corresponding to the OD value of the sample to be tested on the standard curve is the actual content of IgE in the sample.

3. Reference value

The total IgE content in normal people's peripheral blood serum measured by this method, ranges from 20 IU/ml to 200 IU/ml.

[Notes]

(1)Before adding the reagents, the bottle should be turned over several times to mixed well, and the bottle body should be kept vertical when adding the reagents.

(2)When washing the plate, each well must be fully filled to prevent the free enzymes in the well can not be washed away.

(3)You are advised to use double wells for standard products and take the average OD value.

(4)When the total IgE content is greater than 400 IU/ml, it is non-linear, and appropriate dilution of the sample is required to obtain an accurate value.

(5)This experiment involves human blood components, so we need to follow the pollutant treatment procedures strictly.

[Experimental Report]

(1)Describe the principle and method of quantitative detection of total IgE in serum by ELISA.

(2)According to your standard curve, calculate the IgE content of the sample.

[Questions]

Some people have much higher serum IgE levels than normal. Do you know of any possible immunological mechanisms?

(Xingyuan Pan, Zhijie Lin)

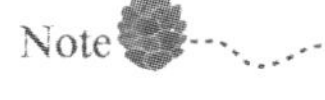

Chapter 2 Basic Experiments of Pathogenic Biology

Experiment 1 Physiology of Bacteria

[Experimental Objectives]

(1) To master the inoculation methods of bacteria in different culture media.

(2) To be familiar with the preparation methods of common bacterial culture media and the growth phenomenon of bacteria in different culture media.

(3) To understand the commonly used biochemical reactions of bacteria and their significance in the process of bacterial identification.

[Experimental Materials and Equipment]

(1) Bacterial media of plates, slants, solids, semi-solids and liquids.

(2) Bacterial agar slant cultures.

(3) Glucose fermentation tubes, lactose fermentation tubes, peptone water medium, lead acetate medium, urea medium, plain agar plate medium, etc.

(4) Indole reagent (Kovac's reagent), methyl red reagent and VP reagent.

(5) Sterile cotton swabs, inoculation loop, inoculation needle, physiological saline, alcohol lamp, constant temperature incubator, etc.

[Experimental Contents]

1. Preparation of bacterial medium

(1) Broth/liquid medium: it can be used for general bacterial culture or bacterial enrichment culture and can also be used to prepare carbohydrate fermentation tube and agar medium.

①Add 3-5 g of yeast extract, 10 g of peptone and 5 g of sodium chloride into 900 ml of distilled water and stir to dissolve.

②Adjust the pH to 7.4-7.6, and then set the volume to 1000 ml.

③Dispense into appropriate containers, autoclave at 121 ℃ and 103 kPa for 20 min, carry out sterility test and then put in a 4 ℃ refrigerator for spare.

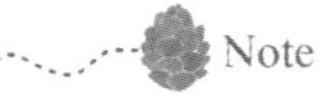

(2) Plain agar medium: it can be used for general bacterial isolation culture and can also be used as a sugar-free medium.

①Take 4.5 g of agar powder into 1000 ml of broth medium.

②Adjust the pH to 7.6, and autoclave at 121 ℃ and 103 kPa for 20 min.

③After the agar cooled down to 50-60 ℃, if it was dispensed into sterile test tubes and placed at an angle, it was prepared as agar slant medium after solidification; if it was poured into sterile Petri dishes, it was prepared as agar plate medium after solidification. After the sterility test, put it in a 4 ℃ refrigerator for spare.

Note: the agar plate medium should be stored in an inverted position, which is easy to pick up and put down. This avoids the evaporation of water and maintains sterility.

(3) Semi-solid agar medium: it can be used to preserve bacterial strains or transport bacteria over short distance and to detect the power of bacteria.

①Dissolve 0.25-0.5 g of agar powder in 100 ml of broth medium.

②Autoclave at 121 ℃ and 103 kPa for 20 min.

③Dispense the agar into test tubes before it solidifies, and place them upright. When the agar solidifies, it will become a semi-solid agar medium. After the sterility test, place it in a 4 ℃ refrigerator for storage.

(4) Blood agar medium: it is used for the cultivation and isolation of pathogenic bacteria with high nutritional requirements.

①100 ml of autoclaved plain agar medium (pH 7.6) was cooled to 50-55 ℃, and 8-10 ml of aseptic defibrinated sheep or rabbit blood (pre-warmed for 30 min in the 37 ℃ incubator before use) was added by aseptic technique. Gently shake (to prevent the production of air bubbles) and pour them into sterilized Petri dishes or test tubes to prepare blood agar plates or blood agar slant medium.

②After the solidification of the medium, randomly select some media to conduct aseptic incubation at 37 ℃ for 18-24 h; if there is no bacteria growth on the medium, that is, the remaining media can be used or stored in a 4 ℃ refrigerator standby.

2. Inoculation methods for bacteria

Bacteria are widely distributed in nature and the human body, and there are many kinds of bacteria. When testing whether a certain pathogenic bacterium is present in various specimens in the clinic, it is necessary to separate different bacteria to obtain a certain pathogenic bacterium, and this process is called the isolation and cultivation of bacteria.

(1) The plate zoning demarcation method: this method is mainly used for the isolation and purification of specimens containing more bacteria, such as feces, pus and other specimens.

①Hold the inoculation loop with the right hand (like holding a pencil/brush), cauterize the inoculation loop and the metal rod with the outer flame of the alcohol lamp, and when it cools down (method of determining whether the inoculation loop has cooled down: wait for 3-5 s, then you can touch the edge of the plate medium in the blank space with the inoculation loop, and if the agar does not dissolve, it indicates that the inoculation loop has cooled down), use the inoculation loop to touch the specimen to be tested gently.

②Hold up the agar plate with your left hand and open it near the flame of the alcohol lamp; hold the inoculation loop with bacteria with your right hand and make the inoculation loop surface and the surface of the agar plate at an angle of 30°-40°; draw a line back and forth on the agar plate densely, with no crossings between the line and the line. When drawing the line, make a brisk sliding motion on the surface of the plate with finger force, and the inoculation loop should not be embedded in the medium.

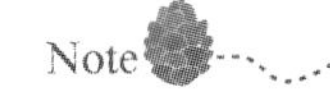

③Cauterize the inoculation loop to kill the bacteria left on it, and leave it to be cooled down; for the second zone, the inoculation loop should be contacted with the first zone 1-2 times, and the line should be drawn continuously and then individually. The area of the second zone of the line should account for 1/5-1/4 of the total area of the plate. After the second zone is finished, sterilize the inoculation loop by flame, and then draw the line in the third and the fourth zones in the same way.

④After the delineation is completed, return the inoculation loop to its original place after sterilization and cover the plate with a lid. After labeling, invert the plate (to prevent condensation water from dripping down from the plate cover during the incubation process and disperse the colonies) and put it into the incubator at 37 ℃ for incubation.

⑤Remove the plate after 18-24 h of incubation and observe the various colonies formed on the surface of the agar plate, paying attention to their size, shape, edge, transparency, color and other traits.

The diagram of the plate zoning demarcation method is shown in Fig. 2-1-1.

(2) The plate continuous demarcation method: this method is mainly used for specimens containing less bacteria, such as throat swab specimens and cerebrospinal fluid specimens.

①Hold the inoculation loop with the right hand (like holding a pencil/brush), cauterize the inoculation loop and the metal rod with the outer flame of the alcohol lamp, leave it to cool down (wait for 3-5 s), and gently touch the specimen to be tested with the inoculation loop.

②Hold up the agar plate with the left hand and open it near the flame of the alcohol lamp. Apply the specimen to 1/5 of the medium, then use the inoculation loop or directly use a throat swab to draw a continuous line on the plate and gradually move it downward until it fills the surface of the plate.

The diagram of the plate continuous demarcation method is shown in Fig. 2-1-2.

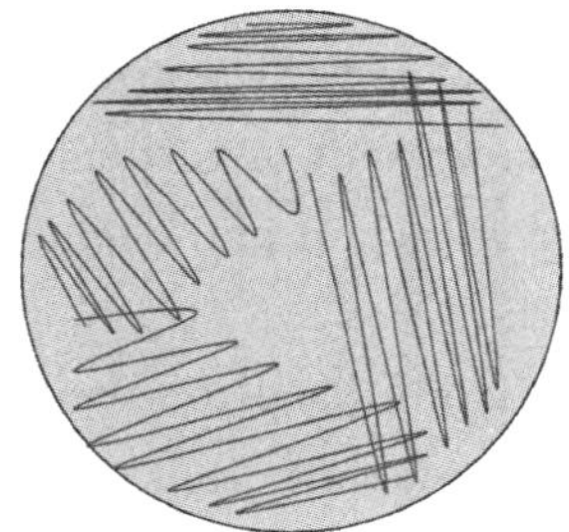

Fig. 2-1-1 The diagram of the plate zoning demarcation method

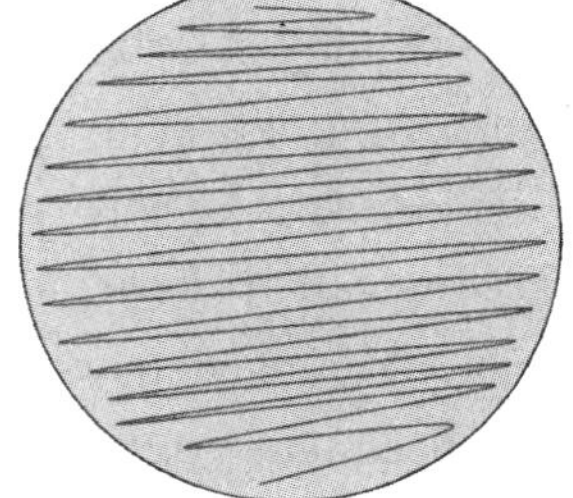

Fig. 2-1-2 The diagram of the plate continuous demarcation method

(3) The slant medium inoculation method: this method is mainly used for pure cultivation and preservation of strains.

①The left thumb and forefinger, middle finger and ring finger hold the strain tube and the medium tube to be inoculated, respectively, with the strain tube located on the left side and the medium tube located on the right side. The medium should slant up (do not become horizontal) to avoid the bottom of the tube's condensate infiltrating the surface of the medium or even wetting the rubber stopper.

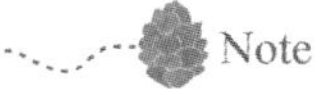

Note

②Use the right thumb and forefinger to loosen the plugs of the two test tubes, so that they are easy to be pulled out during inoculation.

③Hold the inoculation loop with the right hand, and put the part of the inoculation rod that is to be inserted into the test tube through the flame of the alcohol lamp 2-3 times quickly to kill the stray bacteria of the surface. Do not touch the sterilized inoculation loop again.

④Use the palm of the right hand and the little finger, little finger and ring finger to pull and hold the rubber plug of the two test tubes, respectively, and let the mouths of the two test tubes quickly through the flame of the alcohol lamp several times for sterilization.

⑤Extend the inoculation loop into the strain tube and slowly exit after picking a little bit of the bacteria moss from the slant. And then extend it into the tube of medium to be inoculated; gently draw a straight line from the bottom of the slant to the top, and then dram an upward meandering line from the bottom. Be careful not to scratch the surface of the medium during the operation, and do not touch the inner wall of the test tube when the inoculation loop is in and out of it.

⑥After inoculation, the inoculation loop will be sterilized and returned to its original place. The mouths of the two test tubes will be quickly passed through the flame of the alcohol lamp 2-3 times. Stuff the rubber stopper back, and then put the medium tube in a 37 ℃ incubator to culture for 18-24 h to observe the growth of bacteria.

(4) The semi-solid medium inoculation method (puncture inoculation method): this method is mainly used for kinetic testing and strain preservation.

①Hold the strain tube and the semi-solid agar medium tube with the left hand in the same way as the slant medium inoculation method.

②Hold the inoculation needle with the right hand, and after sterilization and cooling, insert it into the strain tube to pick up a small amount of bacteria moss. Then, withdraw from the strain tube and vertically pierce into the center of the semi-solid agar medium until close to the bottom of the tube (but do not touch) and then exit along the original path.

③After inoculation, the inoculation loop will be sterilized and returned to its original place. After plugging the rubber stopper, put the semi-solid agar medium tube in a 37 ℃ incubator for 18-24 h to observe the growth of bacterial.

(5) The liquid medium inoculation method: this method is mainly used for pure cultivation and biochemical tests.

①Hold the strain tube and the liquid medium tube with the left hand in the same way as the slant medium inoculation method.

②Hold the inoculation loop with the right hand, and after sterilization and cooling, insert it into the strain tube to pick up a small amount of bacteria moss. Then, withdraw from the strain tube and insert it into the liquid medium tube. Gently grind on the wall of the tube close to the liquid surface, dip a little liquid medium and mix it to make the bacteria mixed in the liquid medium.

③After inoculation, the inoculation loop will be sterilized and returned to its original place. After plugging the rubber stopper, put the liquid medium tube in a 37 ℃ incubator for 18-24 h to observe the growth of bacterial.

3. Observation of bacterial culture characters

(1) Characteristics of bacterial culture on a solid medium.

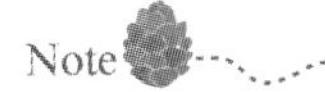

On a solid medium, a bacterial group formed after the division and reproduction of a bacterium is called a colony. The colonies fuse to form a moss. The colonies of different bacteria have their characteristics, and the following points should be noted when observing.

①Size: expressed by the diameter (mm), about 1 mm is a small colony, 2-3 mm is a medium colony and over 3 mm is a large colony.

②Shape: round and irregular shape.

③Edge: neat or untidy edge.

④Surface: raised, depressed, flat, smooth, rough, dry, wet, and other different surfaces.

⑤Transparency: transparent, opaque or translucent.

⑥Color: for bacteria producing fat-soluble pigment, the colony has color, and the medium does not, whereas for bacteria producing water-soluble pigment, both the colony and the surrounding medium show color.

⑦Hemolytic: observe the bacterial hemolysis of red blood cells on the blood plate. There are complete hemolysis, incomplete hemolysis and no hemolysis.

⑧Colony type: according to their characteristics, colonies can be divided into smooth colonies (S-type), rough colonies (R-type) and mucoid colonies (M-type). The S-type colonies are round, have a smooth surface, are wet, and have neat and transparent edges, while the R-type colonies are opposite, and the M-type colonies have a moist and sticky surface.

(2) Characteristics of bacterial culture in the semi-solid medium.

The semi-solid medium can be used to observe whether the bacteria are dynamic or not: after puncture culture, the bacteria without power grow along the puncture line, and the medium is clear, which is linear growth; while the bacteria with power grow outwardly along the puncture line, the puncture line becomes blurred, and the medium becomes turbid, which is turbid growth.

(3) Characteristics of bacterial culture in the liquid medium.

①Turbid growth: the medium is uniformly turbid or granular turbid, such as *Staphylococcus and Escherichia coli* (*E. coli*).

②Surface growth: the surface of the medium has a smooth or wrinkled film or stalactite-like sagging, such as *Bacillus subtilis and Mycobacterium tuberculosis*.

③Precipitation growth: the medium is clarified, but there is bacterial precipitation at the bottom of the test tube, such as *Streptococcus*.

4. Observation of biochemical tests

(1) Carbohydrate fermentation test.

①Principle. Different types of bacteria contain enzymes for fermenting different sugars (alcohols and glycosides) and therefore have different metabolizing abilities for various sugars (alcohols and glycosides) and different metabolic products. This test identifies the type of bacteria based on their ability to produce acid or gas after decomposing sugars (alcohols and glycosides) in the medium. A certain amount of indicator and an inverted test tube are added to the medium, and the final concentration of sugar is 0.5%-1%. After inoculation and incubation for a certain period, if the bacteria have an enzyme that decomposes a certain type of sugar, it will decompose the sugar to produce acid which will cause the indicator to change color. If the indicator is methyl red, it turns red; if it is bromocresol purple, it turns yellow. If gas is produced, bubbles are produced in the inverted test tube. Most bacteria can utilize sugars as a carbon and energy source, but they vary greatly in their ability to decompose sugars: some bacteria can decompose certain sugars and produce acid and gas, while others only produce acid

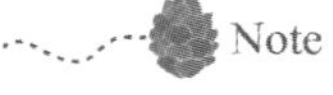

and no gas. For example, *E. coli* can decompose lactose and glucose to produce acid and gas; *Salmonella typhi* (*S. typhi*) can decompose glucose to produce acid but can not produce gas or decompose lactose; *Proteus vulgaris* (*P. valgaris*) can decompose glucose to produce acid and gas but can not decompose lactose.

② Method. Inoculate *S. typhi*, *E. coli* and *P. vulgaris* in two kinds of carbohydrate fermentation tubes respectively, and observe the results after incubation at 37 ℃ for 18-24 h.

③ Results. If the medium does not change color and there are no bubbles in the inverted test tube, it indicates that no acid or gas is produced and the sugar is not decomposed, and the result of the experiment is reported as "−"; if the medium turns red (or yellow) and there are no bubbles in the inverted tube, it indicates that acid is produced, but gas is not produced, and the result of the experiment is reported as "+"; if the medium turns red (or yellow) and there are bubbles in the inverted tube, it indicates that acid and gas are produced, and the result of the experiment is reported as "⊕".

(2) VP test.

① Principle. Some bacteria decompose glucose to produce pyruvic acid; pyruvic acid is further decarboxylated to produce neutral acetyl methyl alcohol; the latter can be oxidized under alkaline conditions to produce diacetyl, and the diacetyl reacts with the guanidinium of arginine in peptone to produce red compounds, which is a positive VP test.

② Methods. *E. coli* and *S. typhi* were inoculated in peptone water medium respectively, and incubated at 37 ℃ for 18-24 h. VP reagent was added to the culture solution respectively and then left to observe after mixing.

③ Results. If the reagent turns red, it is a positive result; if it turns yellow or a copper-like color, it is a negative result.

(3) Methyl red test.

① Principle. Some bacteria decompose glucose to produce pyruvic acid; pyruvic acid is further decomposed into formic acid, acetic acid, lactic acid, etc., so that the pH of the medium is less than 4.5, which will make the methyl red indicator red; if pyruvic acid is further decarboxylated to produce neutral acetyl methyl alcohol, so that the pH of the medium is greater than 5.4, which will make the methyl red indicator orange.

② Method. Inoculate *E. coli* and *S. typhi* in peptone water medium respectively, and incubate at 37 ℃ for 18-24 h. Add a few drops of methyl red indicator and observe the color of the culture solution.

③ Results. If the culture solution is red, it is positive; if the culture solution is orange-red, it is weakly positive; if the culture solution is orange-yellow, it is negative. If the result is negative, the bacteria should be cultured for 4-5 d and then tested again.

(4) Indole test.

① Principle. Some bacteria have tryptophanase which can decompose tryptophan in peptone to form indole. Indole is colorless and not easy to be observed directly, but after adding Kovac's reagent, the *p*-dimethylaminobenzaldehyde in the reagent reacts with indole to form a red rose indole which is easy to be observed.

② Method. Inoculate *E. coli* and *S. typhi* in peptone water medium and incubate at 37 ℃ for 18-24 h. Add a few drops of Kovac's reagent in each tube to make a thin layer on the surface of the liquid, and then gently shake the tube to observe the color.

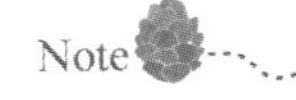

③Results. The surface reagent showing red is a positive result, while showing yellow is a negative result.

(5) Hydrogen sulfide test.

①Principle. Some bacteria can decompose the sulfur-containing amino acids in the medium to produce hydrogen sulfide. When hydrogen sulfide meets ferrous ions (e. g. ferrous sulfate) or lead ions (e. g. lead acetate), a black-brown ferrous sulfide or lead sulfide precipitate is formed, and the more black-brown precipitate there is, the more hydrogen sulfide is generated. The medium used in hydrogen sulfide test contains sodium thiosulfate which is a reducing agent that can maintain the reducing environment so that the formation of hydrogen sulfide is no longer oxidized.

②Method. Inoculate *E. coli* and *P. vulgaris* in lead acetate medium by puncture against the inner wall of the test tube respectively, and observe the color at the puncture line after incubation at 37 ℃ for 18-24 h.

③Results. Positive results were obtained if the puncture line was black-brown, and negative results were obtained if there was no black-brown.

(6) Urease test.

①Principle. Bacteria with urease can decompose urea to produce ammonia, which forms ammonium carbonate in the medium. This makes the medium alkaline, and the phenol red indicator turns red in this environment.

②Method. *E. coli* and *P. vulgaris* were inoculated in urea medium, and cultured at 37 ℃ for 18-24 h to observe the medium's color.

③Results. The medium turns to red is a positive result and yellow for a negative result.

(7) Citrate test.

①Principle. Some bacteria utilize citrate as the only carbon source, they can decompose citrate to produce carbonate and decompose ammonium salts in the medium to produce ammonia, which increases the medium's alkalinity and changes the bromothymol blue indicator from light green to dark blue.

②Method. *E. coli* and *Enterobacter aerogenes* (*E. aerogenes*) were inoculated on sodium citrate agar slant, and cultured at 37 ℃ for 24-48 h to observe the medium's color.

③Results. If the medium changes to dark blue, the result is positive; if the medium still does not change color after 7 d of culturation, a negative result can be issued.

(8) Digital classification and identification system.

①Principle. The database consists of a number of bacterial entries, each representing a bacterial species or a bacterial biotype. Coding is the conversion of bacterial biochemical reaction results into mathematical patterns, which can then be converted into corresponding bacterial names by consulting a codebook or computerized analysis system. The code can be searched in the codebook to find digital information (code checking), such as the name of the bacterium, evaluation of the identification results, biochemical results, percentage of positives, additional tests that must be added, and points to note. If a code corresponds to only one type of bacteria, the likelihood (ID%) of being that type of bacteria is 99.99%, regardless of the odds. If a code corresponds to two or more species of bacteria, calculate the ID% of each species of bacteria. If ID% ≥ 99%, the probability of being that species is very high; if 90% ≤ ID% < 99%, the probability of being that species is high; if 80% ≤ ID% < 90%, the probability of being that

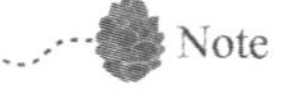
Note

species is also high, but additional tests are needed to confirm further; if ID% < 80%, it is generally impossible to accurately differentiate between species, and more than one additional test must be added before accurate results can be obtained, and this is the explanation.

②Composition. This system is a complete microbial identification system consisting of identification cards, additive reagents (some tests require the addition of reagents after incubation to show a color change, either in the form of a kit or as a single reagent) and search tools (automatically processed and reported by computer). Identification cards contain commonly used biochemical reactions, such as fermentation tests, assimilation tests, assimilation or fermentation inhibition tests, enzyme tests, and others.

(9) Automatic bacterial identification system.

The automatic bacterial identification system is a system that combines photovoltaic technology, computer technology and digital identification of bacteria. The system makes the traditional bacterial test method to be significantly improved, and provides more informative test data for the clinic than the traditional manual test. Commonly used automatic bacterial identification systems include MicroScan, Vitek-AMS and PHOENIX™ 100. Now take MicroScan automatic bacterial identification system as an example and briefly describe it.

①Principle. Photoelectric colorimetry is used to determine the different colors produced by the pH change caused by the decomposition of the substrate by the bacteria, and at the same time, using the 8-bit digital bacterial identification principle, the final identification results are obtained through matrix analysis. Part of the identification system can increase the identification speed by 4-8 times due to the fluorescence technology. MicroScan is one of the commonly used identification systems at present, which can identify nearly 500 kinds of bacteria and has a good computer interface, providing an accurate and convenient test method for the diagnosis and treatment of infectious diseases. It can also use the software statistical function to count the detection rate of bacterial strains in different specimens, the monthly trend report of isolates in the ward, the isolation rate of different bacterial strains, etc.

② Method. The specimens to be examined were zoned, delineated, and inoculated in appropriate media for microscopic examination by Gram staining. Use the quantitative bacterial needle to collect 1-3 colonies placed in the strain dilution solution. Pour the diluted bacterial suspension into the injection tank, install the 96-well inoculation plate with a vacuum inoculator, and suck the bacterial suspension from the injection tank. Add the bacterial solution into the corresponding reaction plate and place the reaction plate into the reaction plate position in the host. The instrument can automatically keep warm, add reagents, and read and process the results.

③Results. The system can print the report automatically. After activating the prompting system, when abnormal situations occur in the results, important tips will appear in the report for clinicians and examiners to refer to.

[Experimental Report]

(1) Draw the results of the cultivation of bacteria in plate, slant, semi-solid and liquid media.

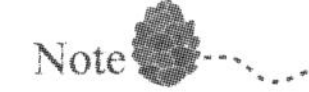

Note

(2) Write the principles of biochemical metabolism and draw the results of biochemical metabolism of different bacteria.

[Questions]

(1)What should be paid attention to when preparing different cultural media? How to isolate suspected pathogenic bacterium from a specimen containing a large number of stray bacteria?

(2)When inoculating by different methods, how can we better ensure that the bacterial strains are not contaminated? Why should plates be inverted after inoculation?

(3)What biochemical tests are commonly used to identify *E. coli* and *E. aerogenes*?

(4)Can all bacteria be successfully cultured? Can all pathogenic bacteria be isolated and cultured?

(Guimei Kong, Chengfeng Gao)

Experiment 2 The Distribution of Bacteria and the Effect of External Factors on Bacteria

[Experimental Objectives]

(1)To master the common methods of disinfection and sterilization.

(2)To master the paper-disc agar-diffusion method of detecting bacterial susceptibility to drugs.

(3)To master the detection methods of minimum inhibitory concentration and minimum bactericidal concentration of drugs.

(4) To understand the distribution of bacteria and their examination methods and to establish the concept of aseptic operation.

[Experimental Materials]

(1)LB agar plate, LB liquid medium and gentamicin.

(2)*Staphylococcus aureus and Salmonella*.

(3) Alcohol lamp, inoculation loop, tweezer, susceptibility paper, sterile black paper, UV lamp, etc.

[Experimental Contents]

1. Bacterial examination of air and finger skin

(1)Principle. A large number of microbes are parasitized in the air and on the human body surface. These microbes grow to colonies after being cultured, but there are very few colonies in the disinfected parts.

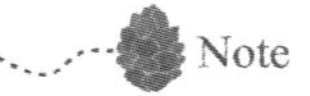
Note

(2)Method.

①Five sterile LB agar plates are placed in the four corners and the middle of a 10 m^2 room.

Open the lid for 30 min, and observe the growth of bacteria after incubation at 37 ℃ for 24 h.

②Take two sterile LB agar plates. Smear the unsterilized finger on the surface of one of the LB agar plates. Disinfect the finger with 2% iodine tincture, remove the iodine tincture with 75% alcohol, and smear the disinfected finger on the surface of the other LB agar plate. Observe the results after incubation at 37 ℃ for 24 h.

(3) Results. Several colonies with different sizes, shapes, and pigments are present on the surface of the media. Pay attention to distinguish the growth of bacteria before and after disinfection.

2. Ultraviolet sterilization test

(1) Principle. All ultraviolet rays with wavelength between 210 nm and 310 nm have bactericidal ability, among which the bactericidal ability of 260 nm is the strongest. The bactericidal mechanism of ultraviolet rays is mainly due to the induction of the formation of thymine dimer in bacteria, which inhibits the replication of DNA.

(2) Method.

①The bacterial solution of *Staphylococcus aureus* is dipped with the inoculation loop, and successive lines are drawn on LB agar plates.

②Open the plate. Place the sterile black paper in the middle of the LB agar plate within 1.2 m from the UV lamp for 30 min with an aseptic tweezer. Then, remove the black paper and burn it, cover the plate, and observe the growth of bacteria after incubation at 37 ℃ for 24 h.

(3) Results. There is bacterial growth on the surface of the medium covered with black paper, and there is no bacterial growth on the uncovered surface of the medium, indicating that the bacteria have been killed.

(4) Notes.

①The penetration of ultraviolet rays is not strong, so it is only suitable for air and object surface sterilization in an aseptic room and an operating room.

②The distance between the UV lamp and the irradiated object should not exceed 1.2 m.

3. The susceptibility of bacteria to drugs detected by the paper-disc agar-diffusion method

(1) Principle. The susceptibility paper containing quantitative antimicrobials is adhered to the agar plate that has been inoculated with bacteria. After the drugs contained in the susceptibility paper are dissolved by the water in the agar, a decreasing concentration gradient is formed around the paper. The growth of bacteria is inhibited in the range of bacteriostatic concentration around the paper, thus forming an inhibition zone. The size of the inhibition zone reflects the susceptibility of bacteria to antimicrobial agents.

(2) Method.

①Take two agar plates and label *Staphylococcus aureus* and *Salmonella* on the bottom of the plates respectively.

②The above two kinds of bacterial solution were inoculated on the surface of two agar plates by continuous scribing respectively.

③The susceptibility paper is clamped with a sterile tweezer and attached to the surface of the bacteria-coated agar plate individually.

④After incubating at 37 ℃ for 18-24 h, observe whether there is an inhibition zone around the susceptibility paper, and compare the size of the inhibition zone to judge the susceptibility of bacteria to drugs.

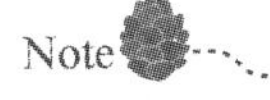

(3)Result. Use a vernier caliper to measure the diameter of the inhibition zone. By looking at Tab. 2-2-1 and Tab. 2-2-2, we can find out whether the bacteria is sensitive (S), medium sensitive (I) or resistant (R) to these drugs.

Tab. 2-2-1 Criteria for judging the diameter of inhibition zone of Enterobacteriaceae

Antibiotics	The amount of medicine per susceptibility paper/μg	Diameter of inhibition zone/mm		
		R	I	S
Ampicillin	10	≤13	14-16	≥17
Streptomycin	10	≤11	12-14	≥15
Gentamicin	10	≤12	13-14	≥15
Tetracycline	30	≤11	12-14	≥15
Kanamycin	30	≤13	14-17	≥18
Chloromycetin	30	≤12	13-17	≥18
Sulfonamides	250/300	≤12	13-16	≥17

Tab. 2-2-2 Criteria for judging the diameter of inhibition zone of Staphylococcaceae

Antibiotics	The amount of medicine per susceptibility paper/μg	Diameter of inhibition zone/mm		
		R	I	S
Oxacillin	30	≤21	—	≥22
Gentamicin	10	≤12	13-14	≥15
Erythrocin	15	≤13	14-22	≥23
Tetracycline	30	≤14	15-18	≥19
Chloromycetin	30	≤12	13-17	≥18
Sulfonamides	250/300	≤12	13-16	≥17

(4)Significance. Drug susceptibility testing is suitable for understanding the sensitivity of pathogenic microorganism to various antibiotics, which can guide the rational selection of antibiotics in the clinic.

(5)Attentions. The criteria for judging the sensitivity of different bacteria to the same kind of antibiotics are different.

4. Detection of minimum inhibitory concentration and minimum bactericidal concentration of drugs

(1)Principle. The drug is diluted twice with the liquid medium, packed in a 1.5 ml EP tube in turn, and then bacteria are inoculated to the EP tube. After incubation for 24 h, the growth of the test bacteria in each EP tube is observed and the minimum inhibitory concentration (MIC) of the drug is obtained.

(2)Method.

①12 sterile EP tubes are labeled from 1 to 12 (the 11th tube is a negative control, and the 12th tube is a positive control).

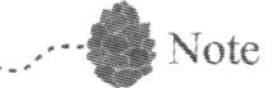
Note

②Add 500 μl LB liquid medium to each EP tube, respectively.

③Add 500 μl gentamicin (the concentration is 800 μg/ml) to the 1st tube, mix and absorb

500 μl into the 2nd tube, and so on until the 11th tube.

④500 μl LB liquid medium and 50 μl *Salmonella* solution with a concentration of 5×10^5 CFU/ml are added to each tube, except the 11th tube.

⑤Culture at 37 ℃ for 18-24 h and observe the results.

(3) Results. In normal tests, the 11th tube should have no bacteria, and the 12th tube should have bacteria. The growth of bacteria in other test tubes should be observed.

Determination of the minimum inhibitory concentration: if the medium in the EP tube is clear and still clear after shaking, it is considered aseptic growth; if it is turbid, it indicates bacterial growth. The lowest drug concentration in the EP tube with no bacterial growth is the minimum inhibitory concentration.

Detection of the minimum bactericidal concentration: when the drug concentration is slightly higher than the MIC, the drug's bacteriostatic effect is irreversible, which is called bactericidal action. Sequentially, 0.1 ml of culture is aspirated from EP tubes with no visible bacterial growth inoculated on agar plates and incubated at 37 ℃ for 18-24 h. The drug concentration at the largest dilution with less than 5 colonies on the plate is taken as the minimum bactericidal concentration.

(4) Attentions.

①The units of minimum inhibitory concentration and minimum bactericidal concentration are shown with μg/ml.

②The minimum inhibitory concentration and minimum bactericidal concentration can be the same or different.

[Experimental Report]

(1) Draw the test results of bacteria in the air and on the finger.

(2) Draw the result of ultraviolet sterilization.

(3) Draw the result of the drug susceptibility testing.

(4) Write results of minimum inhibitory concentration and minimum bactericidal concentration.

[Questions]

(1) What is the main principle of ultraviolet sterilization? What problems should be paid attention to in the course of operation? What is the practical significance?

(2) What is the main principle of the drug susceptibility testing? What problems should be paid attention to in the course of operation? What is the practical significance?

(3) What are the criteria for determining the minimum inhibitory concentration and minimum bactericidal concentration?

(4) What problems do you think may exist in the use of antimicrobials? What is the relationship between these problems and bacterial resistance?

(5) What are the research strategies for bacterial drug resistance and resistance mechanisms?

(Yinyan Yin, Cuicui Liu)

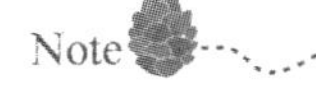

Experiment 3 Examination of Bacterial Morphology and Structure

[Experimental Objectives]

(1)To be familiar with the basic morphology and structural characteristics of bacteria.

(2)To master the principle and method of Gram staining.

[Experimental Materials]

(1)Instructional smears.

Coccus: instructional smears of *Staphylococcus*.

Bacillus: instructional smears of *Escherichia coli*.

Vibrio: instructional smears of *Vibrio cholerae*.

Capsule: instructional smears for showing capsule of *Streptococcus pneumoniae*.

Flagella: instructional smears for showing flagella of *Proteus vulgaris*.

Spore: instructional smears for showing spore of *Clostridium tetani*.

(2)Agar slant cultures (18-24 h) of *Staphylococcus* and *Escherichia coli*.

(3) Gram staining reagents: crystal violet, Lugo's iodine solution, 95% alcohol, and carbolfuchsin dilution.

(4) Inoculation loop, slides, physiological saline, alcohol lamps, light microscope (oil immersion lens), etc.

[Experimental Contents]

1. Observation of bacterial morphology and special structure

(1)The basic morphologies of *Staphylococcus*, *Escherichia coli* and *Vibrio cholerae* were observed under an oil immersion lens, and their shapes, sizes, arrangements and staining properties were compared.

(2)Observation of the special structure of bacteria under an oil immersion lens. The size and color of capsule and its relationship with *Streptococcus pneumoniae*; the shape and position of spore of *Clostridium tetani*; the shape, number and position of flagella of *Proteus vulgaris*.

2. Gram staining

(1)Principle. Gram staining was founded in 1884 by the Danish physician Gram and is one of the most important staining methods in bacteriology. This method can divide bacteria into two categories, i. e. Gram-positive bacteria and Gram-negative bacteria, according to different staining characteristics. It is generally believed that the principle of Gram staining is related to the composition and structure of bacterial cell wall. After primary staining with crystal violet and Lugo's iodine solution, water-insoluble complex of crystal violet and iodine is formed in the bacterial cell wall. The isoelectric point (pI 2-3) of Gram-positive bacteria (such as *Staphylococcus aureus*) is lower than that of Gram-negative bacteria (such as *Escherichia coli*).

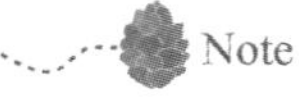
Note

Gram-positive bacteria have more negative charge than Gram-negative bacteria under the same pH condition, that is why Gram-positive bacteria is firmly bound to positively charged crystal violet. The iodine of Lugo's iodine solution combines with crystal violet in the bacteria and then bounds with the magnesium ribonucleic acid salt-polysaccharide complex of Gram-positive bacteria, so that the colored bacteria are not easy to de-colorize. The peptidoglycan network in the cell wall of Gram-positive bacteria has more layers and dense cross-links, while the content of lipids is low. When treated with alcohol, the pore size of peptidoglycan network of the Gram-positive bacteria becomes smaller due to dehydration, and the permeability is reduced, so that the crystal violet-iodine complex is retained in the bacteria and is not easy to de-colorize. Therefore, the Gram-positive bacteria appears blue-purple. The content of peptidoglycan in the cell wall of Gram-negative bacteria is low, and the content of lipids is high. When treated with alcohol, lipids are dissolved, the permeability of the cell wall is increased, and the crystal violet-iodine complex is easy to be extracted by alcohol and de-colorizes, so that it can be stained with the color of carbolfuchsin in the next counterstaining process, and shows red.

(2) Methods.

①Smear preparation: two drops of physiological saline was added to two parts of a clean slide (one drop for each part) first, and *Staphylococcus* and *Escherichia coli* was added to physiological saline respectively and mixed.

② Primary staining: add 2-3 drops of crystal violet to the smear, incubate at room temperature for 1 min, rinse with thinly running water, and dry.

③Mordant staining: add a few drops of Lugo's iodine solution on the smear, incubate at room temperature for 1 min, rinse with thinly running water, and dry.

④De-colorization: add a few drops of 95% alcohol, shake gently and incline the smear till the alcohol flow is not purple (about 30 s), rinse with thinly running water, and dry.

⑤Counterstaining: add a few drops of carbolfuchsin dilution, incubate for 30 s, rinse with thinly running water, and dry.

⑥Observation: add one drop of cedar oil on the top of the smear and observe with the oil immersion lens(10×100) after the water was absorbed by absorbent paper or naturally dried.

(3) Results: those staining with purple are called Gram-positive bacteria, and those staining with red are called Gram-negative bacteria. *Staphylococcus* is Gram-positive coccus, arranged in piles or in grape clusters. *Escherichia coli* is Gram-negative bacillus, arranged irregularly and dispersed.

[Notes]

(1) The amount of bacteria on the smear should be moderate and the smear should not be too thick or too thin. The bacteria should be distributed totally.

(2) The smear should not be overheated during fixation to avoid from destroy of bacterial morphology.

(3) The de-colorization is the key step of the success for Gram staining. The time should be flexibly mastered according to the thickness of the smear. Insufficient de-colorization will cause false positive, while excessive de-colorization will cause false negative.

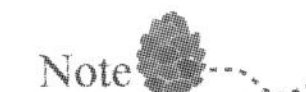

[Experimental Report]

(1)Please draw the basic morphology and special structure of bacteria you observed under oil immersion lens.

(2)Please draw the Gram staining results of two kinds of bacteria you observed under oil immersion lens.

[Questions]

(1)What is the main principle of Gram staining? What issues should need to pay attention to during operation? What is the practical significance?

(2)When you perform a Gram staining for an unknown strain, how to confirm that your staining results are correct?

(Hongmei Jiao, Rihan Wu)

Experiment 4 Pyogenic Coccus

[Experimental Objectives]

(1)To master the morphology and staining and culturing characteristics of pyogenic coccus.

(2)To be familiar with plasma coagulase test and anti-streptolysin O test.

[Experimental Materials]

(1) Instructional smears: Gram-stained specimens of *Staphylococcus*, *Streptococcus*, *Streptococcus pneumoniae*, *Neisseria meningitidis* and *Neisseria gonorrhoeae*, and capsular staining specimen of *Streptococcus pneumoniae*.

(2) Agar plate cultures of *Staphylococcus aureus*, *Staphylococcus epidermidis* and *Staphylococcus saprophyticus*, and blood agar plate cultures of *Streptococcus A*, *Streptococcus B*, *Streptococcus C* and *Streptococcus pneumoniae*.

(3)Rabbit plasma, physiological saline, sample to be tested (containing like-staphylococcal sample) or agar slant cultures of *Staphylococcus*.

(4)Slides, pipettes, microscope, etc.

(5)Serum to be tested, microreaction plate, ASO latex reagent, etc.

[Experimental Contents]

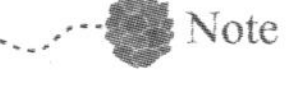

1. Observation of the morphology and staining characteristics of pyogenic coccus under a light microscope

(1)*Staphylococcus* is spherical or slightly oval. It is positive for Gram-staining. The typical arrangement is in clusters of grapes. It is double-balled or short-chained in the pus. It turns to Gram-negative quite frequently, when aging, dying, or being engulfed by neutrophils. It can be induced into an L-shape after the drug treatment such as penicillin.

(2) *Streptococcus* is spherical or oval. It is positive for Gram-staining and arranged in chain, and varies in length. *Streptococcus* is arranged in paired or short chains commonly in clinical specimen. Long chains are formed in liquid medium. Most strains can form hyaluronic acid capsules in the early stage of cultivation, and with the extension of culture time, the hyaluronidase produced by bacteria can make the capsules disappear. It is always show negative for Gram-staining in old media or pus specimen or after being engulfed by phagocytes.

(3) *Streptococcus pneumoniae* is spear-shaped and arranged in pairs, with broad ends facing each other, and tips opposite to each other. It is arranged in single or short chain in sputum specimen, pus specimen, or diseased lung tissue. Capsules can be formed in the host or the blood serum plate, and the capsules can be dyed with color after special-staining.

(4) *Neisseria meningitidis* is Gram-negative diplococcus. It is kidney-shaped or bean-shaped, and the contact surface of the two bacteria is flat or slightly inverted. The arrangement is irregular after artificial cultivation, such as single, double, 4 connected, etc. In the patient's CSF smear specimen, it is often located in neutrophils and the morphology is very typical. Newly isolated strains have capsule and pilus.

(5) *Neisseria gonorrhoeae* is similar to *Neisseria meningitidis* in morphology and staining characteristics. It is Gram-negative diplococcus, and arranged in pairs. The contact surface of the two bacteria is flat, resembling a pair of coffee beans. *Neisseria gonorrhoeae* is usually located in neutrophils in pus specimen, with irregular arrangement. In chronic patients, *Neisseria gonorrhoeae* is mostly distributed outside of the cell. It has capsule and pilus.

2. Observation of culturing characteristics of pyogenic coccus

(1) *Staphylococcus*. Single colony of three types of *Staphylococcus* (*Staphylococcus aureus*, *Staphylococcus epidermidis* and *Staphylococcus saprophyticus*) in medium size, round, raised, smooth surface, moist, neat edge, opaque and fat-soluble pigment was formed after incubated on agar plate for 24-48 h. The colonies are initially white, and then due to different pigment production, *Staphylococcus aureus* is golden, while *Staphylococcus epidermidis* is white, and *Staphylococcus saprophytic* is mostly lemon. The colonies of three types of *Staphylococcus* on blood agar plate are similar with those on regular agar plate. There is an obvious hemolytic ring around *Staphylococcus aureus* colony, while there was no hemolytic ring around colonies of *Staphylococcus epidermidis* or *Staphylococcus saprophytic*.

(2) *Streptococcus*. Colony of *Streptococcus* on blood agar plate is gray-white and needle-point-sized, and different hemolysis can be found around the colony. A narrow grass-green hemolytic ring (incomplete hemolysis, i. e., α hemolysis) may be seen around the colony of *Streptococcus A*. A well-defined, wide and transparent hemolytic ring (complete hemolysis, i. e., β hemolysis) is visible around the colony of *Streptococcus B*. *Streptococcus C* does not produce hemolysin, and there is no hemolytic ring around the colony.

(3) *Streptococcus pneumoniae*. Colony on blood agar plate is small, gray-white, round and slightly flattened, and translucent, with grass-green hemolytic ring (α hemolysis), which is very similar to *Streptococcus A*. If the incubation time is long, it can produce a sufficient amount of

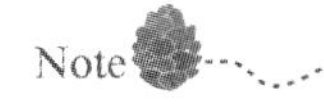

autolysin, which can dissolve the bacteria, making the center of the colony sunken into the shape of the navel.

(4) *Neisseria meningitidis*. Colony is colorless, round, smooth, moist and transparent, neatly edged, and drop-like on the chocolate(colored) blood agar plate.

(5) *Neisseria gonorrhoeae*. A round, raised, colorless or gray-white, and small colony with a diameter of 0.5-1.0 mm is formed after cultured on the chocolate(colored) blood agar plate at 37 ℃ for 48 h.

3. Plasma coagulase test

(1) Principle. Plasma coagulase test is an important test to identify the pathogenicity of *Staphylococcus*. Most strains of pathogenic *Staphylococcus* produce plasma coagulase, while non-pathogenic strains do not. There are two types of plasma coagulase produced by pathogenic *Staphylococcus*. One is free coagulase, which is a protein secreted out of bacteria and can be activated as a thrombin-like substance by co-factors in human or rabbit plasma. It turns liquid fibrinogen into solid fibrin, thereby coagulates plasma. The other is binding coagulase, which is a fibrinogen receptor attached on the surface of bacteria. It can directly interact with fibrinogen in plasma, precipitates it around bacteria and condenses it into lumps.

(2) Methods.

Slide method: it is used for the determination of binding coagulase.

①Take a clean slide, divide it into two zones, and add one drop of physiological saline in the middle of each zone.

②A little of the agar slant cultures of *Staphylococcus aureus* and *Staphylococcus epidermidis* were spread well into the physiological saline respectively by a sterilized inoculation loop.

③One drop of undiluted rabbit plasma was added into the bacterial suspension in each zone and mixed well.

④The results were observed after a few seconds. It is positive if there is granular agglutination and negative if there is no granular agglutination.

Tube-test method: it is used for the determination of free coagulase.

①Add 0.5 ml of fresh 1 : 4-diluted rabbit plasma into each test tube. Tube 1 and 2 were added with 0.5 ml of cultures of *Staphylococcus aureus* and *Staphylococcus epidermidis*, respectively. The third tube was added with 0.5 ml of medium as control.

②Place all tubes into a 37 ℃ water bath for 3 h, and check once every 30 min.

③It is positive for plasma coagulase test if the plasma in the test tube is jelly-like, and negative if the plasma is still liquid in the test tube.

(3) Results. *Staphylococcus aureus* can produce plasma coagulase, which is positive in the test. *Staphylococcus epidermidis* does not produce plasma coagulase and is negative in the test.

4. Thermostable DNase assay

(1) Principle. Pathogenic *Staphylococcus aureus* can produce a thermostable DNase, which can decompose DNA. While non-pathogenic *Staphylococcus epidermidis* and *Staphylococcus saprophyticus* also produce DNase, but the DNase is not heat-tolerant. Therefore, thermostable DNase assay can be used as a method to identify pathogenic *Staphylococcus*.

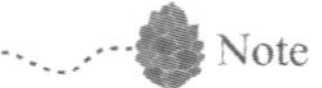
Note

(2) Methods.

Slide method: holes were punched on toluidine blue nucleic acid agar, with the pore diameter of 3-5 mm. Each hole was added with one drop of bacteria (*Staphylococcus aureus*, *Staphylococcus epidermidis* or *Staphylococcus saprophyticus*) cultures, which were pretreated by boiling water for 15 min. Results were observed after 3 h inoculation at 37 ℃.

Plate method: label the colony desired for test on the *Staphylococcus aureus* plate. Put the plate into a dry heat sterilizer at 60 ℃ for 2 h, and then pour 10 ml of melted toluidine blue nucleic acid agar on the plate. Observe the result after incubating the plate at 37 ℃ for another 3 h.

(3) Results. The colony of *Staphylococcus aureus* producing thermostable DNase was surrounded by pink circle.

5. Anti-streptolysin O test (anti "O" test, ASO test)

(1) Principle. The ASO latex reagent is cross-linked by hemolysin "O" and polystyrene latex and the sensitivity of the ASO latex reagent is increased to 200 IU/ml in the test. The agglutination particles appear visible to the naked eyes at 200 IU/ml or above without dilution for serum sample. It can assist in the diagnosis of rheumatic fever, glomerulonephritis and other diseases caused by *Streptococcus*.

(2) Methods. One drop of serum to be test, positive serum control and negative serum control was added to the microreaction plate, respectively, and then one drop of ASO latex reagent was added to each sample. Gently shake for 2 min to mix well, and observe the results after another 2 min.

(3) Result. Those with clear agglutination are positive and can be determined as ASO > 200 IU/ml. Those without clear agglutination are negative and can be determined as ASO < 200 IU/ml.

[Notes]

(1) The reagent should be set to room temperature and shake well before use.

(2) The kit should be stored at 2-10 ℃, and do not freeze.

(3) When adding reagents, and negative and positive controls, make sure that the droplet size is same.

[Laboratory Report]

(1) Please draw out the morphology and staining characteristics of pyogenic coccus under oil immersion lens.

(2) Please briefly describe the principle, methods and results of plasma coagulase test.

[Questions]

(1) What are the common pyogenic coccus? What are the characteristics of their morphology, staining and culturing?

(2) How to distinguish pathogenic *Staphylococcus* from non-pathogenic *Staphylococcus*?

(3) What is the principle of ASO test? How to determine the result?

(4) What is the current situation and development trend of drug resitance of pathogenic coccus?

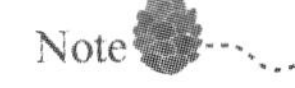

(Hongmei Jiao, Rihan Wu)

Experiment 5　Enterobacteriaceae

[Experimental Objectives]

(1)To be familiar with the isolation and identification of pathogenic Enterobacteriaceae.

(2)To master the principle, methods and results analysis of Widal test.

[Experimental Materials]

(1) Gram-stained instructional smear of *Escherichia coli*, *Bacillus typhi*, *Bacillus dysenteriae*, and *Bacillus proteus*.

(2)SS agar plates inoculated with Enterobacteriaceae, and disaccharide iron, indigo matrix, semi-solid and urea media inoculated with *Escherichia coli*, *Bacillus typhi*, *Bacillus paratyphosus B*, *Bacillus dysenteriae*, and *Bacillus proteus*, respectively.

(3)Patient's fecal (mimic) specimens, SS agar medium dry powder, distilled water, beakers, glass rods, microwave oven, sterilized flatware, Enterobacteriaceae slant cultures, Enterobacteriaceae diagnostic sera, etc.

(4)Typhoid patient's serum (1 : 10 diluted), physiological saline, *Salmonella typhi* O antigen diagnostic bacterial solution, *Salmonella typhi* H antigen diagnostic bacterial solution, *Salmonella paratyphi* A and B diagnostic bacterial solutions, microreaction plates, micropipettes and dropper tips, oscillator, thermostat, etc.

[Experimental Contents]

1. Major bacteria of Enterobacteriaceae

(1) Morphology and Gram-staining characteristics. Observe the basic morphology of *Escherichia coli*, *Bacillus typhi*, *Bacillus dysenteriae*, and *Bacillus proteus* under oil immersion lens, and compare their shapes, sizes, arrangements and staining characteristics.

(2)Isolation and cultivation of Enterobacteriaceae.

①Principle. SS agar medium is a strong selective identification medium for the isolation of Enterobacteriaceae. In addition to nutrients, the medium contains chemicals such as bile salts, brilliant green, sodium thiosulfate and sodium citrate, which can inhibit the growth of non-pathogenic bacteria (such as *Escherichia coli*), while bile salts have the effect of promoting the growth of *Salmonella* and *Bacillus dysenteriae*. In addition, SS agar medium is also added with lactose and neutral red indicator (red in acidic environment, while yellow in alkaline environment). Pathogenic Enterobacteriaceae do not decompose lactose, so the colonies on the SS agar plate are colorless or yellowish, smooth and small. *Bacillus dysenteriae*, *Bacillus paratyphosus B*, and *Salmonella typhimurium* can produce H_2S, so the centers of their colonies are black. *Escherichia coli* generally does not grow on SS agar plate, but if the fecal specimen is inoculated with a large amount of *Escherichia coli*, we can still see its growth on the SS agar plate. Because *Escherichia coli* can ferment lactose to produce acid, so it can form red, larger and

Note

smooth colonies on the SS agar plate, which is easy to distinguish from pathogenic bacteria. Nowadays, SS agar plates are mostly prepared with commercialized SS agar medium dry powder.

②SS agar plate preparation. Weigh 48 g of SS agar medium dry powder in a beaker, add 1000 ml of distilled water, place the beaker in a microwave oven and heat for 1-2 min (be careful not to boil), take out the beaker and stir with a glass rod, then return it to the microwave oven to continue to heat, and repeat the above operation until the medium dry powder is completely dissolved. After the completely dissolved medium is cooled to room temperature, pour it into sterile plates (15-20 ml for each plate), and then use it for bacterial isolation and cultivation after the agar solidifies.

③Specimen inoculation. A small amount of patient's fecal (simulated) specimen was picked with a sterile inoculation loop (note that the inoculation loop should be cooled after sterilization before sampling), and was inoculated on SS agar plate by the plate zoning demarcation method. Specimen number, class, name and date of inoculation were labeled on the plate, and then the plate was inverted and incubated at 37 ℃ for 18-24 h to observe the characteristics of the colonies.

(3) Biochemical reactions of major bacteria of Enterobacteriaceae (demonstration). Enterobacteriaceae have active biochemical reactions, can decompose a variety of sugars and proteins, and form different metabolites, which are commonly used to differentiate between different genera and strains of bacteria.

The results of biochemical reactions of several major bacteria of Enterobacteriaceae are shown in Tab. 2-5-1.

Tab. 2-5-1 The results of biochemical reactions of several major bacteria of Enterobacteriaceae

Bacteria	Kirschner's bisaccharide iron			Indole matrix	semi-solid (motile)	Urea
	Lactose	Glucose	H_2S			
Escherichia coli	⊕	⊕	−	+	+	−
Bacillus typhi	−	+	−/+	−	+	−
Bacillus paratyphosus A	−	⊕	−	−	+	−
Bacillus paratyphosus B	−	⊕	+	−	+	−
Bacillus dysenteriae	−	+	−	−	−	−
Bacillus proteus	−	⊕/+	+/−	+/−	+	+

Notes: ①"−" means no fermentation, "+" means producing acid, and "⊕" means producing acid and gas.

②Kirschner's bisaccharide iron medium uses phenol red as an indicator, which is yellow in acidic environment and red in alkaline environment. If the bacteria can ferment lactose and produce acid and gas, it can make the slant and bottom of the medium become yellow and have bubbles. If the bacteria only ferment glucose but not lactose, because the content of glucose is less (accounting for 1/10 of the amount of lactose), the amount of acid generated is less, and it is oxidized and volatilized after contact with air. Due to growth and reproduction, the bacteria use nitrogenous substances to generate alkaline compounds, so that the slant of the medium turns red. The bottom layer remains yellow because the acid produced by the bacterial fermentation of glucose is not oxidized and volatilized under anoxia. If the bacteria decompose proteins to produce hydrogen sulfide, it interacts with ferrous sulfate to produce black iron sulfide, turning the medium black.

(4) Widal test.

①Principle. By using the diagnostic bacterial solutions with known *Salmonella typhi* body (O) antigen and flagellum (H) antigen as well as H antigens of *Salmonella paratyphi A* and *Salmonella paratyph B*, and different dilutions of serum, the quantitative agglutination test is performed to determine the presence of the corresponding antibody and its titer in the examined

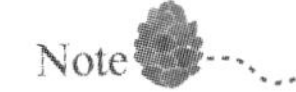

serum, in order to assist in the clinical diagnosis of typhoid fever and paratyphoid fever.

②Methods.

a. Take a microreaction plate, and use 40 wells (10×4) in this experiment.

b. Diluted serum: according to Tab. 2-5-2, firstly use a micropipette to aspirate 50 μl of physiological saline into the first to tenth wells of each row (4 rows in total). Then aspirate 50 μl of 1∶10 diluted patient's serum into the first well of each row, aspirate 50 μl from the first well into the second well after mixing, and then aspirate 50 μl from the second well into the third well after mixing, and so on, until the ninth well of each row. Discard 50 μl after mixing in the ninth well. 50 μl of physiological saline was added into the tenth well without serum as a negative control.

c. Add the ingredients according to Tab. 2-5-2, and incubate the plate at 37 ℃ for 1 h after 3-5 min of shaking (do not shake the plate during incubation to avoid the clots shaking away). Observe the negative control wells first, the correct result should be no agglutination—the liquid in the wells is uniformly turbid or there is a neat and round mass at the bottom of the wells. Then observe the results sequentially from the first well to the ninth well, and according to the strength of the agglutination, the results will be shown as "++++""+++""++""+"and "−", respectively.

Tab. 2-5-2 Antibody dilution method for Widal test

Item	1	2	3	4	5	6	7	8	9	10
physiological saline volume/μl	50	50	50	50	50	50	50	50	50	50
Serum(1∶10) volume/μl	50	—	—	—	—	—	—	—	—	—
Diagnostic bacterial solution volume/μl	50	50	50	50	50	50	50	50	50	50
Dilution	1∶40	1∶80	1∶160	1∶320	1∶640	1∶1280	1∶2560	1∶5120	1∶10240	Control

Note: The diagnostic bacterial solutions were *Salmonella typhi* O antigen diagnostic bacterial solution, *Salmonella typhi* H antigen diagnostic bacterial solution, H antigen diagnostic bacterial solutions of *Salmonella typhi* A and *Salmonella typhi* B, respectively.

③Results. "++++", the upper layer of liquid is clarified, and all bacterial agglutinates sink to the bottom of the hole; "+++", the upper layer of liquid is mildly turbid, and the agglutinates sink to the bottom of the hole; "++", the upper layer of liquid is moderately turbid, and there is obvious agglutination at the bottom of the hole; "+", the upper layer of liquid is turbid, and there is only a small amount of agglutinates at the bottom of the hole; "−", the liquid in the hole is the same as the negative control hole, with uniform turbidity, no agglutination.

④Titer determination. The agglutination titer of the serum is determined by the highest dilution of the serum at which the "++" agglutination occurs.

⑤Analysis of results. The interpretation of the results of the Widal test must be combined with clinical manifestations, course of disease, medical history and regional epidemiology. The following points should be noted.

a. Normal value. The serum of normal people may contain a certain amount of antibody due to hidden infection or vaccination, and its titer varies from region to region. In general, *Salmonella typhi* O antibody agglutination titer ≥1∶80, *Salmonella typhi* H antibody

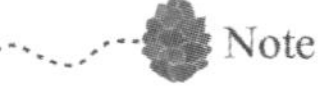
Note

agglutination titer≥1 : 160, and H antibody agglutination titer of *Salmonella paratyphi* A or B ≥1 : 80 to have diagnostic value.

b. Dynamic observation. Antibodies appear about a week after the onset of the disease and increase with the course of the disease. Sometimes a single increase in the titer of an antibody cannot be determined, and it can be reviewed weekly during the course of the disease. If the increase in the titer is progressive or the titer increases 4 times or more during the recovery period, there is a diagnostic significance.

c. The significance of O and H antibodies in diagnosis. After suffering from typhoid fever, paratyphoid fever or vaccination, the appearance and disappearance of O and H antibodies in the body are different. IgM-type O antibody appears early, lasts for a short time, and is not easy to be stimulated by non-specific stimulation to reappear after disappearance, whereas the IgG-type H antibody appears later, maintains for several years, and is easy to be stimulated by non-*Salmonella* and other pathogens to reappear transiently after disappearance (non-specific recollective reaction). Therefore, if both O and H antibodies agglutination titers are above normal, there is a high likelihood of typhoid fever or paratyphoid fever, and if both are low, there is a low likelihood of typhoid fever or paratyphoid fever. If the agglutination titer of O antibody is not high but H antibody is high, it may be a vaccination or non-specific recollective reaction (repeat the test at certain intervals, and if the titer does not increase, then it is a non-specific recollective reaction). If the agglutination titer of O antibody is high but H antibody is not high, it may be an early stage of infection or infection by other *Salmonella* (e. g. , *Salmonella enteritidis*) that have a cross-reactivity with the O antigen of *Salmonella typhi*, as shown in Tab. 2-5-3.

Tab. 2-5-3 Results of Widal test

Results	Clinical significance
O<1 : 80 & H<1 : 160	Normal
O≥1 : 80 & H≥1 : 160	Typhoid fever
O≥1 : 80 & PAH≥1 : 80	Paratyphoid fever A
O≥1 : 80 & PBH≥1 : 80	Paratyphoid fever B
O≥1 : 80 & H<1 : 160, or O≥1 : 80 & PAH/PBH<1 : 80	Early stage of typhoid fever, paratyphoid fever A or paratyphoid fever B; or other *Salmonella* infections
O<1 : 80 & H≥1 : 160, or O<1 : 80 & PAH/PBH≥1 : 80	Vaccination or non-specific recollective reaction

Note: O means *Salmonella typhi* O antibody agglutination titer, H means *Salmonella typhi* H antibody agglutination titer, and PAH and PBH mean H antibody agglutination titers of *Salmonella paratyphi* A and *Salmonella paratyphi* B, respectively.

d. Others. There are a few cases of typhoid fever or paratyphoid fever in which the results of the Widal test are always within the normal range throughout the course of the disease, which may be due to the early treatment with antibiotics or the immunocompromise of the patients.

[Experimental Report]

(1) Briefly describe the principle, method, result judgment and analysis of Widal test.

(2) Illustrate the colony characteristics of Enterobacteriaceae on SS agar plate and the results of slide agglutination test.

(3)Record the results of biochemical reactions of *Escherichia coli*, *Bacillus typhi*, *Bacillus dysenteriae and Bacillus pyogenes* on disaccharide iron, indigo matrix, semi-solid and urea media.

[Questions]

(1) What should be paid attention to in the process of Widal test? How to ensure the accuracy of the results judgment?

(2)If the test serum has a *Salmonella typhi* O antibody agglutination titer of 1 : 160, is the patient infected with *Salmonella typhi* certainly? What is the reason?

(3) How to reduce or exclude the influence of normal flora in the isolation and cultivation of pathogenic Enterobacteriaceae?

(Guimei Kong, Chengfeng Gao)

Experiment 6　Anaerobic Bacteria

[Experimental Objectives]

(1) To master the morphology and culturing characteristics of *Clostridium tetani*, *Clostridium perfringens* and *Clostridium botulinum*.

(2)To be familiar with the principles and common methods of anaerobic culture.

[Experimental Materials]

(1)Bacterial species: meat residue cultures of *Clostridium tetani*, *Clostridium perfringens* and *Clostridium botulinum*.

(2)Observation of bacterial morphology: Gram-stained instructional smears of *Clostridium tetani*, *Clostridium perfringens* and *Clostridium botulinum*.

(3)Cotton, sterile gauze, 10% NaOH solution, solid paraffin, slides, sterile droppers, etc.

[Experimental Contents]

1. Observation of morphology and structure of bacteria

(1) Observe the basic morphology of *Clostridium tetani*, *Clostridium perfringens* and *Clostridium botulinum* under the oil immersion lens, and compare their shapes, sizes, arrangements and staining characteristics.

(2)Observe the special structure of bacteria: the shapes and positions of the spores of *Clostridium tetani* and *Clostridium botulinum*; the size and color of the capsule of *Clostridium perfringens*.

2. "Surge fermentation" test

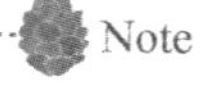
Note

(1)Principle. *Clostridium perfringens* can rapidly decompose lactose in milk to produce a large amount of acid, solidifying casein, and flush vaseline on the surface of the medium to the cotton plug at the mouth of the test tube, which is called "surge fermentation" phenomenon, which generally occurs after 6-12 h of cultivation.

(2) Methods.

① Preparation of bromocresol purple milk medium. Add 0.1 ml of bromocresol purple solution with a concentration of 16 g/L to 100 ml of fresh skim milk, 5 ml for each tube was packed separately, and the melted vaseline was added to the surface, with the thickness being about 5 mm, and conduct intermittent steam sterilization: 75 ℃, 30 min on day 1; day 2, 80 ℃, 30 min; day 3, 85 ℃, 30 min.

② *Clostridium perfringens* was inoculated into bromocresol purple milk medium and cultured at 37 ℃ for 12-24 h.

(3) Results. The bacteria decompose lactose to produce acid and gas, and casein solidifies and forms sponge-like fragments.

3. Anaerobic culture of pork medium

(1) Principle. Pork medium is suitable for the cultivation of anaerobic bacteria because it does not contain saturated fatty acids and can consume oxygen when oxidizing, resulting in an anaerobic environment.

(2) Methods.

① Preparation of pork medium: take 0.5 g of beef residue, put them in a test tube of 15 mm × 150 mm, then add 7 ml of broth medium with pH 7.6, add 3-4 mm thick melted vaseline, and reserve after high-pressure steam sterilization.

② *Clostridium tetani* was inoculated into pork medium and cultured at 37 ℃ for 24-48 h.

(3) Results. The medium is partly cloudy, and the meat is partly digested and turns black and slightly smelly.

[Experimental Report]

Draw the basic morphology and special structure of *Clostridium tetani*, *Clostridium perfringens* and *Clostridium botulinum* observed under the oil immersion lens.

[Questions]

(1) What is the main principle of anaerobic culture? What are the methods of anaerobic culture?

(2) What are the biosafety issues that should be considered in anaerobic culture?

(Yinyan Yin, Cuicui Liu)

Experiment 7 *Mycobacterium*

[Experimental Objectives]

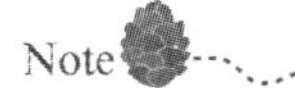

(1) To master the morphology and staining characteristics of *Mycobacterium tuberculosis*.

(2) To master the methods of acid-fast staining.

[Experimental Materials]

(1)Instructional smears for acid-fast staining of *Mycobacterium tuberculosis*.

(2)Sputum (simulated) samples of tuberculosis patient.

(3)Acid-fast staining solutions: carbolfuchsin dilution, 3% hydrochloric acid with ethanol solution, and Loeffler methylene blue solution (appendix A).

(4)Slides, inoculation loop, alcohol lamp, microscope, etc.

[Experimental Contents]

1. Observation of morphology and staining characteristics of *Mycobacterium tuberculosis*

Mycobacterium tuberculosis is slender and slightly curved, arranged in a single or branched shape. It is positive for Gram staining, but not recommended. Acid-fast staining is commonly used for *Mycobacterium tuberculosis*, and showing red in results, while other non-acid-fast bacteria and cell plasma, etc. are blue. In the old lesions or cultures, the morphology of *Mycobacterium tuberculosis* is often untypical, and can be granular-, spherical-, or short rod-shaped.

2. Observation of culturing characteristics of *Mycobacterium tuberculosis*

Mycobacterium tuberculosis was inoculated in modified Lowenstein-Jensen solid medium and cultured at 37 ℃, checking it once a week. *Mycobacterium tuberculosis* grows very slowly, and its colony will be visible to the naked eyes after growing for 2-4 weeks. The colony is dry, hard, granular in surface, milky white or beige in color, and raised on the surface of the medium, resembling cauliflower-like. It grows superficially in liquid medium, forming coarse and wrinkled membrane.

3. Acid-fast staining (Ziehl-Neelsen staining)

(1)Principle. The cell wall of *Mycobacterium tuberculosis* contains a large number of lipoid (such as mycolic acid), which is not easy to colored generally. The mycotic acid is bound tightly with carbolfuchsin under the heated staining or prolonging the staining time. The complex can resist the de-colorization of strong decolorizing agent (3% hydrochloric acid with ethanol solution), hence it is called acid-fast staining. When counterstained by Loeffler methylene blue solution, *Mycobacterium tuberculosis* are still red and positive for acid-fast staining, while other microorganisms and tissue cells are blue and negative for acid-fast staining.

(2)Methods.

①Use the inoculation loop to take sputum and evenly coat it into a thick smear, and fix it with flame after natural drying.

②Hold the smear with a slide holder, and add the carbolfuchsin dilution on the smear. Heat it slowly at a high flame. Temporarily leave from the flame when there is vapor (not boiling). The staining solution should be supplemented appropriately to avoid drying up when the staining solution is reduced by evaporation. Maintain this operation for 3-5 min, and wash with water after the smear cooled down.

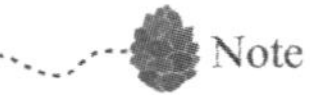

③Add 3% hydrochloric acid with ethanol solution to de-colorize for 1 min. Gently shake the smear during de-colorization, until no red ethanol flow out, and wash with water.

④Add Loeffler methylene blue solution to counterstain for 1 min, wash with water and dry it, and observe with an oil immersion lens.

(3) Results. Under the oil immersion lens, *Mycobacterium tuberculosis* spreads out, appears elongated or slightly curved rod-shaped, and is stained red, which is called positive for acid-fast staining, while non-acid-fast bacteria and other components are stained blue.

[Notes]

To improve the detection rate, a thick smear (i. e., five times thicker than a normal smear) is recommended. The de-colorization time depends on the thickness of the smear. The de-colorization time can be appropriately extended in the thick smear until without red ethanol flow out.

[Experimental Report]

(1) Please draw the morphology and staining characteristics of *Mycobacterium tuberculosis* observed under the oil immersion lens.

(2) Please briefly describe the principle, methods, results and significance of acid-fast staining.

[Questions]

(1) How to do a microbiological test for a patient suspected to have tuberculosis?

(2) What are the screening methods for *Mycobacterium tuberculosis* infection? Describe the principle of each method.

(3) What scientific spirit does the development history of *Mycobacterium tuberculosis* detection and prevention technologies reflect, and how to cultivate an innovative consciousness and a scientific attitude?

(Hongmei Jiao, Rihan Wu)

Experiment 8 Other Bacteria

[Experimental Objectives]

(1) To master the morphological characteristics of "sulfur granule" of *Actinomycetes*.

(2) To be familiar with the morphology and culturing characteristics of *Brucella*, *Bacillus anthracis*, *Yersinia pestis*, *Actinomycetes*, *Mycoplasma*, *Rickettsia*, *Chlamydia* and *Spirochaeta*.

(3) To be familiar with the serological test of *Treponema pallidum*.

[Experimental Materials]

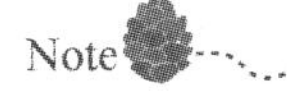

(1) Instructional smears: *Brucella*, *Bacillus anthracis*, *Yersinia pestis*, *Actinomycetes*, *Mycoplasma*, *Rickettsia*, *Chlamydia* and *Spirochaeta*.

(2)Reagents for serological test of *Treponema pallidum*.

[Experimental Contents]

1. *Brucella*

(1)Observe the morphology of *Brucella*: Gram-negative bacillus.

(2)Observe the colonial morphology of *Brucella* on the biphasic liver immersion medium: tiny, transparent, non-pigmented and smooth colonies.

2. *Bacillus anthracis*

(1)Observe the morphology of *Bacillus anthracis*: Gram-positive bacillus, "bamboo like", having capsules, and having oval spores in the middle of the bacterium.

(2)Observe and compare the non-toxic *Bacillus anthracis* colonies on common agar plate and blood agar plate. On the common agar plate, *Bacillus anthracis* forms rough colonies which are flat, off-white, dry, non-transparent and matte. When visualized under microscope, the edges of the colonies are wavy. On the blood agar plate, the colonies are rough, off-white and matte, and have uneven edges. Usually no hemolysis, slight hemolysis can be observed when the bacterium is cultured for a long time.

3. *Yersinia pestis*

(1)Observe the morphology of *Yersinia pestis*: after methylene blue staining, the bacilli are blue, oval and stubby, and both ends are heavily stained.

(2) Observe the morphology of *Yersinia pestis* colonies: on common agar plate, the surroundings of the colonies are thin and the center is raised. In the broth medium, colonies grow turbidly at the beginning and gradually form flocculent precipitates. After 48 h, the mycoderm can be formed. After 4-5 d, filaments droop from the mycoderm, like stalactites, which is a typical characteristic that helps identify *Yersinia pestis*.

4. *Actinomycetes*

Demonstration teaching of sulfur granule: sulfur granules are made into tablets, and radial mycelia are visible under a microscope, with a diameter of 1 μm. The end of the mycelium is rod-shaped and chrysanthemum-like.

5. *Mycoplasma pneumoniae*

(1)Observe the morphology of *Mycoplasma pneumoniae*: without cell wall, pleomorphic.

(2)Observe the morphology of *Mycoplasma pneumonia* colonies: they have high nutrition demand and grow slowly. When cultured in the soft agar medium with high nutrition for 5 d, it will form typical "fried-egg" colonies on agar, which is a typical characteristic that helps identify *Mycoplasma*. Due to the different time of appearance for different *Mycoplasma* colonies, continuous observation should be performed for 8 d. If no colony appears after 8 d, a negative result can be reported.

6. *Chlamydia*

Chlamydia has a unique life cycle, and has two different granular structures that can be seen. One is elementary body, which is small and compact, round, infectious, and stained purple by Giemsa staining solution and red by Macchiavello staining solution. Another is reticulate body, which is large and loose, round or oval, non-infectious, and stained red by Giemsa staining solution and blue by Macchiavello staining solution.

Note

Giemsa staining is as follows.

(1) Preparation of Giemsa staining solution: see Appendix A.

(2) The sample was fixed with methanol for 5 min, and the buffer solution and Giemsa staining solution were mixed at a ratio of 20 : 1. Then stain for 10-30 min, wash with running water, and observe under the oil immersion lens. The nucleus is red, the cytoplasm is blue, and the pigment particles are brown.

7. *Rickettsia*

Rickettsia typhi can be stained purple or blue by Giemsa staining solution, and usually have heavy stained poles, while be stained red by Macchiavello staining solution.

8. *Spirochaeta*

(1) Morphology and staining characteristics of *Leptospira*: After Fontana silver staining, *Leptospira* can be stained into dark brown, one or both ends are curved in a "C", "S" or "8" shape.

Fontana silver staining is as follows.

①Dry the smear.

②Fix with fixative for 2 min.

③Rinse with absolute ethanol.

④Incubate with mordant for 2 min.

⑤After washing with water, incubate with silver solution for 2 min.

⑥Microscopic examination after washing.

(2) Morphology and staining characteristics of *Treponema pallidum*.

①Silver staining for *Treponema pallidum*. The genital secretions of patients with syphilis are stained with silver, and 8 to 14 spirochetes can be visible, with the ends being sharp. They are stained brown and the tissue is claybank.

②Serological test of *Treponema pallidum*. There are two types of antigens commonly used in serological test of *Treponema pallidum*. One is the cardiac lipids of normal bovine myocardium, and the other is the *Treponema* antigen. Here we introduce a rapid plasma reagin (RPR) test that is currently used internationally for the initial screening of *Treponema pallidum*.

a. Principle. The standard myocardial antigen is adsorbed on special activated carbon particles. After mixing this carbon-containing antigen with patient's serum, it can react with anti-*Treponema pallidum* antibodies in the serum to form black aggregate particles on white cards which are visible by naked eyes. Furthermore, semi-quantitative determination of antibody levels can be conducted by this test.

b. Methods. Lyophilized positive control serum is dissolved with 0. 2 ml of physiological saline 5 s before the test. Pipette 50 μl of serum to be tested into the card. Add one drop of RPR antigen vertically in each serum to be tested and the positive control serum. Shake the card by hand to fully mix the serum and antigen, and observe the result after 8 min.

c. Results. The results should be judged according to the following criteria within 3 min after shaking the card.

Positive reaction: medium or large black agglutinations. Weak positive reaction: small, black and scattered agglutinations. Negative reaction: no agglutinations, or only rough carbon particles in the middle.

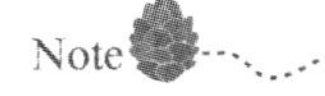

[Experimental Report]

Draw the morphology of *Bacillus anthracis*, *Spirochaeta*, *Treponema pallidum* and the sulfur granule of *Actinomycetes* under the oil immersion lens.

[Questions]

(1) What is RPR test? Describe its principle and application briefly.

(2) What is the significance of accurate diagnosis of *Treponema pallidum* infection to the prevention and treatment of syphilis?

(Yinyan Yin, Cuicui Liu)

Experiment 9 Virus

[Experimental Objectives]

(1) To understand the viral morphology under electron microscope.

(2) To know the viral CPE and inclusion body.

(3) To master the principle and the determination methods of ELISA.

[Experimental Materials]

(1) Photographs of viral morphology taken by electron microscope, instructional films of viral inclusion body, and microscope.

(2) Serum to be tested, ELISA kit for the detection of HBsAg, and 37 ℃ incubator.

[Experimental Contents]

1. Observation of photographs of viral morphology taken by electron microscope and instructional films of viral inclusion body

(1) Basic forms of virus.

①Spherical (nearly spherical): such as viruses in human and animal.

②Rod-shaped (filament): such as the plant viruses.

③Bullet-shaped: such as the rabies virus.

④Brick-shaped: such as poxvirus.

⑤Tadpole-shaped: such as bacteriophage.

(2) Observation of viral CPE and inclusion body. Host cell will be round, aggregated, necrotic, dissolved or fall off from the plate after infected by some viruses, such as enterovirus, while some will fuse into one multinucleated giant cell after infected by the other sets of viruses (measles virus, cytomegalovirus, etc.), but the multinucleated cell has individual nuclear. Inclusion body (Negri body) formed by rabies virus is located in the cytoplasm of nerve cells,

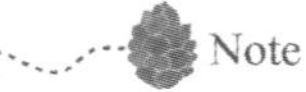
Note

and is eosinophilic and round or oval in shape.

2. Detection of HBsAg by ELISA

(1)Principle. HBsAg is detected by double antibody "sandwich" method. The "first" anti-HBs is coated at slats, while the "second" anti-HBs labeled by HRP is used as enzyme marker. The tetramethyl-benzidine (TMB) and peroxide are used as substrates for reaction. The HBsAg included in the serum to be tested will bind to the anti-HBs coated at slats first and another side will be bind to the HRP-labeled anti-HBs to form the anti-HBs-HBsAg-anti-HBs-HRP "sandwich" complex. The "sandwich" complex will be colored by adding substrates, while the reagent will be colorless or weak signal in negative sample.

(2)Methods.

①50 μl of the sample to be tested, positive control and negative control were added to A1, A2 and A3 of a 96-well plate which is coated with anti-HBs, respectively. Well A4 as blank control.

②50 μl of anti-HBs labeled by HRP was added to each well (except blank control).

③The reaction plate was covered after mixing for 5 min, and incubated at 37 ℃ for 30 min.

④Discard the supernatant and wash the plate with detergent for five times.

⑤50 μl of substrate A and 50 μl of substrate B were added into each well (including the blank control), and incubate the plate at 37 ℃ for 10 min.

⑥50 μl of stop solution was added into each well to terminate the reaction. Then the colors will be compared by spectrometry or eyes.

(3)Results.

①Visual results: the results will be observed by eyes directly under a white background. The stronger color indicates positive reaction; colorless or extremely lighter color indicates negative as well. Mark as "+" or "−" to each well according to the color of reaction.

②Comparing by spectrometry: set up the blank control as "0" first, and read the depth of color of each well at 450 nm by the ELISA reader. The OD_{450} of sample greater than that of standard (mean OD_{450} of negative control×2.1) is positive, otherwise is negative.

[Experimental Report]

Please describe the principle, methods and results of the detection of HBsAg by ELISA.

[Questions]

(1)What are the principles for collection of virus samples? What is the differences from collection of bacterial samples?

(2) What are the commonly methods for the detection of virus? Please describe the advantages and disadvantages of those methods.

(3)If there is a suspected noval virus infection, how to accurately and quickly determine the type of pathogen?

(Hongmei Jiao, Rihan Wu)

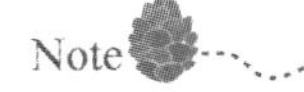

Experiment 10　Fungi

[Experimental Objectives]

(1)To master the morphology and culturing characteristics of common fungi.

(2)To learn the preparation techniques of specimens for examination of fungi without staining.

[Experimental Materials]

(1)Instructional smears for *Candida albicans*, *Cryptococcus neoformans*, dermatophytes, and spore and hypha of yeast.

(2)Slant cultures of *Candida albicans*, *Cryptococcus neoformans*, and dermatophytes.

(3)Lactophenol cotton blue staining solution, high-quality ink, and fungal fluorescence staining solution, etc.

(4)Small tweezers, cover glass, slides, microscope, etc.

[Experimental Contents]

1. Observation of morphology and staining characteristics of fungi

The *Candida albicans* is round or oval. Some have spore, and bud elongation to produce pseudohypha. Gram staining is positive (coloring is not uniform). The *Cryptococcus neoformans* is round or oval, with a wide capsule. Microscopic observation with ink negative staining shows that the round or oval fungi are wrapped in a wide blank band. Dermatophyte is a type of multicellular fungus with spore and hypha.

2. Inspection of fungi without staining

(1)Methods. Skin scrap, nail scrap or a hair of patient with fungal infection was loaded to a clean slide by tweezer, and add 1-2 drops of 10% KOH solution. After a few minutes, cover glass was added on the top of sample, and the slide was heated by the flame until tissue or keratin was dissolved, but do not overheat to avoid bubbles or dried. Cold down the slide, and the cover glass was pressed tightly to disturb the dissolved tissue and expel all bubbles, then wipe the surrounding solutions with paper towels. The presences of hypha and spore of fungi were observed with a low-power microscope firstly. Second, the characteristics of hypha and spore were checked with a high-power microscope. Weak light was recommended when using microscope.

(2)Results. Under the low-power microscope, the hypha shows as strong refraction and green fibrous branched filaments. Under the high-power microscope, the hypha is separated, and the end of the hypha has thicker and shorter articular spores sometimes. If hypha or spore is found during microscopic observation, the initial diagnosis can be made, but the strain is not determined.

3. Staining of fungi

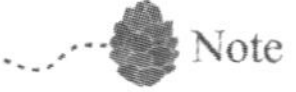

(1)Lactophenol cotton blue staining.

①Principle: lactophenol cotton blue staining solution can interact with fungi and color it to blue. Lactic acid has killing effect on fungi. This method is used for staining and observation of fungi usually.

②Methods:2-3 drops of lactophenol cotton blue staining solution were added to the center of the slide,and a small piece of yeast colony with particles or partial color was picked up by sterilized inoculation loop. Mix well in the staining solution. Add a cover glass and gently press to make a tablet (heated or not),and observe under a low-power,high-power microscope or oil immersion lens.

③ Results: cells, hyphae and spores of yeast can be colored bright blue, while the background is dull blue.

(2)Ink negative staining.

① Principle: the capsule of *Cryptococcus neoformans* is thick, and not easy to stain. Meanwhile,the fungus has strong refraction. So the fungus can be seen in a black background by ink negative staining.

②Methods: mixone drop of high-quality ink with sample to be tested on a slide, and observe under microscope.

③Results:the broad and thick capsule of *Cryptococcus neoformans* can be observed under the microscope after ink negative staining.

(3)Fungal fluorescence staining.

①Principle:most fungi contain chitin. The recombinant chitinase of the fungal fluorescent staining solution can bind to the chitin in the fungal cell wall. It makes the hypha and spore of fungi emit bright blue-green fluorescence under the fluorescence microscope at 340-380 nm wavelength to achieve rapid detection of fungi.

②Methods:the cell culture or scrap was placed on the slide,and staining solution A and solution B were dropped. Then,the slide was covered with a cover glass and directly observed.

③Results:unicellular or hypha and spore of fungi will show blue-green fluorescence.

4. Fungal culturing methods

(1)Plate culture method: the inoculation method is similar to that of bacteria. It is a method adopted by most laboratories,mainly used for the isolation and cultivation of yeast and yeast-like fungi.

(2)Inclined culture method: the inoculation method is similar to that of bacteria, mainly used for primary cultivation of clinical specimens,secondary cultivation of filamentous fungi,and storage of strain. It is most commonly used for mycotic cultivation.

(3)Small culture method:it is the best method for observing the structure of filamentous fungi,mainly used for the identification of filamentous fungi. ①Use an inoculation knife to mark a 1 cm^3 "井" on the agar plate,and take a block and place it on the center of a sterile slide. ②Inoculate the fungi to be tested on the center of the four sides of the agar block,cover them with sterile cover glass,place them on a U-shaped glass rod in a sterile plate,and add a small amount of sterile water to the plate for moisturizing and incubation. ③After the fungal colonies growing up,remove the cover glass and add a drop of lactophenol cotton blue staining solution to the slide for staining. Cover the cover glass and use absorbent paper to absorb excess staining solution from the surrounding area. Observe the characteristics of hypha and spore under the microscope for identification.

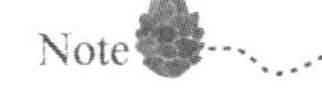

5. Observation of fungal colonies

(1)Colony of *Cryptococcus neoformans* belongs to yeast-type colony. Its surface is round, smooth, moist and milky white or creamy, and it is mucus-like sometimes.

(2) Colony of *Candida albicans* belongs to yeast-like colony with a smooth, moist and milky white surface. Its nutritious hypha protrudes into the medium, and the surroundings of the colony can be seen to be feathery under light observation.

(3) Colony of *Epidermophyton floccosum* is a filamentous colony. The surface of the colony is composed of a large number of hypha, which looks like cotton wool, villi or powder. There are wrinkles in the center and radial grooves in the periphery. The medium is always cracked. The back of the colony is brown.

[Experimental Report]

(1) Please illustrate the morphology of hypha or spore of fungi in non-staining specimens.

(2) Please record the characteristics of the fungal colonies you observed.

[Questions]

(1) Why do we need to do small cultivation for fungus sometimes?

(2) Is the culture temperature of superficial and deep fungi same? Why?

(3) What are the rapid detection methods of fungal infection and the corresponding application ranges?

(Hongmei Jiao, Rihan Wu)

Experiment 11　Test of Endotoxin (Limulus Amoebocyte Lysate Test)

[Experimental Objectives]

(1) To master the determination method of bacterial endotoxin in drugs.

(2) To be familiar with the principle of limulus amoebocyte lysate test.

[Experimental Materials]

Limulus amoebocyte lysate (LAL), bacterial endotoxin standard, bacterial endotoxin test water, pyrogen-free glass test tube, 1 ml pyrogen-free syringe, needle, test tube holder, vortex mixer, constant temperature incubator, sealing film, alcohol cotton ball, grinding wheel, test products (water for injection), etc.

[Experimental Contents]

1. Principle

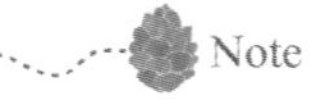

LAL is a biological reagent which is derived from the deformable cell lysate extracted from the blue blood of limulus and freeze-dried at low temperature to detect bacterial endotoxin. Gel

LAL test is a qualitative or quantitative method to detect trace bacterial endotoxin *in vitro*. In this method, the LAL contains coagulase which can be activated by trace bacterial endotoxin, so LAL can be coagulated with the bacterial endotoxin to form a gel under appropriate conditions. Biological products, injectable agents, chemicals, radiopharmaceuticals, antibiotics, vaccines, dialysate and other preparations as well as medical equipment (such as disposable syringes and implanted biological materials) must pass the LAL test before use.

2. Method

(1) Preparation of bacterial endotoxin positive control solution. Dilute the bacterial endotoxin standard with bacterial endotoxin test water to make a 4λ or 2λ bacterial endotoxin standard solution, and set aside.

For example, the concentration of bacterial endotoxin standard is 10 EU/ampoule, and the sensitivity (λ) of LAL is 0.125 EU/ml. The steps for preparation of bacterial endotoxin standard solution are as follows.

①Take an ampoule of bacterial endotoxin standard, open the bottle after sterilizing the neck with alcohol cotton ball, add 1 ml of bacterial endotoxin test water, seal the bottle with sealing film and then put it on the vortex mixer for 15 min. The concentration of bacterial endotoxin at this time is 10 EU/ml.

②Take 3 test tubes, mark them and place them on the test tube holder. Prepare 4λ and 2λ bacterial endotoxin standard solutions by referring to the dilution method in Tab. 2-11-1.

Tab. 2-11-1 Preparation of bacterial endotoxin positive control solution

Items	Standard solution	1	2	3
Bacterial endotoxin	1 ampoule(10 EU)	0.2 ml	1.0 ml	1.0 ml
Bacterial endotoxin test water	1 ml	1.8 ml	1.0 ml	1.0 ml
Concentration/(EU/ml)	10	1.0	0.5(4λ)	0.25(2λ)

(2) Preparation of the test solution. MVD=cL/λ. c, the concentration of the test solution; L, the limit units of bacterial endotoxin of the test product, expressed as EU/ml, EU/mg or EU/U. When L is expressed as EU/ml, c is 1 ml/ml; When L is expressed as EU/mg or EU/U, the unit of c is mg/ml or U/ml (note: when L is expressed as EU/ml, the value of c is not the concentration of the sample but 1). EU, bacterial endotoxin unit; λ, marked sensitivity of LAL; MVD, maximum effective dilution multiple of the test product.

For example, the test product is water for injection, and its bacterial endotoxin limit L is 0.25 EU/ml (*Chinese Pharmacopoeia* stipulates that the amount of bacterial endotoxin per 1 ml of water for injection should be less than 0.25 EU).

The sensitivity of LAL (λ) is 0.125 EU/ml, so MVD $= cL/\lambda = 1 \times 0.25/0.125 = 2$. Therefore, the original test product should be diluted twice as the test solution, that is, 0.5 ml water for injection + 0.5 ml water for inspection.

(3) Preparation of the test positive control solution. Take 4λ bacterial endotoxin standard solution, add the same volume of the test solution and mix well. For example, when preparing the test positive control solution for water for injection, use 0.5 ml of 4λ (0.5 EU/ml) bacterial endotoxin standard solution, add 0.5 ml of water for injection, and mix evenly.

(4) Preparation of LAL. Take 8 tubes of LAL ampoules of 0.1 ml/ampoule and mark them. Flick the bottle wall to make the powder fall into the bottom of the bottle, gently scratch the bottle neck with the grinding wheel, disinfection with 75% alcohol and then open it for later

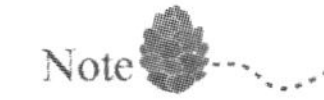

use. Please pay attention to prevent glass debris from falling into the bottle when opening. Add 0.1 ml of liquid to each ampoule, gently rotate the ampoule to fully dissolve the contents, and avoid violent vibration to produce bubbles.

(5) Sample addition and incubation. Add the reagents to each ampoule as shown in Tab. 2-11-2. Seal the mouth of the ampoule with sealing film and incubate at 37 ℃ for about 60 min.

Tab. 2-11-2 Method of adding reagents for LAL test Unit: ml

Reagents	Positive control tube (A)		Negative control tube (B)		Test positive control tube (C)		Test tube (D)	
	1	2	1	2	1	2	1	2
Bacterial endotoxin positive control solution (No. 3 tube)	0.1	0.1						
Bacterial endotoxin test water			0.1	0.1				
Test positive control solution (No. 5 tube)					0.1	0.1		
Test solution (No. 4 tube)							0.1	0.1

(6) Judgment of the results.

① To determine whether the experiment is valid. Gently take each ampoule, slowly invert 180°, and observe. As shown in Tab. 2-11-3, the test is valid when the two parallel tubes of positive control tube (A) are positive, the two parallel tubes of negative control tube (B) are negative, and the two parallel tubes of test positive control tube (C) are positive.

Tab. 2-11-3 Judgment of the validity of LAL test result

Tube number	Phenomena		Judgment
A	+	+	Experiment valid
B	−	−	
C	+	+	

② Judgment of the test tube. As shown in Tab. 2-11-4, if the two parallel tubes of test tube (D) are negative, the result is judged to be compliant; if the two parallel tubes of test tube are positive, the result is judged to be non-compliant; if one tube is positive and the other tube is negative, the experiment needs to be retested. When retesting, 4 test tubes are required (if all 4 test tubes are negative, the result will be judged as compliant; otherwise, it will be non-compliant).

Tab. 2-11-4 Judgment of the LAL test tube

Tube number	Phenomena				Judgment
D		−	−		Compliant
		+	+		Non-compliant
		+	−		Retest
Retest (4 tubes)	−	−	−	−	Compliant

(7) Precautions.

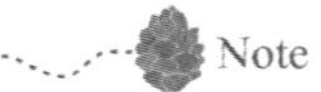

① Microbial and bacterial endotoxin contamination should be prevented during the operation. Before the test, wash hands with soap and disinfect with 75% alcohol.

②Glass test tubes, syringes and needles should be washed clean and then repeatedly rinsed with distilled water for more than three times. Dry bake (250 ℃ for 30 min) to remove pyrogen and then use.

③Since the gel reaction is reversible, be careful not to subject the tubes to vibration during the thermostatic reaction process and observation of the results, so as not to break the gel and produce false-negative results.

④When dissolving the LAL and mixing the test product with the LAL, do not vibrate violently to avoid bubbles.

[Experimental Report]

(1) Describe the detection methods and principle of bacterial endotoxin.

(2) Write down the bacterial endotoxin test results and analysis the results.

[Questions]

(1) Why is it necessary to perform bacterial endotoxin testing for biological products and medical equipment? What should be paid attention to in the process of bacterial endotoxin testing?

(2) What should be done with bacterial endotoxin contaminated samples? What are the common methods to remove bacterial endotoxin?

(Guimei Kong, Chengfeng Gao)

Experiment 12 Parasitic Relationships and Parasite Evolution

[Experimental Objectives]

To understand parasitic relationships and the evolution of parasites.

[Experimental Materials]

Specimens.

[Experimental Contents]

1. Free living

Such as locusts, their motor organs and sensory organs are developed, and their mouthparts are chewable.

2. Commensalism

Echeneis naucrates is adsorbed on the surface of the large fishes by it's sucker. It's not good or bad for the large fishes, but it's good for *Echeneis naucrates*.

3. Mutualism

The sea anemone lives on the surface of the hermit crab's carapace. The hermit crab can carry the sea anemone around, allowing the sea anemone to expand its foraging area while the sea anemone uses its spines and secretions to protect the hermit crab. Both benefit from each other.

4. Parasitism

The parasite changes in morphology and physiology to adapt to parasitic life.

(1) Changes in body shape: schistosoma parasites in blood vessels, so it's body is slender; the body of flea is flattened on both sides in order to move between hairs.

(2) Organ changes: such as parasitic pork tapeworm in the digestive tract, its head segment has four suckers and small hooks which give it strong attachment ability, so as not to be discharged by the host. It absorbs nutrients through the body wall, and the digestive organs are completely degraded. But to increase its chances of survival, its reproductive organs are developed and hermaphrodite.

[Experimental Report]

Briefly describe the three relationships between living things.

(Fang Tian, Feng Lu)

Experiment 13 Trematode

[Experimental Objectives]

(1) To realize the life cycle of trematode. To be familiar with the main morphological characteristics of *Clonorchis sinensis* (liver trematode), *Fasciolopsis buski* (intestinal trematode), *Paragonimus westermani* (lung trematode) and *Schistosoma japonicum* (schistosome) at each developmental stage.

(2) To master the morphological characteristics of adults and eggs of liver trematode, intestinal trematode, lung trematode and *schistosome*.

(3) To realize morphological characteristics of intermediate hosts of *Clonorchis sinensis*, *Paragonimus westermani*, *Fasciolopsis buski* and *Schistosoma japonicum*.

[Experimental Materials]

Teaching specimens (slices), microscopes, cedar oil, xylene, lens wipping paper, etc.

[Experimental Contents]

Teaching content

Ⅰ The developmental stage of trematode

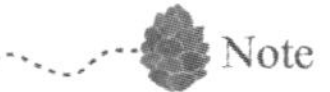

1. Egg

Except for schistosome eggs, they all have egg covers, and contain developed miracidia or undeveloped yolk cells and egg cells (egg specimens of *Clonorchis sinensis*).

2. Miracidium

It's pear-shaped, ciliated, active in water and must enter the snail for further development (stained specimens of miracidium of *Schistosoma japonicum*).

3. Sporocyst

Sporocyst is developed from miracidium which drilled into the snail body. It is ovoid sac when it is immature, and then it gradually changes into long sacs. The embryoid cell masses with different development degree could be seen in the body (stained specimens of sporocyst of *Schistosoma japonicum*).

4. Redia

Mature redia is oval cyst with an obvious muscular pharynx and a short primitive digestive tract at one end. Black matter is usually seen in the primitive digestive tract. The redia contains mature or immature cercariae (stained specimens of rediae of *Clonorchis sinensis*).

5. Cercaria

Cercaria escapes from the snail and is divided into the body and the tail. Cercaria swings in the water to find a second intermediate host or final host by the swing of the tail. The morphology varies with species (stained specimens of cercariae rediae of *Clonorchis sinensis*).

6. Metacercaria

Metacercaria always parasite in the second intermediate host. It has a distinct wall enclosing the larvae. Black excretory vesicles are seen in living metacercariae, which vary in shape from species to species (slide specimens of metacercarie of *Clonorchis sinensis*).

7. Adult

Observe bottled gross specimens of four main parasitic trematodes in the human body, which are *Clonorchis sinensis* (liver trematode), *Fasciolopsis buski* (intestinal trematode), *Paragonimus westermani* (lung trematode) and *Schistosoma japonicum* (schistosome).

Ⅱ *Clonorchis sinensis* (liver trematode)

1. Adult in preserved specimen (naked eye observation)

The worm is long and narrow, flat thin and translucent, and looks like sunflower seeds. The front end is slightly narrow, and the back end is blunt and round, 1-2 cm long. The uterus, testis, and vitelline glands are faintly visible.

2. Adult in stained specimen (observation with low-power microscope)

(1) The oral sucker at the top is slightly larger than the ventral sucker located in the anterior 1/5 part of the body.

(2) This worm is hermaphroditic. Two deeply branched testes in tandem locate in the posterior 1/3 part of the body.

(3) The only one ovary is shallowly lobed and locates in front of testis. The uterus coils forward and opens into the genital lumen.

(4) The oval seminal receptacle and Laurer's canal are clearly visible. Vitelline glands are in the lateral fields.

(5) The excretory vesicle is a long S-shaped pouch structure located in the middle of the posterior 1/3 part of the body.

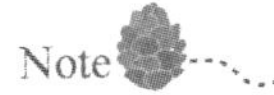

3. Egg specimen (observation with low-power and high-power microscopes)

The liver trematode egg is the smallest worm egg.

(1)(27-35)μm×(12-20)μm.

(2)Yellow-brown.

(3)Egg looks like a sesame seed under the low-power microscope and a watermelon seed under the high-power microscope.

(4)Eggshell is thicker, with operculum resting on a rim which takes the shape of distinct shoulders.

(5)There is an asymmetrical miracidium inside the egg.

4. Fresh specimen of metacercaria digested with artificial digestive fluid (observation with low-power microscope)

The metacercaria is ellipsoidal shape, 138 μm×115 μm, with two suckers (oral sucker and ventral sucker) and excretory vesicle containing black granules.

5. The first intermediate hosts (naked eye observation)

Observe *Parafossarulus striatulus* and *Alocinma longicornis*.

6. The second intermediate hosts (naked eye observation)

Observe fresh water fish and crayfish.

Ⅲ *Fasciolopsis buski* (intestinal trematode)

1. Adult in preserved specimen (naked eye observation)

It is the largest parasitic human trematode.

(1)Long elliptic, flesh-colored, and looks like a slice of raw meat.

(2)(20-75)mm×(8-20)mm×(1-3)mm. The ventral sucker is significantly larger than the oral sucker.

2. Adult in stained specimen (observation with low-power microscope)

(1)The ventral sucker is near by the much smaller oral sucker.

(2)The bowel curves in waves.

(3) The two testes in tandem is highly branched and is coral-like, accounting for the majority of the posterior body.

(4)The ovary is located in the middle of the body, divided into 3 petals, with each petal branching again. The uterus is coiled between the ventral sucker and Mehlis' gland.

(5)There is no seminal receptacle. The vitelline glands are located in the both sides of the body.

3. Egg specimen (observation with low-power and high-power microscopes)

(1)Large size, (130-140)μm×(80-85)μm. It is the largest worm egg.

(2)Pale yellow in color.

(3)Oval shape.

(4)Thin shell, small operculum, with a germinal cell surrounded by ventral granules.

4. Redia in stained specimen (observation with high-power microscope)

It is long bagged, with mouth, pharynx and problastic cell mass.

5. Cercaria in stained specimen (observation with high-power microscope)

Body part has not eyespot, with long tail, no membrane wrapped.

6. Metacercaria in stained specimen (observation with high-power microscope)

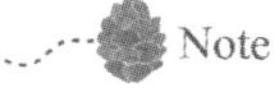

Two layers of capsule wall, the outer layer is easy to break, while the inner layer is tough. There are larvae in cyst, and the excretory vesicle contains refraction particles which is irregularly arranged on both sides of the capsule and is easy to identify.

7. Intermediate hosts (naked eye observation)

Planorbis caenosus, with flat coil shell, light yellow, and translucent.

8. Plant vector

Aquatic plants (caltrop, water chestnut, etc.).

Ⅳ *Paragonimus westermani* (lung trematode)

1. Adult in preserved specimen (naked eye observation)

(1) The body is elliptic, dorsally convex, and ventrally flattened reddish-brown.

(2) (7.5-12) mm × (4-6) mm × (1-3) mm. It looks like half a peanut. The middle part of the abdomen is a uterus filled with yellow eggs.

2. Adult in stained specimen (observation with low-power microscope)

(1) The sizes of two suckers are sub-equal. The oral sucker is located at the anterior end of the body. The ventral sucker is located in front of the midline of the body.

(2) The digestive tract is divided into two ceca and is wavy curved.

(3) The two testes are located in the posterior part of the body. The ovary and the uterus are situated side by side.

(4) The vitelline glands are branchlike, which locate in both sides of the body.

(5) The excretory vesicle extends forward to the level of the pharynx.

3. Egg specimens (observation with low-power and high-power microscopes)

(1) (80-118) μm × (48-60) μm.

(2) Golden-yellow.

(3) Ellipsoidal shape.

(4) Thickness of eggshell is uneven, thicker at the back end.

(5) There are a germinal cell and more than ten yolk cells inside the egg.

4. Redia in stained specimen (observation with high-power microscope)

It is cylindrical. There are mouth, pharynx and gastrocoel at the front of radia. There are embryonic cell mass and short cercariae inside radia.

5. Cercaria in stained specimen (observation with high-power microscope)

It is round or oval. The whole body has fine spines. The front end has a small thorn, and the tail is very short and spherical.

6. Metacercaria in stained specimen (observation with high-power microscope)

It is global with distinct wall. The larva in the cyst is spiral curved, and the oral and ventral suckers and large and distinct excretory vesicle can be seen.

7. The first intermediate hosts (naked eye observation)

Semisulcospira spp. is large, brownish-yellow, and tower-shaped. The top of the shell is often worn by collision with rocks.

8. The second intermediate hosts (naked eye observation)

Stone crab and river crab grow in mountain streams. Crayfish are mostly found in northeast of China, and are crustaceans.

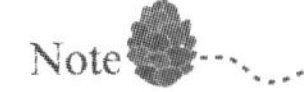

9. Pathological specimen

Pathological changes of lung or brain are caused by *Paragonimus westermani* infection.

Note the nodular ridges on the surface. The adult parasite in the sac, surrounded by fibrous thick wall.

Ⅴ *Schistosoma japonicum* (schistosome)

1. Adult in preserved specimen (naked eye observation)

Adults are dioecious, with a male and a female living together.

2. Adult in stained specimen (observation with low-power microscope)

(1)It is elongated cylindrical in shape.

(2)Two sexes are separate.

(3)The male usually embraces the female into its gynecophoric canal, which appears "K" like.

(4)Male: (10-20) mm × (0.5-0.55) mm, seven testes are situated one by one. Just behind the ventral sucker, there is a longitudinal groove-gyncophoral canal.

(5)Female: dark colored thread-like, (12-28) mm × 0.3 mm. The unbranched oval ovary lies in the mid-portion of the body. The uterus lies in the anterior portion of the body.

3. Egg specimen (observation with low-power and high-power microscopes)

(1)(70-106) μm × (50-80) μm.

(2)Light yellow.

(3)Ovoidal.

(4)Thin eggshell and lacking the operculum, with a small spine on the side near one end.

(5)There is a miracidium inside the egg. The soluble egg antigen (SEA) is secreted by miracidium.

4. Miracidium

(1)Miracidium stained specimen (observation with low-power microscope).

It is pear-shaped, and slightly protrude at the front. Cilia outside the body may fall off in the process of making. Gastrocoel and a pair of head gland are in the front of the body, and embryo cells are in the back of the body.

(2)Living miracidium (observation with naked eye or magnifying glass).

They hatch from mature eggs. The triangular flask containing miracidium was placed in a bright place during observation. So that the light source from the side of the front shot into flask with dark things as the background, mainly to see the bottleneck. The miracidium is white elongated dots in the water and swims in straight lines.

5. Sporocyst stained specimen (observation with low-power microscope)

It was extracted from the liver of infected *Oncomelania hupensis* and divided into the first and second generations. The second generation of sporocyst is observed, and the long pouch structure would be noted, lacking pharynx and intestine, and containing cercariae and embryo cell mass with different maturity.

6. Cercaria

(1)Cercaria stained specimen (observation with low-power microscope).

There are 5 pairs of puncture glands on both sides of the ventral sucker, and the tail ends bifurcate.

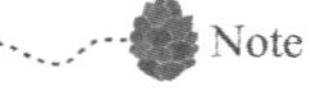

(2)Living cercaria(observation with magnifying glass).

The body part is floating on the water, and the tail is suspended under the water and bent forward. The body is slightly comma-like, and the tail twists and swings when active. Do not touch with hands during observation to prevent infection.

7. Intermediate hosts (observation with naked eye)

Oncomelania hupensis is about 1 cm long, and the operculum shell is tower-shaped with 6-7 spirals. Mountain-type snail shells are more slippery, while plain-type snail shells are rough (with wheel ridge). They are different shades of brown.

8. Pathologic specimen

(1) Mesentery with parasitic adult: parasitic adults in the mesentery vein, with part of the black female deep into the intestinal wall blood vessels.

(2) Rabbit liver of egg deposition: egg nodules infestation.

(3) Healthy rabbit liver: smooth surface without lesions.

Individual observation

(1) Observe the adult slide specimens of *Clonorchis sinensis*, *Fasciolopsis buski*, *Paragonimus westermani* and *Schistosoma japonicum*.

(2) Observe the egg slide specimens of *Clonorchis sinensis*, *Fasciolopsis buski*, *Paragonimus westermani* and *Schistosoma japonicum*.

(3) Observe trematode eggs mixed drop specimens.

(4) Observe the squashes of liver tissue of rabbits with schistosome and intestinal mucosa tissue of rabbits with schistosome.

(5) Rabbits with schistosomiasis were dissected to observe the parasitic sites of adult, liver and intestinal lesions, and egg nodules.

Video

Watch video of *Schistosoma japonicum*.

[Experimental Report]

Draw eggs of *Clonorchis sinensis*, *Fasciolopsis buski*, *Paragonimus westermani* and *Schistosoma japonicum* in detail.

[Questions]

(1) What are the similarities and differences in the life history of liver trematode, intestinal trematode, lung trematode and schistosome? And infer the similarities and differences of its prevention and control measures.

(2) What are the main morphological differences of adult and egg of between schistosome and the other three species of trematode?

(3) Why can fecal precipitation incubation be used to diagnose schistosomiasis japonica?

(4) Can the presence of eggs of schistosome in intestinal mucosa biopsy confirm the presence of schistosomiasis? How to analyze?

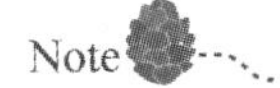

(Fang Tian, Feng Lu)

Experiment 14　Tapeworm

[Experimental Objectives]

(1) To master the diagnostic methods of taeniasis and morphological characteristics of adults, eggs and cysticerci of *Taenia solium* and *Taenia saginata*.

(2) To be familiar with the morphology of eggs of *Echinococcus granulosus* and *Hymenolepis nana*.

(3) To understand the morphology of adults of *Echinococcus granulosus* and *Hymenolepis nana*.

[Experimental Materials]

Teaching specimens (slices), microscopes, cedar oil, xylene, lens wipping paper, etc.

[Experimental Contents]

Teaching content

Ⅰ *Taenia solium*

1. The specimen of adult (naked eye observation)

It is flattened ribbon-like, segmented, creamy white in color, and measures 2-4 m. It consists of three parts: scolex, neck and strobila. The strobila has 700-1000 proglottides. Proglottides bear the reproductive organs (both male and female). There are three types of proglottides: immature, mature and gravid proglottides.

2. The stained specimen of scolex (observation with low-power microscope)

It is spherical with four suckers and rostellum armed with two rows of small hooklets. The number of small hooklets is 25-50.

3. The stained specimen of mature proglottides (observation with magnifying glass)

Each mature proglottid has 2 full sets of reproductive organs, in which one is male and another is female. The testes are follicular, about 100 in number. The ovary has three lobes.

4. The stained specimen of gravid proglottides (observation with magnifying glass)

Count the number of lateral branches of uterus on one side. 7-13 lateral branches on each side of uterus are unequal in length.

5. Bottled specimen of cysticercus (naked eye observation)

The cysticercus has the size of a soybean and is milky white. The capsule is translucent and filled with liquid, and the white dot on the inner surface of the capsule wall is the scolex. Let living cysticercus in bile and heating, scolex turned out, and its shape is the same as adult scolex after staining.

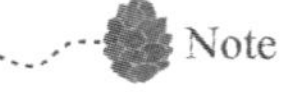
Note

6. Pathological specimen

Cysticercus parasitizes in pork. The cysticercus is white and bubble-like, surrounded by a connective tissue fiber membrane.

Ⅱ *Taenia saginata*

1. The specimen of adult (naked eye observation)

The morphology is similar to that of the adult of *Taenia solium*, but the strobila is hypertrophic and can grow to 4-8 m, with 1000-2000 proglottides.

2. The stained specimen of scolex (observation with low-power microscope)

The scolex is square, with 4 cup-shaped suckers, without rostellum and small hooklets.

3. The stained specimen of mature proglottides (observation with magnifying glass)

The ovaries are only divided into left and right lobes, and the rest are as same as that of *Taenia solium*.

4. The stained specimen of gravid proglottides (observation with magnifying glass)

The uterine branches are orderly, with 15-30 branches on each side.

5. Pathological specimen

Cysticercus parasitizes in beef.

6. Egg specimen (observation with low-power and high-power microscopes)

(1) 31-43 μm.

(2) Spherical.

(3) Brown.

(4) Eggshell is easily ruptured. The embryophore is yellow-brown with radial streaks.

(5) Contain an oncosphere with 6 hooklets.

Ⅲ *Echinococcus granulosus*

1. The stained specimen of adult (observation with low-power microscope)

The body is 2-7 mm. The scolex is pear-shaped, with 4 suckers, and there are 28-48 small hooklets on the rostellum. The strobila usually has only one immature proglottid, one mature proglottid and one gravid proglottid. The structure of the mature proglottid is similar to that of *Taenia solium*. The uterus of the gravid proglottid forms pouch branches on both sides and contains 200-800 eggs.

2. Pathological specimen

Echinococcus is parasitic in livers of human and animals. Its outer layer is the tissue envelope of the host and its inner wall is the cyst wall of echinococcus. The cyst wall can be divided into two layers. The outer laminated layer is thicker and looks like powdery skin. The inner layer is the germinal layer, which is very thin. The daughter cyst, brood capsule and protoscolex can be suspended in cyst fluid, which is called hydatid sand.

3. The stained specimen of protoscolex (observation with low-power microscope)

The protoscolex is oval, and the suckers and the rostellum of the hooklets can be seen. Because of the overlap of the suckers, often only two suckers can be seen. A protoscolex in the final host body can develop into a parasite.

4. Eggs

The eggs are basically the same as those of *Taenia solium* and *Taenia saginata* and can hardly be distinguished under an ordinary light microscope.

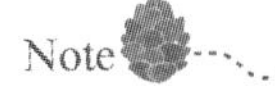

Ⅳ *Hymenolepis nana*

1. The specimen of adult (naked eye observation)

It is milky white and 5-80 mm long with 100-200 proglottides whose width greater than length.

2. The stained specimen of adult (observation with low-power microscope)

(1)Scolex: rhomboid or round, 4 suckers, 1 rostellum, and 1 circle of small hooklets whose number is 20-30.

(2)Mature proglottides: oval, 3 testes arrangement along horizontal line, and 2 ovarian lobes in the center, below which is the vitelline gland.

(3)Gravid proglottides: the uterus is cystic and filled with eggs, with the number being 80-180.

3. Egg specimen (observation with low-power and high-power microscopes)

It is round or oval, colorless and transparent, and contains an oncosphere. The oncosphere is surrounded by an embryonic membrane, which has a very thin eggshell. The two poles of the embryonic membrane are slightly raised, giving birth to 4-8 filaments.

Individual observation

Observe the eggs of *Taenia solium*, *Taenia saginata* and *Hymenolepis nana*, scoleces and gravid proglottides of *Taenia solium* and *Taenia saginata*, and protoscolex.

[Experimental Report]

Draw the eggs of *Taenia solium*, *Taenia saginata* and *Hymenolepis nana*.

[Questions]

(1)Compare *Taenia solium* and *Taenia saginata* based on their morphology and life cycle. Why say the harm of *Taenia solium* is bigger than *Taenia saginata*?

(2)Why echinococcosis is more common in animal husbandry areas in northwest of China?

(3)How to explain the serologic diagnostic result of cysticercosis cellulosae?

(Fang Tian, Feng Lu)

Experiment 15 Nematode

[Experimental Objectives]

(1)To realize the life cycle and common morphology of nematodes.

(2) To study morphological characteristics of eggs of *Ascaris lumbricoides*, *Trichuris trichiura*, *Enterobius vermicularis* and hookworm. To study the microfilaria of *Filaria*.

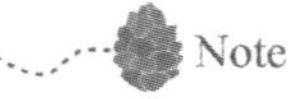

(3)To study the pathogenesis of nematode infection.

[Experimental Materials]

Teaching specimens (slices), microscopes, cedar oil, xylene, lens wipping paper, staining solution, etc.

[Experimental Contents]

Teaching content

Ⅰ *Ascaris lumbricoides*

1. Adult in preserved specimen (naked eye observation)

The female worm is 20-35 cm long. The male worm is rather small and 15-31 cm long, with the tail end turning to the ventral side.

2. Anatomical specimen of adult (naked eye observation)

(1) Digestive organs: they are vertical straight tubes, opening at the top of the insect body, connected with a short rod-shaped esophagus, followed by the midgut and rectum. Rectum of female worm is connected to the anus at the back end, rectum and ejaculatory duct of male worm are connected to the cloaca.

(2) Reproductive organs: the reproductive organs of female worm are two groups of the same tubular structure. The ovary is as long as a line, in which one end is free, and the other end is gradually expanded to form fallopian tube and uterus. The uterus is the largest part, which is filled with eggs. The end of the uterus of the two groups merges into a vagina, and the vaginal door opens at the junction of anterior 1/3 and middle 1/3 of the insect body abdomen. The reproductive organs of male worm are a single group of tubular structure, which are testis, vas deferens, seminal receptacle (the largest), and ejaculatory duct. There are two mating spines at the tail end extending into the cloaca and out of the body.

3. Slide specimen of roundworm head (observation with low-power microscope)

On the tip of the head, there are three lips arranged as a Chinese word "品".

4. Morphology of egg (observation with low-power and high-power microscopes)

Fertilized egg: ①(45-75) μm×(35-50) μm; ② broad oval; ③ yellow-brown; ④ thicker egg shell and outer albuminous coats; ⑤ the content is a fertilized ovum. A crescent-shaped clear space at each end inside the shell.

Unfertilized egg: ①(80-94) μm×(39-44) μm; ② long and slender; ③ yellow-brown; ④ thin egg shell and an irregular outer layer; ⑤ granular contents.

The albuminous coats of fertilized egg and unfertilized egg can be shed, that is, deproteinized egg. The color of this egg becomes colorless and the internal structure remains unchanged. Infection stage egg (containing larva): the appearance is the same as the fertilized egg, but inside of the egg is a curly larva.

5. Pathological specimen (naked eye observation)

Observe the gross pathological specimen of roundworm parasitism in the biliary tract, intestine, appendix and trachea.

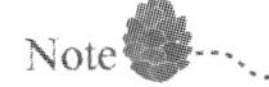

Ⅱ *Trichuris trichiura*

1. Adult in preserved specimen (naked eye observation)

It looks like a buggy whip. The anterior 3/5 is slender and the posterior 2/5 is thick. The female worm is 30-50 mm in length, and the male worm is smaller and 30-45 mm long, with a curved tail.

2. The stained specimen of male (observation with low-power microscope)

There is a copulatory spicule at the tail, and there is a telescopic spicular sheath at the outside of the copulatory spicule.

3. The stained specimen of female (observation with low-power microscope)

The vulva is located behind the middle part of the body and ventral in front of the coarse part, and the end of the tail is blunt and round.

4. Morphology of egg (observation with low-power and high-power microscopes)

①(50-54) μm × (22-23) μm; ② barrel-shaped; ③ yellow-brown; ④ smooth shell, with a translucent polar plug at each end; ⑤the content is an undeveloped cell.

5. Pathological specimen (naked eye observation)

Parasitism on the intestinal wall, invasion of the intestinal mucosa with the slender anterior end of the parasite, and free in the intestinal lumen with the short posterior end of the parasite.

Ⅲ *Enterobius vermicularis*

1. Adult in preserved specimen (naked eye observation)

It looks like a pin and is white. The female worm is 8-13 mm long and the male worm is only 2-5 mm long. The tail of the male is curled to the abdomen, while the tail tip of the female is slender.

2. The stained specimen of adult (observation with low-power microscope)

The anterior end tapers are flanked on each side by cuticular extensions which is called "cephalic alae". The esophagus is slender, terminating in a prominent posterior bulb, which is called esophageal bulb.

3. Morphology of egg (observation with low-power and high-power microscopes)

①(50-60) μm×(20-30) μm; ②persimmon seed-shape; ③colorless and transparent; ④thick and asymmetric shell, flattened on the ventral side; ⑤the content is a larva.

Ⅳ *Ancylostoma duodenale* and *Necator americanus*

1. Two adult species in preserved specimen (naked eye observation)

The body of hookworm is thin and long, about 1 cm long, and milky white. The female is thicker and longer than the male, and the tail of the male is straight. The male has a characteristic copulatory bursa at the tail end, which looks like an opened umbrella, the ribs of which are called rays. *Ancylostoma duodenale* is larger and looks like "C". *Necator americanus* is smaller and looks like "S".

2. Specimens of adult mouth capsule(observation with low-power microscope)

There are two pairs of hooklets in the mouth capsule of *Ancylostoma duodenale*, but one pair of cutting plate in the mouth capsule of *Necator americanus*.

3. Copulatory bursa of two adult species in preserved specimen (observation with low-power microscope)

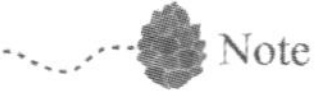
Note

The copulatory bursa of *Ancylostoma duodenale* is round, but that of *Necator americanus* is transversely elliptical. The female of *Ancylostoma duodenale* has a small mucro at the tail end. In the female of *Necator americanus*, no spine exists at the tail end.

4. Morphology of egg (observation with low-power and high-power microscopes)

①(57-76) μm×(36-40) μm;②oval in shape;③shell is thin and colorless;④the content is 2-8 cells;⑤advanced cleavage.

5. The stained specimen of rhabtidiform larva (observation with high-power microscope)

The front end is blunt and round, and the back end is tapery. The front end of the esophagus is thick, the middle is narrow, and the back end is slightly spherical. The length of the esophagus is equal to 1/4 of the body length.

6. The stained specimen of filariform larva (observation with high-power microscope)

The mouth is closed, the front end of the esophagus is long and slender, the back end is not obvious, and the tail end is thin. The length of the esophagus is equal to 1/4 of the body length.

7. Gross specimens of adult parasite in the small intestine (naked eye observation)

Observe gross specimens of adult parasite in the small intestine.

Ⅴ *Wuchereria bancrofti* and *Brugia malayi*

1. Two adult species in preserved specimen (naked eye observation)

Adults look like thin and long threads. The adults of *Wuchereria bancrofti* resemble that of *Brugia malayi* in morphology, but is thinner and shorter. The female is 58. 5-105 mm long and the male is 28. 2-42 mm long. The length of female *Brugia malayi* is 40-69 mm, and the male is 13. 5-28. 1 mm in length.

2. Morphology of unstained microfilaria (observation with low-power and high-power microscopes)

Microfilariae are slender and filamentous, colorless and transparent, highly reflective, with a blunt front end and a tapered back end.

3. The stained specimen of two kinds of microfilariae (observation with high-power and oil immersion lens microscopes)

The microfilaria of *Wuchereria bancrofti* is graceful and sweeping curves; the size is (244-296) μm×(5. 3-7) μm. The cephalic space is shorter. Its body nuclei are equal sized, clearly defined, and countable without caudal nucleus.

The microfilaria of *Brugia malayi* is irregular and stiff curves; the size is (177-230) μm×(5-6) μm. The cephalic space is longer. Its body nuclei are unequal-sized, coalescing, and uncountable with two caudal nuclei (Tab. 2-15-1).

Tab. 2-15-1 Morphological differences of microfilariae between *Wuchereria bancrofti* and *Brugia malayi*

Species	*Wuchereria bancrofti*	*Brugia malayi*
Size/μm	(244-296)×(5. 3-7)	(177-230)×(5-6)
Appearance	graceful, sweeping curves	irregular, stiff curves
Cephalic space (length : width)	shorter (1 : 1 or 1 : 2)	longer (2 : 1)
Body nuclei	equal-sized, clearly defined, countable	unequal-sized, coalescing, uncountable
Terminal nuclei	no	two

4. Slide specimens of filariform larva (L3) in mosquito mouthparts

Observe slide specimens of filariform larva (L3) in mosquito mouthparts.

5. Pathological specimen

Observe pathological specimen of elephantiasis of scrotum.

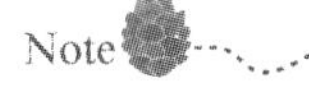

Ⅵ *Trichinella spiralis*

1. The stained specimen of adult (observation with low-power microscope)

It is small. The front end is thinner than the back end, and the esophagus is composed of long single-cell. The female is 3-4 mm long, and the tail is blunt round. The male is 1.4-1.5 mm long and has mating appendages at the tail end.

2. The stained specimen of larva (observation with low-power microscope)

It is elongated and curled into a spiral shape, with a wall forming an oval or prismatic cyst, containing 1 or 2 larvae. The cyst is arranged in parallel with the striated muscle fibers.

Individual observation

Fertilized egg and unfertilized egg of *Ascaris lumbricoides*. The eggs of *Trichuris trichiura*, *Enterobius vermicularis* and hookworm. The microfilaria of filaria.

[Experimental Report]

Draw fertilized egg and unfertilized egg of *Ascaris lumbricoides*. Draw the eggs of *Trichuris trichiura*, *Enterobius vermicularis* and hookworm. Draw the microfilaria of filaria.

[Questions]

(1) Can early infection of roundworm be ruled out with failure of fecal examination to detect roundworm eggs?

(2) Could oral ingestion of roundworm eggs cause roundworm infection?

(3) What are the similarities and differences between the life cycles of whipworm and roundworm?

(4) Description the main identification points of *Ancylostoma duodenale* and *Necator americanus*.

(5) Can filariasis be caused by transfusion of blood containing microfilariae? Why is that?

(6) How is filariasis diagnosed? Why would you do that?

(7) How to identify human infected filariasis body? What is the clinical value of species identification of filaria?

(Fang Tian, Feng Lu)

Experiment 16 Examination of Helminths

[Experimental Objectives]

Note

(1) To learn methods commonly used in feces examination.

(2) To be familiar with the techniques of transparent adhesive paper method, larva of hookworm culturing method, quantitative transparency method (modified Kato's method),

water washing precipitation method, miracidium hatching method and circumoval precipitin test.

(3) To learn the morphological characters of helminths eggs.

[Experimental Contents]

Method for examination of helminths in fecal specimens

Ⅰ Collection of fecal specimens

(1) Provide client with a waxed paper box or a cup (container must be clean and dry) to collect feces. Instruct client to dispose feces directly into container or a piece of paper and transfer feces to container with bamboo stick, and prevent contamination. Feces should not mix with urine and other body fluids, etc.

(2) The feces must be fresh and the inspection time should not exceed 24 h.

(3) The following information should be clearly marked on containers containing fecal specimens: patient's name, specimen number, date of collection, and time of patient's defecation.

(4) In order to obtain satisfactory results, fecal specimens must be sufficient (pigeon egg size). Specimens should not be mixed with urine and other dirt.

(5) If the specimen cannot be examined immediately, put the paper box containing the specimen in a refrigerator. Do not put the specimen in a warm place or in the sun.

Ⅱ Check for common helminths eggs

Methods: transparent adhesive paper method, larva of hookworm culturing method, quantitative transparency method (modified Kato's method), water washing precipitation method, and miracidium hatching method.

Self operation: feces direct smear method, NaCl saturated solution floatation method.

1. Feces direct smear method

Feces direct smear method is the most common method for examining helminths eggs in feces. In order not to change the osmotic pressure of the smear, physiological saline is used as the diluent of feces, so that the parasites and parasitic eggs stuck together with feces are dispersed in the smear through the dilution effect of physiological saline, which does not hinder the transmission of light, but also exposes the morphological structure of parasites and parasitic eggs. So it is easy to identify in microscopic examination. This method is the most widely used method.

Materials: microscope, slide, bamboo stick or toothpick, physiological saline, etc.

Method: transfer a small amount of fecal sample to 3 drops of physiological clean saline on a clean slide. Mix to obtain a fairly dense uniform smear free of large lumps. An oval fecal film about 4 cm long and 1.8 cm wide was applied for microscopic examination.

Matters needing attention:

(1) To judge the thickness of fecal film: one can see the words printed in the newspaper through the fecal film.

(2) If there is pus and blood in the feces, this part should be taken for smear.

(3) The fecal smear takes up about 2/3 of the slide. The feces should not be close to the edge. The coarse particles on the smear should be removed to avoid fouling the platform and fingers.

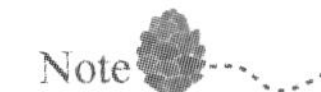

(4)The microscope must be placed flat on the table and must not be tilted. The order of microscopic examination is to observe with a low-power microscope first and turn to a high-power microscope when suspicious.

(5)Three smears per specimen can improve the detection rate. Identify parasitic egg and distinguish them from food residues such as various kinds of plant cells, yeast, pollen, plant fiber, etc. The fecal smear must be kept wet during examination.

(6)Pay attention to prevent the smear being dry. When necessary, add physiological saline again.

2. Floating clustering method

Using a liquid with high relative density, the helminths eggs were raised and concentrated on the liquid surface for examination. There are two commonly used methods: NaCl saturated solution floatation method and zinc sulfate flotation method.

(1)NaCl saturated solution floatation method: NaCl saturated solution is a liquid with high relative density, so that the helminths eggs float up and focus on the liquid surface for inspection. This method is mainly used for the inspection of hookworm eggs.

Materials: floating cup (or penicillin bottle), bamboo stick, glass slide, dropper, microscope, NaCl saturated solution (relative density is 1.20). NaCl saturated solution preparation: slowly add salt into a container filled with boiling water, constantly stirring, until salt is no longer dissolved and there is salt precipitation on the bottom of the container.

Method: mix small lumps of fecal material (about peanut-sized) with small amount of NaCl saturated solution in a floating cup. Then add up to the rim of the cup, cover with a glass slide and allow to contact with it (avoid any air bubble). After 15-20 min, lift the glass slide vertically and turn it over for microscopic examination for eggs.

Matters needing attention: ①This method is suitable for the eggs with low relative density, and has the best effect on checking the hookworm eggs. It can also be used to check other nematode eggs and tapeworm eggs, but it is not suitable for the examination of fluke eggs. ②Coarse slag floating above the liquid surface should be removed. ③When the glass slide is placed over the cup, avoid bubbles. ④The turning speed should not be too fast to prevent the fecal liquid from falling here and there.

(2)Zinc sulfate flotation method.

Materials: centrifugal tube, centrifuge, 33% zinc sulfate solution (relative density is 1.18), pipette, 40-60 mesh metal screen, etc.

Method: the filtered feces were poured into the centrifugal tube and centrifuged at 1500-2000 r/min for 2 min, repeat for 3-4 times, until the water was clear. Finally, the supernatant was poured out and zinc sulfate solution was added to the sediment. After homogenization, add zinc sulfate solution to 1 cm from tube mouth and centrifuge at the same speed for 2 min. Pick the fecal liquid from the surface with a metal ring and place it on a glass slide for microscopic examination.

Matters needing attention: ①This method is suitable for the examination of protozoa cysts, nematode eggs and *Hymenolepis nana* eggs. ②When examining cysts, drop 1 drop of iodized solution and cover coverslip.

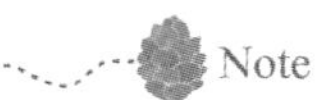
Note

3. Sedimentation

The relative density of helminths eggs is high and can be deposited on the bottom, which is helpful for the concentration of worm eggs and improve the detection rate. However, the effects of this method for hookworm eggs and some protozoa cysts with low relative density are poor.

(1) Water washing precipitation method: it is a traditional method for the examination of intestinal parasite eggs, which is suitable for the examination of many kinds of helminths eggs.

Materials: 500 ml or 1000 ml triangulation cup or enamel cup, 40-60 mesh metal screen, glass stick, straw, etc.

Method: take about 30 g of feces (the size of an egg), screen it through a metal screen into a triangulation cup or enamel cup filled with clear water, let it stand for 20-30 min, pour away the upper layer of feces water, retain the sediment, and then add clear water again, and change the water every 20 min until the water is clear (3-5 times). Finally, the upper layer was poured out, and the sediment was retained. The bottom sediment was absorbed by capillary to make 1-3 smears for microscopic examination.

Matters needing attention: ①There should not have a break when pouring water, so as not to float or dump sediment. ② The operation process should absolutely prevent mutual contamination, and the equipment used should be repeatedly cleaned. ③ When inspecting schistosoma eggs, the precipitation time should not be too long, especially when the room temperature is higher than 15 ℃, because the miracidium inside the eggs are easy to hatch. ④Increasing the number of smears can increase the detection rate.

(2) Centrifugal precipitation: the above fecal solution was centrifuged at 1500-2000 r/min for 1-2 min, remove the supernatant, inject water and centrifuge. The sedimentation was repeated for 3-4 times until the supernatant was clarified. Finally, the supernatant was removed and the sediment was taken for microscopic examination. This method is time- and labor-saving and suitable for clinical examination.

(3) Merthiolate-iodine-formaldehyde centrifugation (MIFC) sedimentation method: this method can be used to concentrate, fix and stain feces, and is suitable for the examination of protozoa cysts, trophozoites, and helminths eggs and larvae.

Reagent formula: ① Liquid A (merthiolate-iodine-formaldehyde solution): 200 ml 1/1000 thiomersal tincture, 25 ml formaldehyde, 5 ml glycerin, 200 ml distilled water. ②Liquid B (5% Lugo's solution): 5 g iodine, 10 g potassium iodide, 100 ml distilled water. During the inspection, 2.35 ml of liquid A and 0.15 ml of liquid B were mixed and reserved.

Method: a mixture of 5 ml above-mentioned mixed solution with 1 g of feces were taken, and the coarse residue was filtered out. 4 ml diethyl ether was added, and the mixture was fully shaken. The mixture was placed in a centrifugal tube for 2 min and centrifuged for 1-2 min at 1500-2000 r/min to divide into 4 layers of diethyl ether, fecal residue, merthiolate-iodine-formaldehyde solution and precipitate.

Matters needing attention: ① This method not only has good concentration effect, but also does not damage the morphology of cysts and eggs, and is easy to observe and identify. ②The effect of this method is better than zinc sulfate flotation method for feces containing more fat.

4. Quantitative transparency method (modified Kato's method)

The thick fecal smear was transparentized with glycerin, and the visual field background was light green.

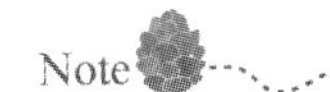

Materials: ①100 mesh metal screen, scraper, cellophane, polystyrene quantitative plate (size 40 mm×30 mm×1.37 mm, mold hole is a long round hole or strip hole, and the average fecal sample taken is 41.7 mg). ②Glycerin-malachite green solution: glycerin 100 ml, 3% malachite green aqueous solution 1 ml, distilled water 100 ml. ③Cut the cellophane into 24 mm×50 mm and soak it in glycerin-malachite green solution for 24 h.

Method: a quantitative plate was placed on a glass slide, and the metal screen was covered on the feces sample. About 50 mg of feces was scraped from the screen with a scraper, and both ends of the quantitative plate were pressed with two fingers of one hand to fill the mold hole with the feces on the scraper and scrape away the excess feces. Remove the quantitative plate, leaving a long form of feces on the slide, and then cover the feces with a cellophane strip containing glycerin-malachite green solution, flatten and press, so that the feces under the cellophane spread into an oval shape. The feces was transparentized for 1-2 h and examined and counted eggs under a microscope.

Matters needing attention:

(1) This method is suitable for the detection of helminths eggs because of the large amount of feces samples, thus improving the detection rate.

(2) It is necessary to master the appropriate thickness and transparent time of fecal film. If the fecal film is thick and transparent time of fecal film is short, it is difficult to find eggs. If the transparent time is too long, the egg is deformed, the egg shell is broken, and it is not easy to identify. The transparent time was 30 min during the inspection of hookworm eggs.

(3) The quantitative plate with two strip holes is easier to press out the proper thickness of fecal film.

(4) Eggs per gram (EPG) = number of eggs on each smear×24×fecal trait coefficient. Fecal trait coefficient: formed feces was 1, semi-formed feces was 1.5, soft and wet feces was 2, and watery feces was 4.

5. Larva of hookworm culturing method

It is designed according to the principle that the larva in the hookworm eggs can hatch in a short time under the appropriate temperature and humidity.

Materials: 1.2 cm×12 cm tube, filter paper strip (filter paper was cut into about 1.5 cm×10 cm T-shaped strip), constant temperature incubator, etc.

Method: fold the filter paper strip in half into an angle, take a clean test tube, and add 2-3 ml cold boiled water or distilled water, so that the lower end of the filter paper strip can just immerse in the water after inserted into the test tube. Take 0.2-0.4 g feces, evenly coat in the middle of the filter paper strip, and insert the filter paper strip into the test tube, but do not contact the bottom, pay attention not to make feces mixed with water, and culture at 20-30 ℃. 3-5 d later, the water at the bottom of the tube was examined with naked eyes or magnifying glass for milk white larva of hookworm with serpentine movement.

Matters needing attention:

(1) Before operation, write patient's name or number on the horizontal section of the filter paper strip with pencil.

(2) Water is added daily along the tube wall during cultivation to maintain water level.

(3) When inserting the filter paper strip into the test tube, do not touch the water with the feces.

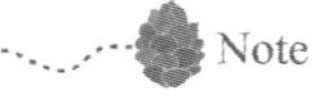

(4) If no larva was found after 3 d, cultivation and observation should be continued until day 5.

6. Miracidium hatching method

According to the characteristics that the miracidium in the eggs of *Schistosoma japonicum* can hatch in a short time in clean water with appropriate temperature, the method combined with water washing precipitation method is suitable for the feces examination of early schistosomiasis patients.

Materials: triangle flask, 500 ml or 1000 ml conical measuring cup, 40-60 mesh metal screen, glass rod, straw, etc.

Method: about 30 g of feces(the size of an egg) were collected and concentrated by water washing precipitation method. The sediment was absorbed by capillary tube, and 3 smears were made for microscopic examination. If no egg was found, all the sediment was poured into a 500 ml triangle flask, and water was added to the mouth of the flask, and incubated at 20-30 ℃. The results were observed with naked eyes or magnifying glass at 4 h, 12 h and 24 h later. If white dots are seen swimming in a straight line below the surface of the water, they are known as miracidia.

Matters needing attention:

(1) The feces must be fresh, not fresh or too little feces can affect the detection rate.

(2) The upper layer of precipitation must be cleared when changing water, otherwise the observation results will be affected.

(3) When the temperature is high, the miracidium can hatch in a short time, so the feces should be washed with 1.2% salt water or ice water in summer, and the room temperature water should be used for the last time.

(4) When the water is poured, there can not have interruption, so as not to float or dump the sediment.

(5) Hatch water must be clear water, and the appropriate pH is 7.2-7.6. If it contains too much salt or residual chlorine or contains NH_2, it will affect hatching.

(6) The operation should be absolutely protected from mutual contamination. The equipments should be cleaned repeatedly and the eggs should be killed with boiling water.

(7) The results should be carefully identified with water worms. The miracidia are the size of a needle tip, long round, gray white, refraction, and the size is same. They usually swim quickly in a straight line at a distance of 1-4 cm from the water surface and then turn when hitting the wall. If necessary, it can be absorbed on a slide and observed under a microscope.

7. Nylon bag egg collection method

This method is mainly used for concentration examination of schistosoma eggs.

Materials: 60 mesh copper screen, 120 mesh nylon bag (inner bag, with the depth of 10 cm, and the mouth diameter of 8 cm), 260 mesh nylon bag (outer bag, with the depth of 15 cm, and the mouth diameter of 9 cm), triangle measuring cup. Put a nylon bag of 120 mesh(aperture slightly larger than schistosoma egg) into a nylon bag of 260 mesh (aperture slightly smaller than schistosoma egg) for later use.

Method: add water to the feces first, after 60 mesh copper screen filtering the coarse fecal slag, pour filter waste into two sets of nylon bag together, remove the copper screen, continue to pour water flushing bag waste slag, and put the bag gently vibration to speed up filtering, until leaching liquid was clean, and then collect fecal slag inside the 260 mesh nylon bag for microscopic examination or miracidium hatching.

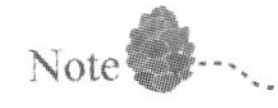

Matters needing attention: compared with the precipitation method, this method has the advantages of shorter time, less egg loss, less equipment used and convenient for mobile survey, but the nylon bag must be strictly cleaned to prevent cross-contamination.

8. Tapeworm examination

In order to evaluate the efficacy of tapeworms repellent, worms are often identified and counted by panning from feces. The method is to take all feces of the patient 24-72 h after taking medicine, add water to stir, filter out the feces residue with a 40 mesh screen or gauze, rinse with water repeatedly, and pour into a large glass dish filled with water. Check the worms with black paper lining the glass dish.

9. Taenia tapeworm gravid proglottid examination method

After the tapeworm proglottides being detected in the feces, clothes, and bedding, they were washed with clean water, placed between two slides, and gently pressed. The internal structure was observed by light, and the species of tapeworm was identified according to the number of uterine branches. If the number of uterine branches on one side is less than 15, it was *Taenia solium*; otherwise, it was *Taenia saginata*. If the above method can not recognize, slowly inject carbon ink or ink or cargored liquid (potassium alum saturated liquid 100 ml, cargored 3 g, glacial acetic acid 10 ml. After mixing, it was placed in a 37 ℃ incubator overnight, and applied after filtration) into the uterus by a small syringe, and count after uterine branches appeared. After the inspection, all the utensils used must be disinfected to kill the eggs.

Ⅲ Microscopic examination of helminths mixed eggs specimens

Low-power microscope is used to search for eggs and determine which kind of helminths egg it is.

Nematodes, trematodes and tapeworms are three important medical helminths. The usual diagnostic method is to examine the eggs. The characteristics used to identify various eggs are as follows. ①Size: the length and width of eggs can be measured, and they are always within a certain range. ②Shape: each egg has its own special shape. ③Color: some eggs are colorless, while others are yellow or brown. ④Thickness of egg shell: some species have thick egg shell, while others have thin egg shell. ⑤Characteristic structures, such as egg lid, spines, plugs, and hooks. ⑥Egg contents: when eggs are excreted in feces, the eggs of some species are composed of single cells, while others may be composed of many cells. Some eggs are usually embryonic (i. e. contain one larva). Sometimes fecal specimens have been stored for several hours or 1-2 d as long as the eggs can develop to a later stage. Eggs change as the developmental stage changes. When excreted in feces, an ascarid egg usually only contains 1 egg cell. While the single egg cell could split, so the old samples can be seen eggs with 2 or 4 egg cells. In the fecal samples stored for hours, hookworm eggs may contain 16, 32, or more egg cells. Eggs could develop into embryos within 12-24 h of excretion, and then hatched larvae. Therefore, the ideal samples for diagnosis should be fresh feces.

Method of examination for perianal parasites

Transparent adhesive paper method

This method is mainly used for inspection of pinworm eggs and taenia tapeworm eggs. Pinworms spawn around the anus. Taenia tapeworm eggs often stick to the anus. They are examined with transparent adhesive paper affixed with a glue surface.

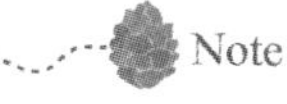

Materials:6 cm long and 2 cm wide of transparent adhesive paper,xylene.

Method:paste the skin around anus using the transparent adhesive paper,stick to the slide and examine by microscope.

Matters needing attention:

(1)Uncover one end of the transparent adhesive paper when inspection,add a drop of xylene between the slide and the transparent adhesive paper,and then stick back to the original place for microscopic examination.

(2)The exmination should be carried out before excretion in the morning.

(3) Attention should be paid to distinguish eggs and bubbles during microscopic examination.

Method for examination of helminths in blood samples

1. Examination of microfilariae in blood samples

In China,there are two kinds of parasitic filariae,they are *Wuchereria bancrofti* and *Brugia malayi*. Their microfilariae all appear in peripheral blood at night. Therefore, all blood tests must be conducted after 9 pm. A staining test can used to determine the species.

(1)Microfilariae thick blood film test:take 3 drops (about 60 μl) of blood from earlobe or fingertip. The blood drops were placed in the center of a clean and dry slide,and spread to an oval thick blood film of 1 cm×2 cm by the angle of another slide. Blood film should be uniformly thickness,flat, naturally dry and having neat edge. Hemolysis was carried out with distilled water or cooled boiled water drops to cover blood film. After 5-10 min, the blood water was poured out and water was added to repeat hemolysis once,until the blood film was not red. The hemoglobin was removed from the blood film, so it turned gray and white. Preparation, hemolysis, fixation and Giemsa staining of thick blood film are the same as those of plasmodium. Hematoxylin staining was better. Search for microfilariae under 10×objective lens. At this point, microfilariae are easy to detect. If microfilariae are found, exchange the oil immersion lens to identify the species. Observe the complete slice.

(2)Hematoxylin staining method.

Preparation of staining solution:1 g of hematoxylin was dissolved in 10 ml pure alcohol or 95% alcohol,with saturated ammonium aluminum sulfate (8%-10%) 100 ml,and poured into a brown bottle. The bottle was tightly bound with two layers of gauze,oxidized in sunlight for 2-4 weeks and filtered, and 25 ml glycerin and 25 ml methanol were added. The staining solution should be diluted about 10 times when use.

Staining method: the hemolysed and fixed thick blood film was stained in Delafield hematoxylin solution for 10-15 min, separated in 1% acid alcohol for 1-2 min, washed with distilled water for 1-5 min until the blood film turned blue,and then stained with 1% eosin for 0. 5-1 min,washed with water for 2-5 min,dried and examined under microscope.

Matters needing attention:

①Microfilariae thick blood film test is the most common method for the diagnosis of filariasis. This test can be used for general examination. The species of worms in the positive patients can be identified after staining by this method.

②Due to the large amount of blood, hemolysis should be carried out after the blood film being dried completely,otherwise the blood film is easy to fall off in the process of hemolysis. Generally,it is best to do hemolysis on the third day after blood collection. Do not heat or dry in

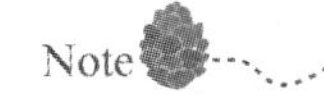

sunlight, in order to avoid the red blood cells from degenerated and insoluble. The blood film is difficult to do hemolysis after placed too long.

③Living microfilariae collection method: fill a half tube of distilled water in a centrifugal tube, add 10-12 drops of blood, add physiological saline to mix, centrifuge for 3 min, and take sediment for examination. Or 1 ml venous blood was taken and placed in a test tube containing 0.1 ml 3.8% sodium citrate, shaken well, and 9 ml water was added. After red blood cells were dissolved, centrifugation was performed at 3000 r/min for 2 min. Remove the supernatant and centrifuge again with water, and sediment was taken for microscopic examination.

2. Circumoval precipitin test (COPT)

In the COPT, a cotton stick was dipped in liquid paraffin to draw two coarse paraffin lines 20 mm apart on a glass slide, and 2 drops of tested serum (equivalent to 0.1 ml) were added between the paraffin lines. A few dried schistosoma eggs (100-150 eggs) were collected by needle tip and mixed evenly in serum, covered with a 24 mm×24 mm coverslip, and sealed with paraffin around. Place the above glass slide in a wet box at 37 ℃ for 48 h, and observe. The results were observed with low-power microscope. If necessary, react for 72 h, and then observe the results. The typical positive reaction was the refraction precipitate in the shape of bubble, finger, sheet or elongated curl, with neat edge and firm adhesion to egg shell. For negative patients, the whole film must be observed. 100 mature eggs were observed in positive patients, and cyclic sedimentation rate and reaction intensity ratio were calculated. Cyclic sedimentation rate refers to the number of eggs with sediment in 100 mature eggs. The cyclic sedimentation rate≥5% can be reported as positive, 1%-4% as weak positive.

[Questions]

(1)What are the main differences in morphology and life history between trematode and nematode?

(2)What are the methods to diagnose hookworm infection? Compare their advantages and disadvantages.

(3)Can feces examination be used to diagnose pinworm infection? Why is that?

(Fang Tian, Feng Lu)

Experiment 17 Amoeba

[Experimental Objectives]

To master the morphological structures of trophozoite and cyst of *Entamoeba histolytica*, and the differentiation with *Entamoeba coli* based on the key points of their morphology identification.

[Experimental Materials]

Teaching specimens (slices), microscopes, cedar oil, xylene, lens wipping paper, etc.

[Experimental Contents]

Teaching specimens

Ⅰ *Entamoeba histolytica*

1. The iron-haematoxylin stained specimen of *Entamoeba histolytica* trophozoites (observation with oil immersion lens)

The worms are dark blue with irregular shape. It is 25-60 μm in diameter. The ectoplasm is lightly colored, and the endoplasm is granular with dark colored. The boundary between endoplasm and ectoplasm is clear. The ectoplasm often shows tongue-like or finger-like pseudopodia. The endoplasm has an arc nucleus, and contains swallowed red blood cells. The nucleus is vesicular, and the inner edge of the nuclear membrane has a circle of uniformly sized and neatly arranged chromatin granules. The nucleolus is smaller, and in the middle mostly. The reticular nuclear fibers are often seen between the nucleolus and the nuclear membrane.

2. The iron-haematoxylin stained specimen of *Entamoeba histolytica* cysts (observation with oil immersion lens)

The cysts are dark blue with spherical shape. It is 5-20 μm in diameter. The cyst wall is thin and stainless with strong refractive, and the blank circle around it is caused by the extension and contraction of the cyst when making specimens. There are 1-4 nuclei in the cyst, and the structure is the same as that of the trophozoite. There are one to several dark blue and rod-like chromatoid bodies. The glycogen is dissolved during staining process and only vacuole is left. In mature cysts, the chromatoid bodies and glycogen vacuoles are often lacking.

3. The unstained specimen of *Entamoeba histolytica* cysts (observation with high-power microscope)

In the physiological saline direct smear of feces, the cyst is spherical and small, the nucleus is not easy to see, and the rod-like and refractive chromatoid bodies can be seen.

4. The iodine stained specimen of *Entamoeba histolytica* cysts (observation with high-power microscope)

The cyst wall is thin and stainless with strong refractive, and the worms inside cysts are yellow. There are 1-4 nuclei in the cyst. The nucleus is small and not easy to see. In the cysts with 1-2 nuclei, there are rod-like chromatoid bodies and brown yellow glycogen vacuole (in mature cysts, most have vanished).

Ⅱ *Entamoeba coli*

1. The iron-haematoxylin stained specimen of *Entamoeba coli* trophozoites (observation with oil immersion lens)

It is slightly larger than the trophozoite of *Entamoeba histolytica* normally. The ectoplasm is less, and the endoplasm is coarse granular. The boundary between endoplasm and ectoplasm is unclear. Food vacuole of the endoplasm contains bacteria, yeasts and starch granules, but no red blood cells. The chromatic granules in the inner edge of the nuclear membrane are uniform in size, and irregular in arrangement. The nucleolus is slightly larger and mostly deviated.

2. The iron-haematoxylin stained specimen of *Entamoeba coli* cysts (observation with oil immersion lens)

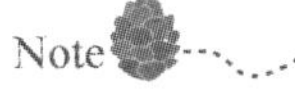
Note

It is spherical and large, 10-30 μm in diameter, with 1-8 nuclei. The structure and morphology are similar to the trophozoite. In immature cyst, there are glycogen vacuoles. Chromatoid bodies are in bundles or fragments with thin and uneven ends.

3. The iodine stained specimen of *Entamoeba coli* cysts (observation with high-power microscope)

It's globular and large, and the cyst wall is slightly thicker with strong refractive. The worms inside cysts are faint yellow. There are 1-8 non-colored and shiny nuclei. The glycogen vacuoles were claybank and dispersed.

Individual observation

(1) Observe the iodine stained specimen of *Entamoeba histolytica* cysts.

(2) Observe the iodine stained specimen of *Entamoeba coli* cysts.

(3) Observe the iron-haematoxylin stained specimen of *Entamoeba histolytica* and *Entamoeba coli* cysts.

Video

Viewing video of amoeba.

[Experimental Report]

Draw the trophozoite and cyst of iodine stained *Entamoeba histolytica* and *Entamoeba coli*.

[Questions]

(1) Describe the morphological characteristics of trophozoites and cysts of *Entamoeba histolytica* and *Entamoeba coli*.

(2) What are the characteristics of the life cycle of *Entamoeba histolytica*?

(Fang Tian, Feng Lu)

Experiment 18 Sporozoa

[Experimental Objectives]

(1) To study the life cycle of plasmodia and understand their pathogenic mechanism.

(2) To study laboratory diagnostic methods of malarial parasites.

(3) To study morphological structures of plasmodia, to identify morphological structures of developing stages of erythrocytic schizogony and gametocytes of *Plasmodium vivax*, and to differentiate the ring form and gametocytes of *Plasmodium vivax* from *Plasmodium falciparum*.

(4) To identify insect vector of malaria.

(5) To learn simple method of experiment with plasmodia.

[Experimental Materials]

Teaching specimens (slices), microscopes, cedar oil, xylene, lens wipping paper, etc.

[Experimental Contents]

Teaching specimens

Ⅰ *Plasmodium vivax* in thin blood film (observation with oil immersion lens)

(1) Early trophozoite (ring form): 2.5 μm in size, vacuole in the center, and peripheral thin rim of blue cytoplasm surrounding the red nucleus. Ring occupies one-third of the size of red blood cells (RBCs).

(2) Late trophozoite (amoeboid): large, amoeboid, with more cytoplasm and prominent vacuole.

(3) Schizont: large, 9-10 μm, and completely fills the enlarged RBC.

(4) Female gametocyte: spherical, larger than male. The cytoplasm was dyed deep blue. Nucleus was dyed dark red and located on the side of the worm. Pigments is dispersed in distribution.

(5) Male gametocyte: same as female but smaller. The cytoplasm was dyed pale blue and nucleus was dyed pale red.

Ⅱ *Plasmodium vivax* in thick blood film

The morphology is atypical normally, because of protozoa being shrivel and break during the drying process, and also for overlap or erect or tilt of the RBCs, protozoa overlap, fold and deform, which making the parasites present bird-like, exclamation mark or question mark, etc. At the same time, because RBCs are destroyed in the hemolysis process, some characteristics of RBCs parasitized by malaria parasites are almost disappeared. In addition, after Giemsa or Wright staining, there are many other substances in various forms on the thick blood film, which makes the morphological diagnosis be difficult. Therefore, we must grasp the nucleus, cytoplasm, malarial pigments and vacuoles of malaria parasites to observe and analyze repeatedly, and compare them with the morphological characteristics of malaria parasites in thin blood film, to master the microscopic examination technology of thick blood film quickly.

1. Early trophozoite (ring form)

The nucleus is dotted and small. The cytoplasm is few and have different shape. The body can be bird-like, exclamation mark and question mark, etc.

2. Late trophozoite (amoeboid)

It's large and changeable in shape. The malarial pigments are brown-yellow, look like tobacco filaments.

3. Early schizont (immature schizont)

The morphology of the parasite changes greatly, with more than 2 nuclei and brown-yellow malarial pigments.

4. Schizont (mature schizont)

It's large, with 12-24 merozoites, which resemble a bunch of grapes. The brown-yellow malarial pigments are concentrated in lumps.

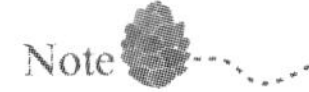

5. Gametocyte

Gametocyte is round or elliptic, with large body and nucleus. The cytoplasm often breaks, sometimes corrodes and disappears completely. The difference between male and female is often not obvious. It should be differentiated from late trophozoite.

Ⅲ *Plasmodium falciparum* in thin blood film (observation with oil immersion lens)

1. Early trophozoite(ring form)

The cytoplasm is few. The ring's diameter is about 1/5 of the diameter of RBC. Sometimes there are two chromatin dots in one ring or multiple rings in one RBC.

2. Gametocyte

Note the particular sausage or crescent shape, position of chromatin, distribution of pigment granules and alteration of infected RBC.

(1) Female gametocyte: crescentic (banana); long slender and pointed tips; larger than RBC. The cytoplasm was dyed blue. Nucleus was dyed deep red.

(2) Male gametocyte: same as female but broader and shorter; rounded tips. The cytoplasm was dyed pale blue with reddish tinges. Both nucleus and pigments are scattered.

Ⅳ Malaria parasites development in mosquitoes (observation with oil immersion lens)

1. Oocysts

The ookinete penetrates into the stomach wall of the mosquito and lies just beneath the basement membrane. It becomes rounded and is covered by a thin elastic membrane to form oocyst. Several thousands of mature oocysts can be found.

2. Sporozoites

Oocysts undergo sporogony (meiosis) to produce thousands of spindle-shaped sporozoites measuring 10-15 μm in length with apical complex anteriorly.

Ⅴ Microscopic examnination of *Toxoplasma gondii* specimens (observation with oil immersion lens)

The trophozoites of Toxoplasma gondii stained with the Giemsa or Wright staining, are examined under oil immersion lens for the parasites. It's banana or crescent-shaped, one end of the organism often appears more rounded, curving than the other end. The size is (4-7) μm × (2-4) μm. It has a single centrally located red nucleus, with a smaller accessory nucleus at one end. The nuclear membrane and nucleoli could be observed after iron-hematoxylin staining.

Individual observation

(1) Observe Giemsa or Wright stained specimens of *Plasmodium vivax* thin blood film.

(2) Observe Giemsa or Wright stained specimens of *Plasmodium falciparum* thin blood film.

Demonstration of the preparation of blood film of malaria parasites and staining

(1) Preparation of both thin and thick blood films at one slide. Collect 2 drops of blood from infected patient and place on one end of a clean slide. Spread one drop of blood near end to the size of two-fen coin with the corner of another slide to make up thick film. Holding another slide at an angle of 30°～45°, and in contact with the other drop of blood, touch the first drop of blood and let it spread along the line of contact between the slides. Then push the slide along with a

smooth and rapid movement, thus drawing the blood out to form a thin film. Let it dry. Its thickness depends on the size of the drop, the angle between the slides and rapidity of which the smear is made.

(2) Giemsa stain. Fix the dried thin blood film with methyl alcohol (avoid fixing the thick blood film) and let it dry. Cover with 2% Giemsa solution on the smears. Let it stay for 30-60 min. Wash by pouring neutral distilled water over the slide until color does not run from it to a noticeable extent. Drain and stand on end to dry.

[Experimental Report]

(1) Draw the morphological structures of *Plasmodium vivax* in RBCs.

(2) Draw ring form, and female and male gametophytes of *Plasmodium falciparum* in a thin blood film (Giemsa or Wright staining), and indicate the structure names of the various parts.

[Questions]

(1) How to identify *Plasmodium vivax* and *Plasmodium falciparum* on thin blood film?

(2) According to the life cycle of *Plasmodium vivax*, explain the paroxysm, recrudescence and relapse.

(3) Describe the morphological characteristics of *Toxoplasma gondii* and its harm to humans.

(Fang Tian, Feng Lu)

Experiment 19 Flagellates

[Experimental Objectives]

(1) To study morphological structures of *Leishmania donovani* and *Trichomonas vaginalis*.

(2) To be familiar with the morphology and inspection methods of *Giardia lamblia*.

[Experimental Materials]

Teaching specimens (slices), microscopes, cedar oil, xylene, lens wipping paper, etc.

[Experimental Contents]

Teaching specimens

Ⅰ *Leishmania donovani*

1. Giemsa or Wright stained specimen of amastigotes of *Leishmania donovani* (observation with oil immersion lens)

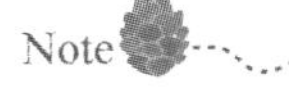

It is round or oval, 2.8-4.4 μm in size. Nucleus measures less than 1 μm, is big and round, and locates in the center or side of the cell. Kinetoplast consists of copies of mitochondrial DNA. It is made up blepharoplast and parabasal body connected by a delicate fibril (cytoskeleton). It lies at right angle to the nucleus. Axoneme extends from blepharoplast to the cell wall. It represents the intracellular portion (root) of flagellum. There is no external flagellum and it is nonmotile. Vacuole is a clear space, and lies adjacent to axoneme.

2. Giemsa or Wright stained specimen of promastigotes of *Leishmania donovani* (observation with oil immersion lens)

This is an extracellular form, which is at the infective stage to humans. It is motile and contains single anterior flagellum. It is 8-15 μm in length. Nucleus is situated centrally and kinetoplast is placed near the anterior end transversely.

Ⅱ *Trichomonas vaginalis*

1. Giemsa or Wright stained specimen of *Trichomonas vaginalis* (observation with oil immersion lens)

It is pear-shaped or round, measures 7-23 μm long and 5-15 μm wide. It bears 5 flagella (4 anterior flagella and 1 lateral flagellum). It doesn't come out free posteriorly. The undulating membrane is supported on to the surface of the parasite by a rod-like structure called as costa. The axostyle runs down the middle of the trophozoite and ends in the pointed end of the posterior pole. It has a single nucleus containing central karyosome with evenly distributed nuclear chromatin and the cytoplasm contains a number of siderophore granules along the axostyle.

2. Living specimen of *Trichomonas vaginalis* (observation with high-power microscope)

Under the suitable temperature (25-30 ℃), the front flagella of *Trichomonas vaginalis* can be seen swinging forward and moving spirally with the vibration of fluctuating membrane. The worm has strong flexibility and can often change its body shape to pass through obstacles. If the movement of the worm is intense and not easy to be observed, one drop of 1 : 10 serum should be added.

Ⅲ *Giardia lamblia*

1. The iron-haematoxylin stained specimen of *Giardia lamblia* trophozoites (observation with oil immersion lens)

The trophozoite has a falling leaf-like motility, usually measures 9-21 μm in length and 5-15 μm in width. In front view, it is inverted pear-shaped (or tear drop or tennis racket-shaped) with rounded anterior end and pointed posterior end. Laterally, it appears as a curved portion of a spoon (sickle-shaped). It is convex dorsally while the ventral surface has a concavity bearing a bilobed adhesive disc. Hence, it appears as sickle-shaped in lateral view. Trophozoite is bilaterally symmetrical. On each side from the midline, it bears one pair of nuclei, one pair of median bodies, four pairs of basal bodies or blepharoplast (from which the axoneme arises), four pairs of flagella (two pairs of lateral, one pair of ventral and one pair of caudal flagella), one pair of parabasal bodies (connected to basal bodies through which the axoneme passes) and one pair of axoneme or axostyle (the intracellular portion of the flagella).

2. The iron-haematoxylin stained specimen of *Giardia lamblia* cysts (observation with oil immersion lens)

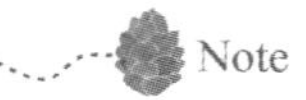

The cyst is oblong or oval, and measures (8-14) μm×(7-10) μm. It usually contains four nuclei and remnants of axonemes, basal bodies and parabasal bodies.

3. The iodine stained specimen of *Giardia lamblia* cysts (observation with high-power microscope)

It is yellow-green, refractive and has non-stained cyst wall. Intracystic nuclei, central corpuscles and flagellar axons are not stained but strong refractive.

Individual observation

(1) Observe Giesma or Wright stained specimen of amastigotes of *Leishmania donovani*.

(2) Examination of living and stained specimens of *Trichomonas vaginalis*.

The vaginal secretions or artificial cultures of patients with trichomonas vaginitis were taken as suspended droplet specimens or smear specimens. Covered with slides, trichomonas were first found under low-power microscope. Then switch to a high-power microscope, and the morphology and movement characteristics were carefully observed.

(3) Examination of iodine stained specimens of *Giardia lamblia* cyst.

Take a drop of *Giardia lamblia* cyst suspension (shake after absorption) on the slide, and cover. Then, a drop of iodine solution was added to the one side of the coverslip to make it gradually permeate to the other side. The cyst was found by low-power microscope, and the structure and morphology of the cyst were carefully observed under high-power microscope.

[Experimental Report]

(1) Draw morphological structures of amastigotes and promastigotes of *Leishmania donovani*, and indicate the structure name of each part.

(2) Draw the iodine stained cysts of *Giardia lamblia* and indicate the structure name of each part.

[Questions]

(1) What are the main types of flagellates that are parasitic in the human body?

(2) Describe the morphological characteristics of common human flagellates.

(3) What are the transmission routes of trichomonas vaginitis? How to prevent it?

(Fang Tian, Feng Lu)

Experiment 20 Ciliates

[Experimental Objectives]

To understand the basic morphological characteristics of *Balantidium coli*.

[Experimental Materials]

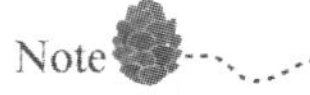

Teaching specimens (slices), microscopes, cedar oil, xylene, lens wipping paper, ect.

[Experimental Contents]

Teaching specimens: the iron-haematoxylin stained specimen of *Balantidium coli* (observation with oil immersion lens).

1. Trophozoite

It is oval shaped, and the average size is about 60 μm × 45 μm. Anterior end bears a groove (peristome) that leads to a mouth (cytostome) followed by a short funnel shaped gullet (cytopharynx) extending up to one-third of the body. The whole body is covered with a row of tiny delicate cilia (organ of locomotion). Cilia near to the mouth part appear to be longer and are called as "adoral cilia". The cytoplasm is divided into outer clear ectoplasm and inner granular endoplasm. The endoplasm contains two nuclei, two contractile vacuoles and numerous food vacuoles.

2. Cyst

It is round, and measures 40-60 μm in size, surrounding by a thick and transparent cyst wall. Cilia may be seen in younger cyst. But as the cyst matures, cilia are absorbed and disappeared.

[Questions]

Try to discuss the morphological characteristics of *Balantidium coli* and its harm to humans.

(Fang Tian, Feng Lu)

Experiment 21 Methods for Protozoa Diagnosis

[Experimental Objectives]

(1) To master the method of fecal direct smear iodine stain.

(2) To master the production and staining technologies of thick and thin blood film slides.

(3) To master the direct examination of vaginal smears to examine *Trichomonas vaginalis*.

[Experimental Materials]

Living *Trichomonas vaginalis* specimen, microscopes, cedar oil, xylene, lens wipping paper, coverslip, slide, etc.

[Experimental Contents]

Fecal protozoan examination

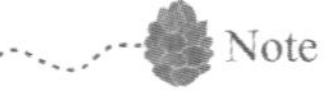

Direct smear method is essential for examining protozoa trophozoites and cysts in feces, because the protozoa trophozoite can be observed by physiological saline smear, such as the movements of pseudopodia, flagella, wave membrane, and cilia. For the cysts, some structures can only be seen clearly in fresh smears, such as the chromosomal chromosome of *Entamoeba histolytica* cyst, and the glycogen block of *Lodamoeba butschlii* cyst. Therefore, protozoa should be treated as a direct smear. For direct smear, it should be noted that the smear should be thin and uniform, and if the smear is thick, the protozoa are too small to be seen easily.

Flagellates and ciliates are easily found in the field of vision due to their faster activity. The amoeba pseudopod stretching activity is not obvious and difficult to be observed, so it is necessary to switch to the high-power microscope to observe carefully to determine whether it is amoeba. But in addition to the *Entamoeba histolytica* trophozoites can be determined for its pseudo-foot expansion and directional movement and red blood cells, many other kinds in the physiological saline smear is difficult to be determined. Therefore, it needs to be identified by iron-hematoxylin staining.

When checking the cyst of the protozoa, first observe its size, shape and refractive power under the low-power microscope, observe whether there is obvious wall structure, and distinguish it from other structures such as white blood cells, human yeast, fat globules and even small bubbles. When switching to a high-power microscope, observe the integrity of the cyst wall firstly, and then observe the difference in the refractive power inside the cyst, such as the parenchyma of *Entamoeba histolytica* cyst is short rod, and its refractive power is stronger than cytoplasm of cyst; the refractive power of the glycogen block of *Lodamoeba butschlii* cyst is also strong. These characteristics can be initially identified. To determine which protozoa it is, it still needs to be dyed with iodine solution, in order to further observe the characteristics of its nuclear and glycogen blocks. If you can not see their structural characteristics, you need to use iron-hematoxylin staining to determine.

Ⅰ Iodine solution staining for protozoal cysts

1. Equipments and medicines

Iodine solution (4 g potassium iodide was dissolved in 100 ml distilled water, and then 2 g iodine was added to be dissolved before use), etc.

2. Method

Use 1-2 drops of iodine solution instead of physiological saline for direct smear, and cover the coated specimen with a coverslip for microscopic examination. If the living trophozoites need to be examined at the same time, a drop of iodine solution can be placed directly on the side of the physiological saline smear. Cover the coverslip again. The cysts were examined on the side of iodine solution in the smear. On the other side, check the living trophozoites.

3. Matters needing attention

(1) After iodine solution staining, the cytoplasm of the cyst was stained yellow or light brown, while the nucleus was stained dark brown, and the perinuclear chromatosome was stained light yellow, but it may not be very clear. The glycogen contained in the cyst was dyed dark brown, and filaments could be seen in the iodine-stained flagellate cyst.

(2) The instruments for collecting specimens are required to be clean and free from contamination by sewage, drugs or aquatic protozoa.

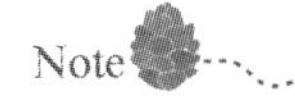

(3) For specimen collection, feces and other specimens should be left in the bedpan and spittoon, but not on wet ground or in public toilets, to prevent contamination.

(4) Protozoal specimens should be checked with fresh materials in time. Do not leave them for too long. The dead protozoa is difficult to identify.

(5) The abnormal parts of feces, such as blood, pus and mucus, should be selected for making smear.

Ⅱ Iron-hematoxylin staining of protozoal trophozoites and cysts

1. Equipments and medicines

22 mm×22 mm coverslips, staining dishes, cover glass forceps, writing brush, etc.

Schaudinns fixative solution: the ratio of saturated mercury chloride aqueous solution and 95% alcohol is 2∶1. Add 5 ml glacial acetic acid for every 100 ml.

Iodine alcohol: 1 g iodine was dissolved in 100 ml 70% alcohol.

4% (2%) ammonium ferric sulfate (alum) solution: 4 g (2 g) ammonium ferric sulfate was dissolved in 100 ml distilled water.

Hematoxylin concentrate: 1 g hematoxylin was dissolved in 10 ml anhydrous ethanol. When used, add 0.5 ml to 100 ml distilled water.

Alcohols: 30%, 50%, 70%, 80%, 90%, 95% and anhydrous ethanols.

Transparent agent: xylene or wintergreen oil.

Sealing tablets: neutral gum or Canadian gum.

2. Method

(1) The feces were thinly and evenly spread on a coverslip with another coverslip or a writing brush, and quickly placed in the fixative solution which had been warmed to 40 ℃. The trophozoite was fixed for 10 min, and the cyst was fixed for 20-30 min.

(2) Pour out the fixative solution, and add iodine alcohol and react for 30 min.

(3) Pour out the iodine alcohol and add 70% alcohol and rinse 2-3 times until the iodine color is exhausted.

(4) Rinse gently in running water for 10 min.

(5) 4% alum solution was added, the trophozoites react for 15 min, and the cyst react for 30 min.

(6) Pour out the alum solution and use tap water for 3 times (pour after filling, repeat 3 times).

(7) Add 0.5% iron-hematoxylin solution, stain for 5-10 min or a little longer. The staining time depends on the performance of the staining solution.

(8) Pour the staining solution and wash it several times with tap water.

(9) Add 2% alum solution to make the specimen fade.

(10) Pour out the alum solution and rinse gently in running water for 20 min.

(11) Use 30% alcohol, 50% alcohol, 70% alcohol, 80% alcohol, 90% alcohol, 95% alcohol, anhydrous ethanol 1, and anhydrous ethanol 2 to dehydration. Each kind of alcohol react 2-5 min.

(12) Put in xylene-anhydrous ethanol mixture or wintergreen oil-pure alcohol mixture for 10 min.

(13) Put in xylene or wintergreen oil for 5 min.

(14) Use neutral gum or Canadian gum to seal.

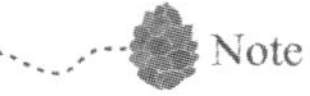
Note

The worm body was blue-black after staining, and the cell structure was clear under optical microscope.

3. Matters needing attention

(1) When applying faeces, it should be thin and not thick.

(2) The staining time depends on the tinting strength of the iron-hematoxylin solution. The staining solution should be placed for a period of time.

(3) The dehydration process should not be too urgent. If the specimen piece is found to be milky white when it is transparent, the new xylene should be used.

(4) Fixative solution, iodine alcohol, and alum solution can be reused.

Ⅲ Culture method of *Entamoeba histolytica*

(1) The composition of nutritional agar biphasic medium is as follows.

Liquid part: NaCl 8 g, KCl 0.2 g, $CaCl_2$ 0.2 g, $MgCl_2$ 0.01 g, Na_2HPO_4 2 g, KH_2PO_4 0.3 g, water 1000 ml.

Solid part: beef extract 3 g, peptone 5 g, agar 15 g.

(2) Disinfected rice flour: dispense rice flour into small tubes and disinfect them in a 180 ℃ oven for 3 times.

(3) Configuration method: at first, 2000 ml of the liquid part was prepared. $CaCl_2$ and $MgCl_2$ were placed in small vials and autoclave sterilized (54.89 kPa, 20 min). After cooling, combined together. 1000 ml of solid part was prepared, which was dissolved completely in a boiling water bath for 2-3 h. If there is any residue, use 4 layers of gauze to filter, divide the filtrate into test tubes while it is still hot, 5 ml for each tube, autoclave, put it on an inclined surface for cooling, and put it in a refrigerator for later use.

Before inoculation, 4.5 ml of liquid part and 0.5 ml of sterile bovine serum were added to each tube, and about 20 mg of disinfected rice flour was added with a platinum ring.

At present, BIS-33 culture medium has a wide range of use and has been applied in *in-vitro* aseptic culture of various parasites.

Vaginal secretion examination

The common parasite in vagina is *Trichomonas vaginalis*. In addition, there are worms that occasionally enter the vagina, such as mites and other nematodes. Containers in which the specimens are kept must be clean to avoid contamination by external worms.

Ⅰ Direct smear examination of vaginal secretions

Use a sterile cotton swab to wipe the secretions from the posterior fornix of vagina, cervix and vaginal wall of the tested subjects, and then put them into a bottle or tube filled with physiological saline. When the weather is cold, pay attention to the specimen insulation. The cotton swab can be taken for direct smear inspection. The active *Trichomonas vaginalis* trophozoite is easier to be identified. If the trophozoite is inactive, it is difficult to distinguish, so it can be used as a smear for staining and then identify. If worms are too less to be found by direct smear, the brine in the bottle can be centrifuged at 1000 r/min for 3 min to absorb the sedimentation for microscopic examination.

Ⅱ *Trichomonas vaginalis* staining test

It is difficult to identify *Trichomonas vaginalis* when it is inactive. It needs to be identified by the staining method. Commonly used methods are Wright staining or Giemsa staining. After the secretions are smeared, let it dry. After staining, the method is the same as the blood film.

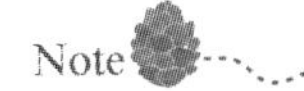

Iron-hematoxylin staining method can also be used and then examine.

Ⅲ *Trichomonas vaginalis* culture test

Because there are too few protozoa in the vagina, it is not easy to find out the *Trichomonas vaginalis* from secretion directly. It can be cultured in culture medium, and the number of protozoa is increased and it is easy to detect. The sampling method of culture test is the same as above, but it is required to take the material and transfer it to the culture medium under aseptic conditions.

There are many kinds of culture medium for *Trichomonas vaginalis*, and it has been considered that the liver dipping soup medium is better.

1. Liver dipping soup medium

Bovine liver or rabbit liver 15 g, peptone 2 g, NaCl 0.5 g, cysteine hydrochloride 0.2 g, maltose 1 g, water 100 ml. Preparation method: at first, grind the liver, immerse it into 100 ml water, mix it well, put it in the refrigerator overnight, heat it for half an hour the next day, filter it with 4 layers of gauze, and complement water to 100 ml. Then add the above ingredients, heat them to dissolve fully, and filter them with filter paper to adjust the pH to 5.5-6.0. Divide the above solution to 15 mm×150 mm test tubes, 8 ml per tube. Seal the tubes with silicone plug, and sterilize at 54.89 kPa for 20 min. Two tubes were cultured in a 37 ℃ incubator for 24-48 h to prove the culture medium is aseptic, others were stored in a refrigerator.

Culture method: before using the culture medium, 2 ml of inactivated sterile bovine serum was added to each tube, a little of penicillin and streptomycin powder (200-400 U/ml) was selected with a platinum ring, and secretions were swabbed from the posterior fornix of vagina, cervix and vaginal wall of the tested subjects with sterile cotton swab and inoculated into the culture medium. After culturing in a 37 ℃ incubator for 24-48 h, the suspension are observed with microscope.

2. 1640 peptone medium

RPMI1640 1.02 g, peptone 0.8 g, NaCl 0.5 g, cysteine hydrochloride 0.2 g, maltose 0.4 g, water 100 ml. Configuration method: heat the above ingredients to fully dissolved, filter with a stainless steel filter, and then dispense the solution into sterilized test tubes, 5 ml per tube. The sterility test was the same as above.

Culture method: 0.5 ml of inactivated sterile bovine serum was added to each tube before use, and the other operations were the same as above.

The 1640 peptone medium was used instead of the liver dipping soup medium to turn the reagent into a finished product, so the medium configuration was convenient and economical.

Preparation and staining of thick and thin blood film smears

See chapter 2 experiment 18 in this book.

[Questions]

What should you pay attention to when vaginal secretions are directly smeared to check *Trichomonas Vaginalis*?

Note

(Fang Tian, Feng Lu)

Experiment 22 Medical Arthropods

[Experimental Objectives]

(1)To study morphological characteristics of different develope stages of mosquitoes.

(2)To understand mosquitoes as vectors of mosquito-borne diseases.

(3)To learn differential characteristics of *Anopheles*, *Culex* and *Aedes*.

(4)To understand the basic morphology of different stages of common flies and their role as vector.

[Experimental Materials]

Teaching specimens (slices), microscopes, cedar oil, xylene, lens wipping paper, etc.

[Experimental Contents]

Ⅰ Mosquitoes

1. Study the specimens of adults of three genera of mosquitoes

(1)A pair of compound eyes, antennae, maxillary palps and a proboscis of head.

(2)The thorax bearing 3 pairs of legs and 1 pair of wings.

(3)10 segmented abdomen (the last 2 segments are modified to male genitalia).

2. Structure of mosquito heads

(1)Study whole mount of head of *Anopheles*.

The mouthpart consists of a tubular labium terminating with two tiny labella, one labium and one hypopharynx, one pair of mandibles and one pair of maxillae. All these form a cannula during blood sucking.

(2)Differentiate the male and female *Anopheles*. Note the plumose antennal hairs of male and pilose hairs of female. Compare the relative length of antenna and proboscis of both sexes.

(3)View *Culex* head, both male and female, and compare.

3. View the egg of *Anopheles*, *Culex* and *Aedes*

Note the shape and size.

4. View the larvae of three genera

Note the siphon or spiracles and resting position of larvae.

5. View the pupae of three genera

They are "comma" shape.

Ⅱ Fly

(1)Study the specimen of housefly: note a pair of compound eyes and proboscis in the head; thorax bearing three pairs of legs and a pair of wings; four longitudinal black strips on the dorsum of thorax, abdomen segmented.

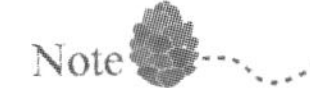

(2)View the specimen of *Chrysomyia megacephala*.

(3)View the specimen of Sarcophagidae species.

(4)Study the external structures of head: note the sucking mouthpart consisting of three parts. The proximal part, that is the rostrum, bears a pair of spin maxillary palps and is considered as a part of head proper; the middle region, that is the haustellum, is supposed to be homologous to labium; the expanded distal part is the oral plates made up of fleshy labella with tracheal structures.

(5)Study the structure of leg: note the hair appearance of leg terminating in pad and claws.

(6)View the fly larvae: note the shape, size and segmentation.

(7)View the preserved specimen of pupae.

(8)See the fly eggs.

Ⅲ Sandfly, fleas, lice and others

(1)View the adult of sandfly.

(2)View the adult of flea.

(3)View the adult of louse.

(4)View the adult of cockroach.

(5)View the adult of tick.

(6)View the adult of mite.

(7)View the adult of bedbug (demonstration).

[Experimental Report]

(1)Compare the differences of three types of mosquito.

(2)Label the head of fly.

(Fang Tian, Feng Lu)

Chapter 3 Comprehensive Experiment

Experiment 1 Preparation and Titer Determination of Polyclonal Antibody

[Experimental Objectives]

(1)To master the principle and the method of preparation of polyclonal antibodies against particulate antigens and deepen the understanding of the factors affecting the immunogenicity of an antigen.

(2)To master the method of titer determination of polyclonal antibody.

[Experimental Materials]

(1)H901 and O901 antigens of *Salmonella typhi*.

(2)Healthy rabbits about 2.5 kg weight, two ears of which are smooth, and the auricular veins and arteries are clearly visible.

(3)Sterile PBS.

(4)Rabbit head holder, centrifuge, water bath, super clean bench, 1.5 ml/15 ml centrifuge tubes, 1 ml/10 ml disposable syringes, etc.

[Experimental Contents]

1. Preparation of immunogens

(1)Principle: use commercial diagnostic agents as immunogens. Because it contains the preservative formaldehyde and is not suitable for direct immunization, we need to use PBS to remove preservative formaldehyde.

(2)Procedures.

①To calculate the amount of bacteria required for immunization.

②Shake the diagnostic solution thoroughly, transfer the required amount of the solution to a 1.5 ml centrifuge tube, centrifuge at 10000 r/min for 1 min, and discard the supernatant.

③Rinse thoroughly with 1 ml sterile PBS, centrifuge at 10000 r/min for 1 min, discard the supernatant, and repeat twice.

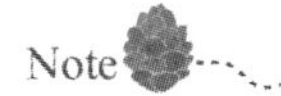

④Resuspend the bacteria in 0.2-0.5 ml sterile PBS.

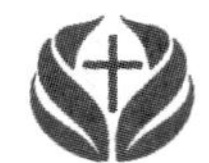

2. Immunization

(1)Principle: the final titer of polyclonal antibody is determined by many factors, including the physical and chemical properties of the antigen itself, the genetic and physiological status of the experimental animals, and the immune procedure and whether adjuvant is used.

①Compared with soluble antigens, particulate antigens are more immunogenic and easier to induce antibodies with high titer, so adjuvants are not necessary.

②The most important thing in the selection of animals is to have enough genetic distance with the species from which the antigen is produced. Other factors, such as genetic background, sex, age, health status, and the number of required antibodies are also important for the selection of animals.

③The immunization procedure affects the production of polyclonal antibodies significantly. Many factors, such as the dosage of immunogens, the route of vaccination, and the times and interval of immunization, must be considered carefully.

a. Too much or too little immunogen can induce immune tolerance rather than immune response, which leads to the failure of antibody preparation.

b. At the same dose, the general antibody production was intradermal $>$ subcutaneous $>$ intravenous $\approx$ intraperitoneal $\approx$ muscular $>$ oral. Nasal drip was mainly used to induce mucosal immunity. However, the amount of immunogen that can be inoculated by different immune routes is different, the intradermal is the least and the intraperitoneal is the most.

c. According to the general rule of antibody production, the second response induces higher levels and affinity of antibodies than the first response, so preparation of antibodies often requires multiple immunizations. The number and interval time of immunization often need to be determined by experiment.

In our experiment, we will compare the results of large-dose and short-interval intra-peritoneal inoculation with those of small-dose and long-interval intra-auricular vein inoculation to illustrate the effect of different immune procedures on polyantibody production.

(2)Procedures.

①Before immunizing animals, remember to collect some normal serum for negative control when testing antibody titers. After the rabbits are stabilized in a new environment for a few days to a week, the blood is taken from the auricular artery. Usually, 5 ml is enough.

②All students are divided into four experimental groups; each experimental group consists of 3 groups as repeats.

a. The first experimental group.

Immunogen: *Salmonella typhi* H901.

Route of vaccination: intra-auricular vein.

Dosage and interval: inoculate 0.2×10^9, 0.5×10^9, 1×10^9, 1.5×10^9, respectively, at days 1, 6, 11, 16.

b. The second experimental group.

Immunogen: *Salmonella typhi* O901.

Route of vaccination: intra-auricular vein.

Dosage and interval: inoculate 0.2×10^9, 0.5×10^9, 1×10^9, 1.5×10^9, respectively, at days 1, 6, 11, 16.

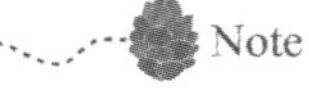

Note

c. The third experimental group.

Immunogen: *Salmonella typhi* H901.

Route of vaccination: intraperitoneal.

Dosage and interval: inoculate 7×10^9 every 2 days for a total of 10 times.

d. The fourth experimental group.

Immunogen: *Salmonella typhi* O901.

Route of vaccination: intraperitoneal.

Dosage and interval: inoculate 7×10^9 every 2 days for a total of 10 times.

3. Titer determination

(1) On the 21st day, blood is taken from the auricular artery to detect the antibody titer.

(2) The blood is collected in a 15 ml centrifuge tube and incubated in a water bath at 37 ℃ for 30 min. Then centrifuge at 2500 r/min for 10 min. Transfer serum into a new 15 ml centrifuge tube, add NaN_3 until the final concentration is 0.02% (W/V) to prevent corrosion, subpackage and store at −20 ℃.

(3) Titer determination: use the Widal test; see Chapter 2 Experiment 5 in this book. Agglutination titer ≥ 1 : 2560 indicates a successful test.

4. Notes

Animal welfare should be fully guaranteed during the experiment.

[Experimental Report]

Compare your serum agglutination titer with those of other groups and analyze the reasons for the differences.

[Questions]

Consider the influence of various factors on the preparation of polyclonal antibodies, and give your suggestion on the optimization of the immune program.

(Xingyuan Pan, Guimei Kong)

Experiment 2 Measure the Proportion of T and B Cells in the Spleen by Flow Cytometry

[Experimental Objectives]

(1) To master the method of preparing mouse spleen single-cell suspension.

(2) To master the basic operation and data analysis of flow cytometry.

(3) To master the normal Proportion of T and B cells in the spleen of mice.

[Experimental Materials]

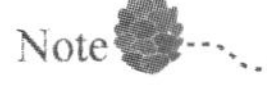

(1) Healthy C57BL/6 mice, 6 weeks old.

(2)75% alcohol, red blood cell lysate, pH 7.2-7.4 sterile PBS, etc.

(3)Ice machine, centrifuge, scissors, tweezers, petri dishes, stainless steel welde mesh, glass syringes, super clean bench, cell counting plate, 1.5 ml/15 ml centrifuge tubes, flow cytometer, etc.

[Experimental Contents]

1. Preparation of mouse spleen single -cell suspension

(1)The mouse is sacrificed after cervical dislocation and soaked in 75% ethanol for 3 min. Take out the spleen and place it in a petri dish filled with 5 ml PBS.

(2)Place the spleen on stainless steel welde mesh (100 or 200 mesh), and press it gently with the needle core of the syringe. Single-cell suspension is obtained by filtration.

(3)Lysis red blood cells and count cell, and adjust to 1×10^6/ml.

2. To label spleen cells by fluorescent antibodies

(1)Prepare four 1.5 ml centrifuges tubes, each containing 100 μl cell suspension (1×10^6/ml).

①Blank tube: no antibodies.

②Single labeled tube 1: add 0.5 μl of mCD3-FITC fluorescent antibody.

③Single labeled tube 2: add 0.5 μl of mCD19-APC fluorescent antibody.

④Double labeled tube: add 0.5 μl of mCD3-FITC and 0.5 μl of mCD19-APC fluorescent antibody.

(2)Incubate on ice in dark for 20 min.

(3)Wash cells with 400 μl PBS. Centrifuge at 6000 r/min for 5 min, discard supernatant, and use 200 μl PBS to resuspend cells.

3. Flow cytometry

(1)Open the analysis software, gate the lymphocytes for analysis through the FSC-SSC scatter diagram (Fig. 3-2-1), and adjust the parameters such as voltage and threshold to ensure the cell is in a proper position and debris interference is eliminated.

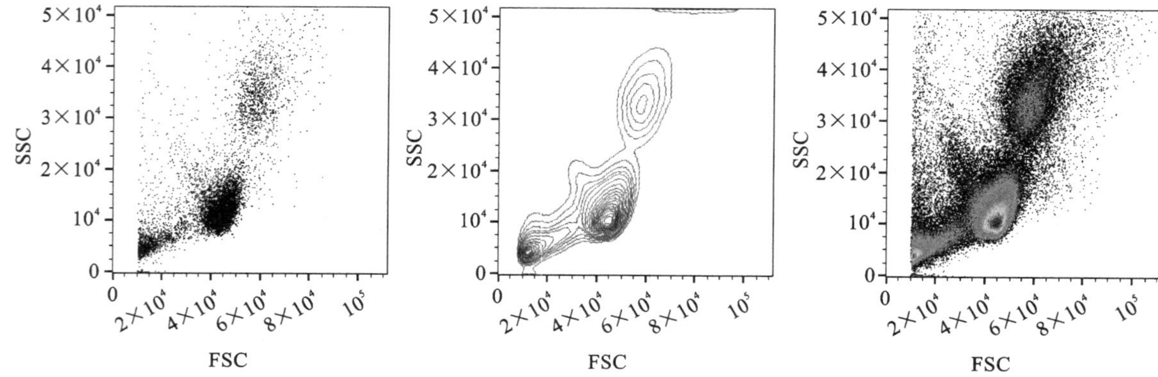

Fig. 3-2-1 Splenic lymphocytes FSC-SSC scatter diagram

(2)Ensure the autofluorescence of unstained cells is completely in the negative region by voltage regulation with blank control and the positive rate of the unstained cells is less than 2%; the unstained cells in the double-fluorescent scatterplot are located in the lower left quadrant.

Note

(3)Adjust fluorescence compensation by single labeled control (Fig. 3-2-2).

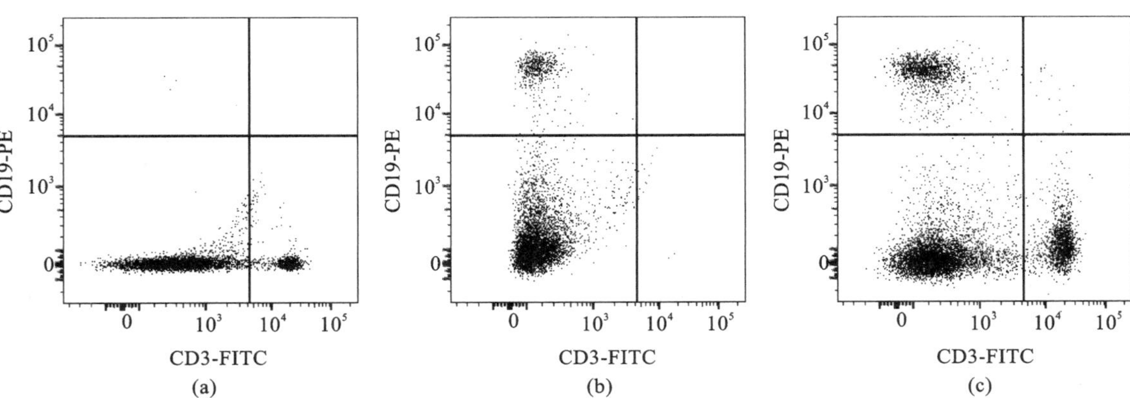

Fig. 3-2-2 Splenic lymphocytes CD3-CD19 stain

(a) CD3 single labeled; (b) CD19 single labeled; (C) CD3-CD19 double labeled

(4) Sample test, get the data.

4. Notes

(1) Red blood cell lysis must be sufficient. Otherwise, it will interfere with the analysis of the results.

(2) Flow cytometer is a valuable instrument that needs to be maintained and recorded in accordance with the specifications.

[Experimental Report]

(1) Explain the functions of 4 centrifuge tubes.

(2) Using your flow chart, calculate the proportion of T and B cells in the mouse spleen.

[Questions]

What is the difference of the proportion of T and B cells in different immune organs and tissues?

(Zhijie Lin, Xingyuan Pan)

Experiment 3 Laboratory Examination of Common Pathogenic Microorganism of Respiratory Tract Infection

[Experimental Objectives]

(1) To master the bacteriological detection methods of respiratory tract specimens.

(2) To learn about other microorganisms in respiratory tract specimens.

[Experimental Materials]

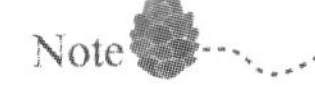

(1) Specimens: simulated sputum, bronchial washing, nasopharyngeal swab or sputum from

suspected respiratory tract infected patient.

(2)Mediums: blood agar plate, chocolate agar plate, MacConkey agar plate, CHROMagar, common biochemical tubes.

(3) Reagents: Gram stain solution, catalase reagent, oxidase reagent, various biochemical reaction related reagents, etc.

(4) Others: disposable sterile syringes, 75% alcohol cotton balls, markers, lens wipping paper, cedar oil, slides.

(5) Apparatus: optical microscope, constant temperature incubator, carbon dioxide (CO_2) incubator.

[Experimental Contents]

Ⅰ Upper respiratory tract specimens

Upper respiratory tract specimens mainly include swabs and extracts of the nose, nasopharynx and oropharynx. Most of them have bacteria of normal oropharyngeal flora.

1. Direct examination

(1)Specimens suspected of *Corynebacterium diphtheriae* infection: make two smears with cotton swabs, one for Gram staining and the other for methylene blue or metachromatic granules staining. If an irregular arrangement of Gram-positive *Corynebacterium* is found and there are obvious blue-black metachromatic granules located at one or both ends of the cell, it can be preliminarily reported that "Gram-positive *Corynebacterium* with metachromatic granules have been found".

(2)Specimens suspected of *Borrelia vincentii* and *Fusobacterium* infection: make the smear with cotton swabs, do Gram staining, and pay attention to prolonging the re-staining time to 2 min. If you see reddish slender *Borrelia* and slightly curved arc-shaped Gram-positive or negative *Bacillus*, it can be reported that "bacteria resembling *Borrelia vincentii* and *Fusobacterium* have been found".

(3) Specimens suspected of *Candida* infection: make the smear with cotton swabs, mix it with a drop of physiological saline, and examine it under a high-power microscope. If yeast-like cells and hyphae are found, it can be reported that "yeast-like fungi, similar to *Candida* have been found". We can also do Gram staining. If Gram-positive, scattered or clustered oval budding yeast-like fungi are found, it can be reported that "yeast-like fungi, similar to *Candida* have been found".

2. Isolation and culture

(1)Culture of common bacteria: in general, inoculate specimens on the blood agar plate, chocolate agar plate or MacConkey agar plate, and culture in CO_2 incubator at 37 ℃ for 24-48 h. The suspicious colonies are identified by smear staining, biochemical reaction, serological test and animal experiments, and then the results can be reported. The drug susceptibility test is performed at the same time.

(2)Culture of special bacteria.

①Specimens suspected of *Corynebacterium diphtheriae* infection: inoculate the specimens on Loeffler serum slant or egg culture medium, and culture at 35 ℃ for 12 h to observe the growth of moss. If there are gray-white, glossy bacterial mosses or round gray-white or yellowish colonies, a microscopic examination of the smear after Gram staining shows typical

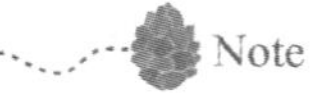
Note

bacterial morphology and metachromatic granules, and then combined with the clinical symptom, a preliminary report can be issued. Steak the colonies on potassium tellurite blood agar plates at 35 ℃ for 48 h for pure culture, and report results after performing biochemical identification and virulence tests.

②Specimens suspected of *Bordetella pertussis* infection: inoculate nasopharyngeal swabs on Bordet-Gengou plates and put them in a glass jar with cover containing a little water at 35 ℃ for 48-72 h. If there are small, raised, gray-white, opaque mercury-like colonies surrounded by narrow hemolytic rings and Gram-negative double or single oval microbacilli after smear observation, a preliminary diagnosis can be issued combined with colony characteristics. After further identification tests such as biochemical reactions, serum agglutination tests and nutritional requirements, if there is no bacterial growth after 7 d of cultivation, a negative report can be issued.

③Specimens suspected of hemolytic streptococcus infection: inoculate the specimens on a blood agar plate and put in a 5%-10% CO_2 incubator at 35 ℃ for 18-24 h. A report can be issued after selecting small β hemolysis colonies for staining, biochemical reaction and serum grouping.

④Specimens suspected of *Haemophilus influenzae* infection: inoculate the specimens on blood agar plate and chocolate agar plate, and inoculate *Staphylococcus aureus* in the center of the blood agar plate linearly, put in a 5%-10% CO_2 incubator at 35 ℃ for 24-48 h. If there are satellite phenomenon and droplet-like colonies, Gram-negative microbacilli, other further identification examinations can be done refer to the relevant chapters of the book.

⑤Specimens suspected of *Neisseria* infection: inoculate the specimens on preheated blood agar plate (or yolk double antibody medium) and chocolate agar plate, and put in a 5%-10% CO_2 incubator at 35 ℃ for 24-48 h. Select the suspected colony for smear staining and oxidase tests. If it is oxidase-positive Gram-negative diplococci, continue to do biochemical reaction and serum identification, and then issue the report.

Ⅱ Lower respiratory tract specimens

Lower respiratory tract specimens mainly include all kinds of sputum and bronchial brushes and washing fluids collected under a bronchoscope. There may be a small amount of normal oropharyngeal flora bacteria in sputum, and there are few or no bacteria of normal flora in specimens collected under a bronchoscope.

1. Specimen observation

The specimens are observed with naked eyes and recorded, including color, viscosity, and whether there is bloodshot or pus and other characteristics. Specimens are examined by direct smear microscopic examination, and the numbers of leukocytes and epithelial cells are observed under a low-power microscope to evaluate whether the specimen is suitable for bacterial culture and to determine whether there are pathogens. The microscopic classification of sputum specimens is shown in Tab. 3-3-1.

Tab. 3-3-1 The microscopic classification of sputum specimens

Classification	Leukocyte numbers	Epithelial cell numbers	Results
A	>25	<10	qualified
B	>25	<25	qualified
C	<10	>25	unqualified

Note: classifications A and B are qualified sputum specimens, suitable for culture. Classification C is unqualified specimens and should be required to re-retain specimens.

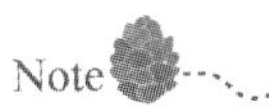

For the specimens confirmed to be from the lower respiratory tract, a preliminary etiological diagnosis will be made according to the staining and morphological characteristics of bacteria observed under the microscope.

2. Direct examination

(1) The purulent or bloody part of the specimens is selected to make smears and examined by Gram staining for microscopic examination in order to issue a preliminary report.

(2) Specimens suspected of *Corynebacterium diphtheriae* infection: make two smears, one for Gram staining and the other for Albert metachromatic granule staining, and then a preliminary report can be issued.

(3) Specimens suspected of or ruled out *Mycobacterium tuberculosis* infection: take caseous or purulent specimens directly or centrifuge to collect bacteria for thick smears, do acid-fast staining, observe the red acid-fast bacilli under an oil immersion lens, and then a preliminary report can be issued.

3. Isolation and culture

(1) Pre-treatment of sputum specimens: sputum specimens should be pre-treated before inoculation.

① Washing: add the specimen to a test tube with 10-20 ml aseptic physiological saline, shake violently for 5-10 s, then use the inoculation loop to pick out the thick sputum stuck to the bottom of the tube. Put it into another test tube and wash it twice by the same way, and finally remove the remaining thick sputum for inoculation. You can also use aseptic plates instead of test tubes.

② Homogenization: add the same amount of 1% pH 7.6 trypsin to the sputum (after washing) and incubate at 35 ℃ for 90 min.

(2) Culture of common bacteria: inoculate the pre-treated sputum or aseptic samples (bronchial brushes or washing fluid, etc.) on blood agar plate, chocolate agar plate, or MacConkey agar plate, and put in a 5%-10% CO_2 incubator at 35 ℃ for 18-24 h. If suspected pathogen colonies are found (Tab. 3-3-2), do smear staining and microscopic examination. Depending on the colony and microscopic characteristics, the corresponding biochemical and serological tests should be selected for identification. The drug sensitivity test is performed at the same time. If there is no colony growth, continue to incubate until 48 h, observe the plate, record and report.

Tab. 3-3-2 Common normal flora and pathogens in respiratory tract specimens

Variety	Gram-positive bacteria and fungi	Gram-negative bacteria
Normal flora	*Streptococcus A*, *Micrococcus*, *Staphylococcus epidermidis*, *Tetracoccus*, *Corynebacterium* except *Corynebacterium diphtheriae*, *Lactobacillus*	*Neisseria* except *Neisseria meningitidis* and *Neisseria gonorrhoeae*
Common pathogens of upper respiratory tract	Group B streptococci, *Streptococcus pneumoniae*, *Staphylococcus aureus*, anaerobes, *Candida albicans*, *Streptococcus* Miller, *Aspergillus*	*Haemophilus influenzae*, *Pseudomonas aeruginosa*, Enterobacteriaceae, *Stenotrophomonas maltophilia*
Occasional pathogens of upper respiratory tract	*Corynebacterium diphtheriae*, *Corynebacterium pertussis*, *Corynebacterium parapertussis*	*Neisseria meningitidis*

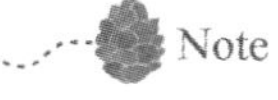
Note

continued

Variety	Gram-positive bacteria and fungi	Gram-negative bacteria
Common pathogens of lower respiratory tract	*Streptococcus pneumoniae*, *Staphylococcus aureus*, β-hemolytic streptococci, *Candida albicans*, *Aspergillus*	*Haemophilus influenzae*, *Moraxella catarrhalis*, non-fermentative bacteria, Enterobacteriaceae, *Pasteurella multocida*, *Haemophilus*, *Neisseria meningitidis*

Identification of common Gram-negative bacilli: take bacteria for oxidase test, catalase test, and nitrate reduction test. If the oxidase test is negative, the catalase test is positive and the nitrate reduction test is positive, it can be judged to be Enterobacteriaceae. Inoculate with KIA, MIU, IMViC and Enterobacteriaceae system biochemical identification tube, finally identify to genus or species. If the biological characteristics are consistent with *Salmonella* or *Shigella*, the diagnostic serum is used for agglutination tests to determine the species or types. If the oxidase test is positive or negative, do not ferment glucose or utilize glucose; it can be judged as non-fermenting bacteria.

Identification of common Gram-positive cocci: take bacteria for a catalase test, the positive bacteria are Micrococcaceae. And O-F experiments are used to identify *Staphylococcus* (type F) and *Micrococcus* (type O). The negative bacteria are often *Streptococcus* or *Enterococcus*.

(3) Culture of common fungi: if specimens are suspected of fungi, inoculate them on Sabouraud medium at 35 ℃. If they do not grow, incubate for 5 d, then record and report. If specimens are suspected of *Candida*, incubate on CHROMagar directly.

(4) Culture of anaerobe: take the trachea or cricothyroid membrane puncture fluid by aseptic operation, and then inoculate on pre-reduced anaerobic blood agar plate or chocolate agar plate, anaerobic culture for 24-48 h, observe and record.

(5) Culture of special bacteria: if specimens are suspected of special bacteria, isolate and culture for special pathogens.

①If specimens are suspected of *Mycobacterium tuberculosis*: refer to relevant chapters for details.

②If specimens are suspected of *Legionella pneumophila*: inoculate organ secretions on buffered charcoal yeast extract (BCYE) agar, put in a 2.5% CO_2 incubator at 35 ℃ for 14 d, and observe the results every day.

③If specimens are suspected of *Nocardia*: Gram-positive or filamentous branches could be observed under the microscope.

④If specimens are suspected of *Mycoplasma*, *Chlamydia*, etc.: refer to relevant chapters for details about isolation, culture and identification.

4. Susceptibility test

Refer to relevant chapters for details.

[Experimental Report]

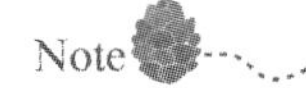
Note

1. Direct examination

(1) For the upper respiratory tract specimens: issue a preliminary report on the bacteria with

special morphology or staining, according to the results of morphological staining. For example, "bacteria resembling *Borrelia vincentii* and *Fusobacterium* have been found", "yeast-like fungi, similar to *Candida* have been found".

(2) For the lower respiratory tract specimens: issue a preliminary report, according to the number of leukocytes and squamous epithelial cells, bacterial morphology and staining characteristics. For example, "Gram-positive cocci, similar to staphylococci have been found", "Gram-negative cocci, suspected to *Neisseria meningitidis* have been found".

2. Culture

(1) Positive: refer to pathogens, report the name and the results of drug susceptible test.

(2) Negative.

①If there is no suspicious pathogenic bacteria growing in the upper respiratory tract, but the bacteria of normal flora of the pharynx grows, report that "no pathogenic bacteria have been detected", or report "*Streptococcus A* (normal flora) grows", "*Neisseria* (normal flora) grows", "culture medium without fungal growth", "culture medium without *Haemophilus* growth". If there are no special pathogens detected on the blood agar plate, while a resident bacterium grows luxuriantly or is close to or even pure culture, it should be considered that this bacterium may be related to the disease, and report that "luxuriant growth of one kind of bacteria".

②If there are no suspicious pathogenic bacteria growing in the lower respiratory tract, report that "no pathogenic bacteria have been detected". The samples from deep sterile parts such as trachea brush or flushing fluid can report no bacterial growth.

[Questions]

(1) How to judge whether the sputum specimens come from the deep part?

(2) How to carry out bacteriological examination of lower respiratory tract specimens?

(3) What biosafety problems may exist in the examination of respiratory specimens? How can these problems be avoided to ensure biosafety?

(Yinyan Yin, Cuicui Liu)

Experiment 4　Isolation and Identification of Enterobacteriaceae

[Experimental Objectives]

To master the bacteriological examination of fecal specimens.

[Experimental Materials]

(1) Fecal specimen or anal swab.

(2) Culture media: SS agar plate, MacConkey agar plate, CAMPY blood plate, China blue plate, eosin methylene blue (EMB) plate, KIA medium, MIU medium, GN bacteriological

enrichment solution, alkaline peptone water, TCBS agar plate and *Vibrio parahaemolyticus* selective plate, CCFA agar plate, etc.

(3) Reagents: indigo matrix reagent, diagnostic serum of *Shigella*, diagnostic serum of *Salmonella*, diagnostic serum of *Vibrio cholerae*, diagnostic serum of enteropathogenic *Escherichia coli* and enteroinvasive *Escherichia coli*, etc.

(4) Others: microscopes, physiological saline, slide, etc.

[Experimental Contents]

1. Direct microscopic observation

(1) Observe by the microscope with direct fecal specimen smear: for patients with inflammatory diarrhea, fecal specimens (anal swabs) can be directly smeared, dried, fixed, and then stained with Gram stain solution for direct observation under the microscope. For diarrhea caused by *Salmonella*, *Shigella*, *Yersinia*, *Campylobacter*, EIEC, and some *Vibrio* spp. leukocytes are often observed in fecal specimen smears, and erythrocytes can be observed in patients with intestinal wall hemorrhage. If "Gram-negative, curved, and accompanied by seagull-winged bacilli" are observed, the patient may be suffering from *Campylobacter* or *Vibrio* spp..

(2) Observation of bacterial dynamics: observe the bacterial dynamics by making wet slides of the fecal specimen or using the suspension method. If the infection is caused by *Campylobacter* or *Vibrio* spp., the characteristic "bid-like" movement can be seen.

2. Bacterial isolation and culture

Identification and selection culture media are commonly used for the isolation of pathogenic bacteria in feces. These media usually contain antimicrobial drugs or chemical inhibitors that can inhibit the growth of normal intestinal flora and favor the growth of intestinal pathogenic bacteria.

(1) MacConkey agar plate: it is used to detect Enterobacteriaceae bacteria and other non-caustic Gram-negative bacilli, and to inhibit Gram-positive bacteria and certain caustic Gram-negative bacilli. On this medium, pathogenic *Salmonella*, *Shigella* (except very few), *Edwardsiella* are clear, colorless or yellowish colonies, while normal intestinal flora, lactose-fermenting bacteria such as *Escherichia*, *Klebsiella*, *Enterobacteria*, and certain *Citrobacter* spp. are dark pink to reddish colonies, and delayed lactose-fermenting bacteria, such as certain *Citrobacter* spp. and *Serratia* are colorless colonies when incubated for 24 h and light pink colonies when incubated for 24-48 h. Bacteria that do not ferment lactose, such as *Proteus*, certain *Citrobacter*, *Providencia* and *Morganella* spp. are transparent, colorless colonies.

(2) SS agar plate: it is used to find bacteria of the *Salmonella* and *Shigella*, inhibits the growth of Gram-positive bacteria and common normal intestinal flora, and detects the production of H_2S by the addition of an indicator. On this medium, *Salmonella* and *Shigella* are transparent or translucent, colorless or yellowish colonies, and the growth of normal intestinal flora is consistent with that on MacConkey agar plate.

(3) CAMPY blood plate: it is a selective medium for the initial isolation of *Campylobacter* from feces. On this medium, *Campylobacter jejuni* are pinkish-gray, moist, flow-like colonies when incubated at 42 ℃.

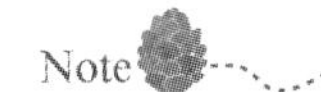

(4) TCBS agar plate: it is a strongly selective medium for the detection of *Vibrio* spp. from fecal specimens. Because of the high pH and high bile salts level of this medium, it inhibits the

growth of most intestinal flora. *Aeromonas* spp. can also be detected on this medium. Because it contains sucrose, *Vibrio* spp. that ferment sucrose such as *Vibrio cholerae* and *Vibrio alginolyticus* have yellow colonies, while *Vibrio parahaemolyticus* and *Vibrio vulnificus*, which doesn't ferment sucrose, has blue-green colonies. Except for occasional blue-green colonies of *Pseudomonas* spp., the majority of the intestinal flora is inhibited.

(5) CCFA agar plate: it is a selective medium for the initial isolation of *Clostridium difficile* from the feces of patients who are suspected antimicrobial drug-associated diarrhea or pseudomembranous enteritis. *Clostridium difficile* exhibits yellow colonies because it can ferment fructose, and this medium inhibits most intestinal flora, including Gram-positive cocci and Gram-negative bacilli.

3. Common pathogenic bacteria in fecal specimens

Gram-positive bacteria: *Staphylococcus* spp., *Candida albicans*, *Clostridium difficile*, *Mycobacterium tuberculosis*, *Bacillus cereus*.

Gram-negative bacteria: *Shigella* spp., *Salmonella* spp., enteropathogenic *Escherichia coli*, *Vibrio cholerae*, *Vibrio parahaemolyticus* hydrophilic *Aeromonas*, *Plesiomonas shigelloides*, *Campylobacter jejuni*, *Yersinia enterocolitica*.

(1) *Shigella* spp. and *Salmonella* spp..

Bacterial culture: these fecal specimens of patients with acute diarrhea should be inoculated with SS (or HE or XLD) agar plate and MacConkey agar plate respectively, and incubated in a 37 ℃ incubator for 18-24 h. Patients or carriers with chronic diarrhea suspected to be infected with *Shigella* spp. should inoculate the specimen with GN bacteriological enrichment solution. Patients or carriers suspected of *Salmonella* spp. infection should inoculate the specimen with selenite bacteriostatic solution, and put it in a 37 ℃ incubator for 6 h, and then transfer to SS agar plate and MacConkey agar plate, and put it in the incubator at 37 ℃ for 18-24 h. Observe whether there are tiny, transparent or semi-transparent, colorless or light-yellow suspected bacterial colonies growing in the SS agar plate, and sometimes the center of the SS agar plate can be seen as a black colony (producing H_2S). On MacConkey agar plates, *Salmonella* spp. and *Shigella* spp. (with very few exceptions) were transparent, colorless or yellowish colonies.

Pick three suspicious colonies and inoculate them with three KIA and MIU media (to do power, indole and urease (MIU) complex test), incubate them at 37 ℃ for 18-24 h, and observe the reaction results. Suspicious colonies can be picked for smear and Gram staining at the same time to observe the morphology and arrangement of bacteria.

If the biochemical reaction results on KIA and MIU media are consistent with the biochemical reaction results of *Shigella* spp. in the Tab. 3-4-1, it is initially recognized that the bacterial strain belongs to *Shigella* spp.. Subsequently, use the diagnostic serum of *Shigella* spp. to identify the serotypes of the bacteria growing in KIA tubes.

Tab. 3-4-1 Preliminary biochemical reaction of *Shigella* spp. and *Salmonella* spp.

Bacteria	KIA				MIU			Nitrate reduction test	Catalase test
	bevel	ground	H_2S	aerogenesis	movement	indole	urease		
Shigella	K	A	−	−/+	−	+/−	−	+	+
Salmonella para-typhi A	K	A	−/+	+	+	−	−	+	+

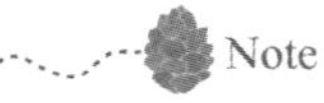
Note

continued

Bacteria	KIA				MIU			Nitrate reduction test	Catalase test
	bevel	ground	H_2S	aerogenesis	movement	indole	urease		
Salmonella para-typhi B	K	A	+	+	+	−	−	+	+
Salmonella typhi	K	A	+/−	−	+	−	−	+	+
Salmonella typhimurium	K	A	+	+	+	−	−	+	+

If the results on KIA and MIU media match the biochemical reaction results of *Salmonella* spp. in the Tab. 3-4-2, it is initially recognized that the bacterial strain belongs to *Salmonella* spp. and needs to be further identified with other Enterobacteriaceae bacteria. After identification as *Salmonella* spp., serologic typing of bacteria grown in KIA tubes was performed with *Salmonella* spp. diagnostic serum.

Tab. 3-4-2 Identification of *Salmonella* from other bacteria in Enterobacteriaceae

Tests	*Salmonella*	*Citrobacter*	*Salmonella Arizonella*	*Edwardsiella*
Lysine decarboxylase test	+	−	+	+
KCN growth test	−	+	−	−
Malonate utilization test	−	+/−	+	+
Indigo substrate test	−	−/+	−	+

(2) Enteropathogenic *Escherichia coli* (EPEC).

Bacterial culture: take the suspicious feces and inoculate them on MacConkey agar plate (or China blue plate or EMB plate), put them in a 37 ℃ incubator for 18-24 h, then pick the red lactose fermentation colonies (blue colonies on the China blue plate, purple-red colonies on the EMB plate), transfer them to KIA and MIU media tubes, and put them in the incubator for overnight at 37 ℃ for observation of the results. Select the suspected bacteria that conform to the culture results of *Escherichia coli*, and further identify them according to the serological and biochemical characteristics of bacteria such as EPEC and EIEC.

(3) *Vibrio cholerae*.

① Direct microscopic examination: take two smears of watery feces or slop-like feces of suspected patients, fix them with ethanol or methanol after drying, stain them with Gram stain solution and phenol fuchsin stain solution (1 : 10 dilution) respectively, and observe whether there are Gram-negative *Vibrio* spp. arranged in the form of schools of fish with an oil immersion lens.

Take another suspicious specimen to make a hanging drop tablet or pressure drop tablet, add a drop of *Vibrio cholerae* multivalent diagnostic serum without preservative in one of the specimens, and observe under the microscope. If the specimen without antiserum is found to have "bid-like" movement of bacteria, and the bacteria in specimen with antiserum stop moving and

clumping indicate that the brake test is positive, it can be reported as "positive *Vibrio cholerae* antisera brake test", which have diagnostic significance.

②Bacterial culture: the fecal specimens of patients suspected of cholera should be inoculated with alkaline peptone water and incubated in a 37 ℃ incubator for 4-6 h, then take the bacterial membrane or culture solution for Gram staining and brake test, and take the bacterial membrane or culture solution and inoculate it on TCBS agar plate (or alkaline agar plate, or gentamicin-potassium tellurite plate), and incubate it in a 37 ℃ incubator for 18-24 h and observe whether there are yellow colonies on TCBS agar plate. Conduct an agglutination test with polyvalent antiserum of *Vibrio cholerae* (physiological saline must be used as a negative control to observe whether there is a self-coagulation phenomenon), if the suspected bacteria antisera agglutination test is positive and physiological saline is not agglutinated, combined with the colonies, the morphology of the bacteria, the oxidase test, etc., it can be preliminarily determined to be *Vibrio cholerae*.

(4) *Vibrio parahaemolyticus*.

Bacterial culture: inoculate the suspicious specimen in *Vibrio parahaemolyticus* selective plate or TCBS agar plate, put it at 37 ℃ for 18-24 h, and then observe the morphology of the colony. *Vibrio parahaemolyticus* formed round, neatly edged, elevated, turbid, green, moist colonies on *Vibrio parahaemolyticus* selective plates, and green or blue-green colonies on TCBS agar plates. Suspect colonies can be further identified by inoculating them in KIA and MIU media containing 3.5% NaCl for salt-tolerant growth tests (Tab. 3-4-3).

Tab. 3-4-3 Preliminary biochemical reaction of *Vibrio parahaemolyticus*

Test	KIA (add 3.5% NaCl)				MIU (add 3.5% NaCl)			Peptone water		
	bevel	ground	gas	H_2S	power	indole	urease	0% NaCl	7% NaCl	10% NaCl
Results	−	+	−	−	+	+	−	−	+	−

(5) *Yersinia enterocolitica*.

Bacterial culture: specimens were streaked and inoculated on *Yersinia*-specific (CIN) medium and MacConkey agar plate, and placed at 37 ℃ for incubation. Feces and anal swabs from carriers were incubated in PBS at pH 7.4-7.8 for 21 d at 4 ℃, and then 0.1 ml of the bacterial solution was pipetted onto selective medium at day 7, 14 and 21 for 48 h. *Yersinia enterocolitica* appeared as lactose-unfermented colonies, hyaline or semi-transparent, small, flattened, colorless, and slightly elevated on MacConkey agar plate, and as red colonies surrounded by an occasional ring of bile salt deposits on CIN medium. Transfer the suspected colonies to KIA, MIU and other biochemical reaction media for further identification.

(6) *Campylobacter jejuni*.

Bacterial culture: liquid or bloody feces was inoculated on *Campylobacter* selective medium (CAMPY-BA, Skirrow blood agar or Butzler blood agar medium), or inoculated in CEM bacterial enrichment solution (after 42 ℃, micro-anaerobic incubation for 18-48 h, and then transplanted to the above selective medium for delineation and isolation), incubated at 42 ℃, under micro-anaerobic (candle jar method is available), preferably using a mixture of gases (85% N_2, 10% CO_2 and 5% O_2) for 24-48 h to observe the bacterial growth and colony characteristics. *Campylobacter* forms translucent, raised, moist, slightly reddish, and glossy

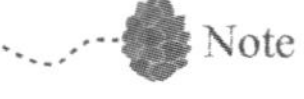
Note

colonies with a diameter of 1-2 mm. If the surface of the medium is moist, *Campylobacter jejuni* and *Campylobacter coli* can spread and grow to form flat large colonies, and all types of colonies are not hemolyzed. Take this kind of colony to do the hanging drop method or pressure drop method to observe the power, which can be seen as an oscillating "bid-like" movement. Gram stain is negative, elongated, and slightly pointed at both ends of the arc-shaped bacteria, there are also S-shaped, spiral or spindle-shaped bacteria. The identification of *Campylobacter* must be determined by a combination of tests.

(7) *Staphylococcus*.

Bacterial culture: take green, seawater-like or pasty feces and inoculate on a high salt mannitol plate or blood plate by line, put it in a 37 ℃ incubator overnight and observe the colonies. Pick the yellow colonies on the high salt mannitol plate for smear, Gram stain, and microscopic examination. If Gram-positive, grape bunch-like arrangement of cocci are seen, coagulase, DNA enzyme and mannitol fermentation and other tests need to be done to determine.

(8) *Clostridium difficile*.

Bacterial culture: take fresh feces with yellow pseudomembrane, immediately inoculate it on cycloserine-cefoxitin-fructose agar (CCFA) plate (inoculate it within 10-20 min), and put the inoculated plate in an anaerobic environment containing 80% N_2, 10% CO_2, and 10% H_2 at 35 ℃ to culture it for 48 h, and then select rough yellow colonies to do suspending-droplet dynamics examination and Gram staining. If microscopic observation of oval or rectangular cells located in the proximal Gram-positive bacilli (in an anaerobic agar plate is more likely to produce cells), further identification can be made.

(9) Fungi.

Fungal culture: fungal diarrhea is mostly secondary to antimicrobial therapy, and the common pathogens are *Candida albicans* and *Candida glabrata*. The specimen is inoculated on Chloramphenicol-containing Sabouraud medium and blood agar medium, and incubated in the air environment at 25-30 ℃ and a biochemical incubator at 37 ℃ for 24-48 h. The subsequent identification method is decided based on the colony morphology and the results of the smear Gram staining.

[Experimental report]

(1) Describe the morphology of Enterobacteriaceae isolated from fecal specimens.

(2) What should be noted during the isolation of Enterobacteriaceae?

[Questions]

(1) What are the differences in colony morphology of different Enterobacteriaceae on identification media?

(2) How the biochemical reactions of *Escherichia coli* and *Shigella* differ?

(3) What biosafety issues may exist in intestinal specimen examination? How to avoid it to ensure biosafety?

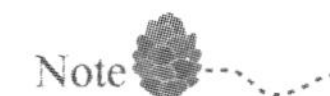

(Guimei Kong, Chengfeng Gao)

Experiment 5 Laboratory Examination of Common Pathogenic Microorganisms of Genitourinary Tract Infections

[Experimental Objectives]

To master the bacteriological examination methods and matters needing attention of genitourinary tract specimens.

[Experimental Materials]

(1)Specimens: urethral or cervical swabs.

(2)Media: blood agar plate, chocolate agar plate, *Ureaplasma urealyticum* and *Mycoplasma hominis* medium, etc.

[Experimental Contents]

1. Smear examination

Do Gram staining on the secretion smear and observe under the oil immersion lens. If the typical Gram-negative renal diplococci are found inside and outside the neutrophils, you can report "Intracellular (extracellular) Gram-negative diplococci are observed, and we suspect it's *Neisseria gonorrhoeae*". If you find small Gram-negative bacilli, sometimes strongly stained at both poles, scattered or clustered, you can report "Gram-negative bacilli are found, similar to *Haemophilus ducreyi*". *Microspironema pallidum* should be examined by darkfield microscope or silver staining method. The inclusion body of *Chlamydia trachomatis* is examined by Giemsa staining method (refer to relevant chapters). *Candida* smear: make wet slides with physiological saline, cover glass slides, and do direct microscopic examination or microscopic examination after Gram staining.

(1) *Neisseria gonorrhoeae*: the specimens are stained with Gram solution and observed under oil immersion lens. Note that they are kidney-shaped and arranged in pairs, and Gram staining is negative. If it is an infectious secretion smear, bacteria are swallowed by neutrophils in the cytoplasm.

(2)*Candida albicans*: the specimens are stained with Gram solution or lactic acid phenol cotton blue solution. Microscopic observation shows that the spores are oval, and Gram staining is positive. Pay attention to whether pseudohyphae formed by budding are present.

(3)Chlamydia: epithelial cells infected with chlamydia are stained with Giemsa solution and observed under oil immersion lens. The cytoplasm of the cell is light red, and the nucleus is purple. The basophilic inclusion in the cytoplasm is dark purple and dense.

(4)Mycoplasma: after Giemsa staining, the colony of mycoplasma shows a typical "fried egg" under low-power microscope. The edge is neat and transparent, and the color is lighter; the center of the colony is dense and blue-purple.

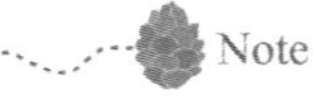
Note

2. Cultivation and identification of common bacteria

Specimens are inoculated on the blood agar plate and the preliminary identification is carried out according to the colony characteristics and bacterial morphology.

3. Isolation, cultivation and identification of *Neisseria gonorrhoeae*

Specimens are inoculated in *Neisseria gonorrhoeae* medium or chocolate agar plate, and cultured in a 35 ℃ and 5%-10% CO_2 incubator for 24-48 h. Protruding, round, gray-white, and smooth colonies can be observed and the diameter is 0.5-1 mm. *Neisseria gonorrhoeae* can produce a large number of oxidases in the growth process, which can oxidize colorless oxidase reagents (5%-10% tetramethyl-*p*-phenylenediamine hydrochloride aqueous solution) into red quinones, and the color of *Neisseria gonorrhoeae* colonies can become fuchsia or black. The suspected colony smears are examined by Gram staining and identified by oxidase test and carbohydrate (glucose, maltose, sucrose, fructose or lactose) fermentation test.

Oxidase test of *Neisseria gonorrhoeae*: the test was performed on *Neisseria gonorrhoeae* plates mixed with stray bacteria. With a 0.5 ml pipette, 2-3 drops of oxidase reagent were added to the suspected small gray-white colonies. The colonies turned red, which was considered oxidase-positive bacteria. Report "*Neisseria gonorrhoeae* is detected" or "*Neisseria gonorrhoeae* is not detected". The oxidase test of *Neisseria gonorrhoeae* is of certain significance for the early and rapid diagnosis of gonorrhea.

4. Isolation, cultivation and identification of *Ureaplasma urealyticum*

Specimens are inoculated in *Ureaplasma urealyticum* medium and cultured in a 35 ℃ incubator for 24-48 h. If the medium changes from clear to purplish red, the experiment is carried out as follows.

(1) 0.1 ml of this medium is inoculated on *Ureaplasma urealyticum* solid medium, and incubate it in a 35 ℃ and 5% CO_2 incubator for 24-48 h. If "fried eggs" or "particle-like" colonies are found under low-power microscope, the identification of *Ureaplasma urealyticum* is carried out according to the relevant chapters.

(2) The above liquid cultures are inoculated in an A7B identification medium and incubated in a 5% CO_2 incubator for 24-48 h. *Ureaplasma urealyticum* produced smaller dark brown or yellow colonies, and other mycoplasmas produced micro-amber colonies, which are larger than *Ureaplasma urealyticum* colonies.

According to the above positive results, report "*Ureaplasma urealyticum* is detected". If there is no colony growth after incubation for 72 h, report "*Ureaplasma urealyticum* is not detected". The type could be identified by PCR method or metabolic inhibition test if it's necessary.

5. Isolation, cultivation and identification of chlamydia

(1) Treatment of the specimen: put the swab into the test tube and wash it out in the transport medium by violent concussion to break up the infected cells and release chlamydia. Inoculate or store in −70 ℃ refrigerator immediately (melt rapidly in 37 ℃ water if inoculation).

(2) Preparation of McCoy cells: McCoy cells form a dense monolayer in a cell bottle. After 0.25% trypsin digestion, the cell concentration is adjusted to 1×10^5/ml, cell climbing slices are placed in a 24-well cell culture plate, and 1 ml cell suspension is added and incubated for 24-48 h in a 5% CO_2 incubator at 35 ℃.

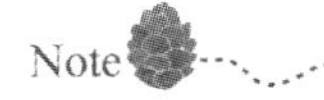

(3) Inoculation of specimens: 0.2 ml of specimens are added to each well, centrifuged at 2000 r/min for 1 h, and then incubated in a 5% CO_2 incubator for 24-72 h.

(4)After discarding the supernatant, wash with PBS for 2-3 times and fix materials with methanol. Giemsa staining, iodine staining (inclusion body is brown) and immunofluorescence are used to detect the inclusion body, and the observation methods of results are the same as previously mentioned.

6. Cultivation and identification of *Candida*

Two Sabouraud medium are inoculated with samples and placed at room temperature (18-25 ℃) and 35 ℃, respectively. The identification methods are referred to the relevant chapters.

[Attentions]

(1) *Neisseria gonorrhoeae* is autolytic and has poor resistance, so samples should be inoculated and smeared as soon as possible after collection. Try to get inoculated at the bedside. If it needs to be transported, the specimen should be placed in the selective transport medium at 35 ℃, and the plate to be inoculated should be preheated.

(2)There are a large number of normal floras in the vagina, so it is necessary to evaluate the pathogenicity of normal flora correctly.

(3)*Chlamydia trachomatis* is an intracellular parasite. When dealing with specimens, the epithelial cells need to be broken so that the *Chlamydia trachomatis* can be released.

(4)Identification of common pathogenic microorganisms of genitourinary tract infections is shown in Fig. 3-5-1.

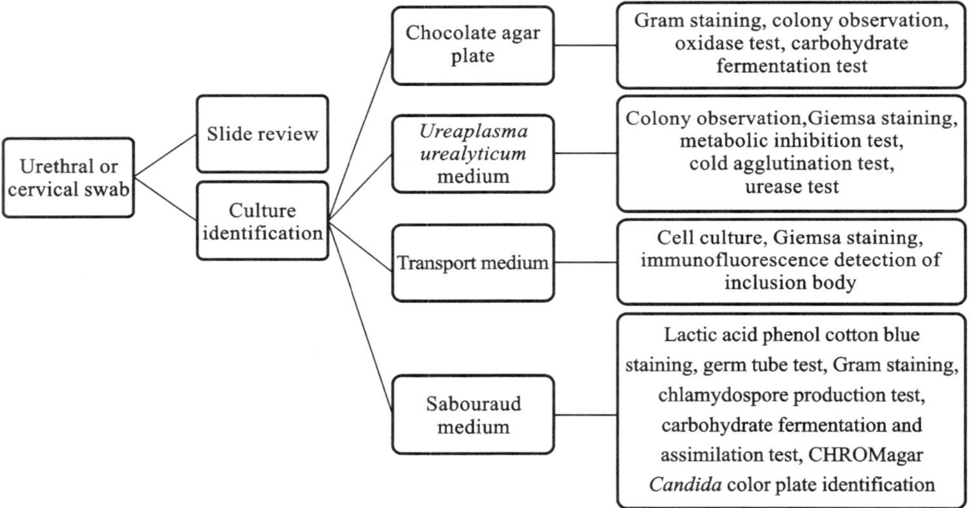

Fig. 3-5-1 Identification of common pathogenic microorganisms of genitourinary tract infections

[Questions]

(1)What are the pathogenic microorganisms that cause sexually transmitted diseases?

(2)What are the characteristics of *Neisseria gonorrhoeae* compared with other pyogenic coccus?

(3)What are the possible biosafety issues in genitourinary tract specimen examination? How can these issues be avoided to ensure biosafety?

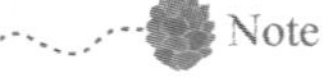
Note

(Yinyan Yin, Cuicui Liu)

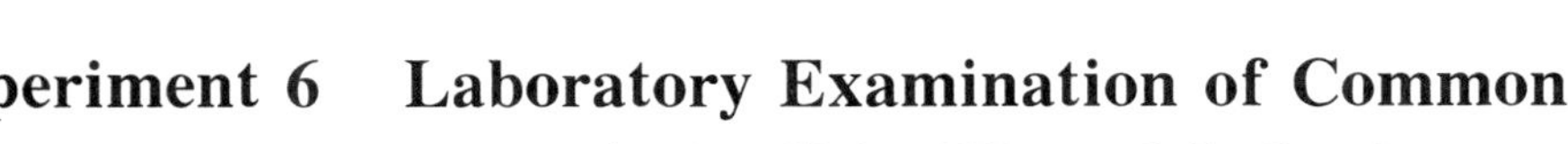

Experiment 6 Laboratory Examination of Common Bacteria in Skin Wound Infections

[Experimental Objectives]

To master the bacteriologic examination of pus specimens.

[Experimental Materials]

(1)Specimens: puncture fluid, pus or wound secretions, or simulated specimen, etc.

(2)Blood agar plates, anaerobic culture bottles, and common biochemical reaction tubes such as O-F tubes, KIA tubes, nitrate biochemical identification tubes and citrate biochemical identification tubes.

(3)Gram staining solution, 3% hydrogen peroxide solution, 1% tetramethyl-*p*-phenylenediamine hydrochloride solution, indole reagent, fresh human or rabbit plasma, etc.

(4)Slides, microscope, etc.

[Experimental Contents]

Pus and wound secretions are the more commonly tested specimens during infection, and examiners and clinicians should work closely together to ensure proper collection and rapid inspection of such specimens. Many types of bacteria can be detected from pus and wound secretions, and the most prioritized pathogenic bacteria are *Staphylococcus aureus* and *Streptococcus pyogenes*, followed by *Pseudomonas aeruginosa* and Enterobacteriaceae, etc.

1. Eye observation

Observe the specimen's character, color and the presence or absence of sulfur granule. If the specimen is green, it may be a *Pseudomonas aeruginosa* infection; if it has a bad smell, it may be an anaerobic or *Bacillus proteus* infection; if there are sulfur granules in the pus, it suggests an actinomycotic infection.

2. Smear examination

(1)General bacterial smear examination. The specimen to be examined should be fixed and then stained with Gram staining solution. Based on the morphology and staining characteristics of the bacteria seen under the microscope, a preliminary report can be made. For specimens suspected to be infected with *Mycobacterium tuberculosis*, acid-fast staining should be performed.

(2)Smear examination of *Actinomyces israelii* and *Nocardia asteroides*. Examine the pus, wound secretions or dressings for grayish-white or sulfur granule less than 1 mm in diameter with the eyes or a magnifying glass. Subsequently, use the inoculation loop to pick the specimen containing sulfur granule and place it on a clean slide, cover with a coverslip, and gently squeeze it; if the structure of the particles is not obvious, add 2-3 drops of potassium hydroxide solution with 50-100 g/L to digest them and then observe them carefully under low-power microscope

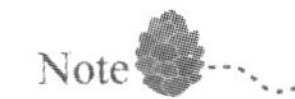

and high-power microscope. Or the specimen can be directly smeared, and after Gram staining (acid-fast staining if necessary), according to the shape and the staining characteristics of the bacteria under the microscope, it can be reported that "Gram-negative/positive bacteria are found in the direct smear". If particles of *Actinomyces israelii* are present, they can be seen in the center of the intertwined filaments. The ends of the filaments are slightly enlarged, rod-like arrangement and radial; sometimes they can be seen embedded in the gelatin-like sheath. *Nocardia asteroids* basically has the same morphology as *Actinomyces israelii*, but the end of the branching mycelium is generally not expanded into a rod-shaped, Gram staining is positive, and acid-fast staining is positive; and *Actinomyces israelii* is positive by Gram staining, and is negative by acid-fast staining. If the middle part of the mycelium stains is Gram-positive, the end part of the mycelium radiating in all directions is Gram-negative, and the acid-fast staining is negative, it can be reported as "Finding *Actinomyces israelii*"; if the Gram staining reaction is the same as that of *Actinomyces israelii*, and the acid-fast staining is positive, it can be reported as "Finding *Nocardia asteroides*"; if the Gram staining is negative, and the acid-fast staining is negative, it can be reported as "Not find *Actinomyces israelii* and *Nocardia asteroids*".

3. Culture examination

(1) General bacterial culture. Take a pus cotton swab or use an inoculation loop to inoculate pus in the blood agar plate, and placed in 37 ℃ incubator for 18-24 h. If the bacteria grow, according to the characteristics of the colony, pick a variety of individual colony to smear respectively, then examine under microscope after Gram staining to initially determine the type of bacteria, and then carry out identification according to the identification point of various types of bacteria.

①Beta-hemolytic *Streptococcus*. If the colony is as small as the tip of a needle, surrounded by a large and transparent hemolytic ring, it may be hemolytic *Streptococcus*, combined with microscopic examination to help identify it. If necessary, culture with serum broth; if there is precipitation and the smear is arranged in a long chain-like after staining, it is suspected to be beta-hemolytic *Streptococcus*.

②*Staphylococcus aureus*. *Staphylococcus aureus* in the blood agar plate grows to medium-sized, raised, moist and golden yellow or white round colonies with β-hemolytic ring. Smear staining microscopic examination for Gram-positive, grape-like or cluster arrangement of cocci. The catalase test, mannitol fermentation test, and plasma coagulase test were positive. *Staphylococcus aureus* was sensitive to neomycin, and the heat-resistant nuclease test was positive. If you see a medium-sized, fat-soluble, golden pigment or no special pigment on the blood agar plate with a transparent hemolytic ring, smear staining microscopic examination for Gram-positive cocci arranged in grape bunches, it can be further confirmed by mannitol fermentation test, plasma coagulase test, and so on.

③ *Streptococcus pneumoniae*. If there are small colonies surrounded by a grass-green hemolytic ring, and microscopy examination of the stained smear is Gram-positive, the short-chain arrangement is mostly alpha-hemolytic *Streptococcus*, the double arrangement is mostly *Streptococcus pneumoniae*. Further identification and differential tests can confirm the diagnosis.

④*Proteus vulgaris*. On the blood agar plate, the colonies are flat with migratory diffuse growth, moist and grayish-white. Due to the action of bacterial protease, a hemolysis-like phenomenon can be seen, with a bad odor. Gram-negative bacilli are polymorphic. The oxidase

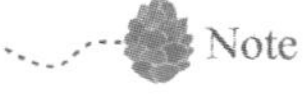

test was negative, the catalase test was positive, and the phenylalanine deaminase test was positive. KIA: K/A, H_2S (+), gas production. MIU: kinetics (+), indigo substrate (+), urease (+).

⑤*Pseudomonas aeruginosa*. The colony on the blood agar plate is flattened, has an irregular edge, is moist, spreads in all directions, and often has water-soluble blue-green pigment on the medium, with β-hemolytic ring and a special smell. They are Gram-negative recto-bacteria. The oxidase test was positive. It can decompose glucose and xylose to produce acid without gas by oxidation. It can reduce nitrate to nitrite and produce nitrogen and utilize citrate. It is positive for arginine double hydrolase, and grows at 42 ℃.

(2) *Bacillus anthracis*. When *Bacillus anthracis* infection is suspected, the patient's pus should be inoculated on the blood agar plate. For a seriously contaminated specimen, it can be first increased in broth medium overnight, then heated at 80 ℃ for 20 min to kill non-spore-forming bacteria, and then transferred to a blood agar plate for isolation culture. After culturing at 37 ℃ for 18-24 h, such as in the blood agar plate, if see the large and flat, plush, gray-white, irregular edge is not neat, curly hair shaped (using low-power microscope to observe more clearly), and not hemolytic colonies, then pick colony to stain for microscopic examination. If it is Gram-positive bamboo-like bacilli arranged in chains, suspension droplet examination without power, then animal inoculation, bead test and phage lysis test are used for differential diagnosis.

(3) Anaerobe. Specimens suspected of anaerobic infection should be inoculated into the culture medium of bovine heart, bovine brain extract or Brucella broth, or directly inoculated into the KVA blood plate (or LKV plate) and placed in an anaerobic environment for culture. When isolating anaerobic bacterial bacteria, such as *Clostridium tetani*, liquid medium which has inoculated with specimens should be first heated in a water bath at 80 ℃ for 20 min to kill non-spore-forming bacteria, and then cultured at 37 ℃ for 24-48 h. According to the growth and smear staining microscopic results, conduct identification by the biological characteristics of the anaerobic bacteria (biochemical reactions and animal testing).

(4) *Actinomyces israelii* and *Nocardia asteroides*.

①*Actinomyces israelii*. For fistula drainage fluid suspected of being contaminated with stray bacteria, the specimen should first be poured into a sterile dish. The blood cells in the solution should be washed with sterile distilled water. Then, the typical or suspected sulfur granule should be selected and crushed and then inoculated into two copies of dextrose broth agar plates and placed at 37 ℃ for aerobic and anaerobic culture respectively. At the same time, inoculate to the Sabouraud glucose agar slant (or plate), and place at 22-28 ℃ for culture. If there is no sulfur granule, you can take the specimen directly inoculated in the above medium.

For specimens not contaminated by bacteria or fungi, sulfur granule or pus can be directly inoculated to sodium thioglycolate broth or deep glucose broth agar plate and placed in anaerobic incubation at 37 ℃, and at the same time, inoculated to Sabouraud glucose agar slant and placed at 22-28 ℃ for culture. After 4 d of incubation, if there were white, rough or nodular colonies on the glucose broth agar plates of anaerobic culture, which were not easy to be removed by an inoculation loop and not easy to be emulsified in physiological saline, and there were no similar colonies on the plates of aerobic culture, it was suspected to be *Actinomyces israelii*.

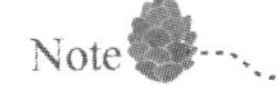

The colonies suspected to be *Actinomyces israelii* were transplanted to the bottom of sodium thioglycolate broth tube and incubated at 37 ℃. After 4-6 d, white fluffy colony material could be seen to grow. The colony material was then crushed by shaking, and the upper culture solution remained clarified. It was transferred to glucose broth agar for deep incubation at 37 ℃ for 4-6 d, and can be seen on the surface of the lower layer of the leaf-shaped colonies in the deep culture tube. After taking the colonies for smear microscopy, there can be intertwined or small fragments of mycelium, and acid-fast staining is negative.

② *Nocardia asteroides*. Smooth, irregularly folded or granular colonies with yellow to orange-yellow color appeared on the weak medium of Sabouraud medium in aerobic culture, and hyphae with fine branched, Gram-positive and reddish in acid-fast staining were detected on microscopic examination of the colonies taken as wet slices.

[Experimental Report]

(1) Describe Gram staining and culture characteristics of staphylococci.

(2) Describe cultural characteristics of *Pseudomonas aeruginosa*.

[Questions]

(1) Describe the significance of sulfur granule in bacterial identification.

(2) What should be done with samples contaminated with stray bacteria?

(3) What biosafety issues may exist in the examination of pus or purulent secretions? How to avoid it to ensure biosafety?

(Guimei Kong, Chengfeng Gao)

Experiment 7 Pathogenic and Immunological Diagnosis of Mice Infected with *Schistosoma japonicum*

[Experimental Objectives]

(1) To understand the infection route, parasitic site and adult morphological characteristics of *Schistosoma japonicum* (*S. japonicum*).

(2) To master the immunological diagnosis of schistosomiasis japonica.

(3) To understand the pathological changes caused by *S. japonicum* eggs.

[Experimental Contents]

Ⅰ Establishment of a mouse model of *S. japonicum* infection

(1) Experimental animals: 20 Kunming mice aged 6-8 weeks.

(2) The positive snail infected with *S. japonicum* were placed in a small beaker with clean and dechlorinated water, and the *S. japonicum* cercariae escaped under the condition of 20-25 ℃ and light. The cercaria were extracted from the surface of the water by an inoculation loop,

Note

moved to the cover glass, and counted under the anatomical mirror, and 30±5 cercariae were collected. After anesthesia, the mice were fixed on the mouse board with their abdomens facing upward. The hair of the abdomen was pulled out, the skin of the abdomen was moistened with dechlorinated water, and the cover glass was directly attached to the skin of the abdomen. The cover glass was removed after being retained for 20 min. The mice were kept until the 6th week.

Ⅱ Observation of pathogenic results of mice infected with *S. japonicum*

1. Adult count of *S. japonicum*

Cardiac perfusion with physiological saline was performed. After the mice were sacrificed for cervical dislocated, the skin was peeled off, the abdominal cavity and chest cavity were opened, and the physiological saline was sucked into the syringe and injected through the left ventricle. After the portal vein was filled, the side was cut open, and the physiological saline was continued to be injected to wash out the worms. After lavage, the whole intestine and mesenteric tissue were removed and pressed between two thick glass plates to count the remaining worms in the mesenteric veins. The final worm count of each mouse was the sum of the number of worms obtained by irrigation and the number of worms obtained by a pressure plate.

2. Egg count of *S. japonicum*

The left anterior lobe of mouse liver was fixed in 10% formaldehyde solution, and the remaining liver was weighed and digested in 10 ml of 5% KOH solution at 37 ℃ overnight. After mixing the digestive fluid well, take 1 ml to a 1.5 ml EP tube, and then take 10 μl from it onto a slide, cover the cover glass, and count the eggs under a 100-fold light microscope.

Number of eggs per gram of liver=(egg count under light microscope/digestive liver mass) ×1000

3. Liver pathology observation

The severely diseased part of the liver was soaked in 10% formaldehyde solution and fixed for more than 12 h. Pathological sections were prepared and stained with hematoxylin and eosin. Under the microscope, observations were made, and photographs were taken. The distribution of egg granuloma was observed.

Ⅲ ELISA was used to diagnose schistosomiasis japonica

1. Experimental principle

ELISA is a commonly used immunological method for the diagnosis of schistosomiasis japonica. The soluble antigen of *S. japonicum* was coated in a special polystyrene reaction hole, and the serum to be tested was added to the reaction hole. If the serum contained a corresponding specific antibody, the antigen-antibody complex could be formed. If the corresponding HRP was added to the reaction hole to label the secondary antibody, the experimental result could be judged by the chromogenic reaction of the substrate.

2. Reagents

PBS (10 mmol/L, pH 7.4), PBST (PBS with 0.05% Tween-20), coated solution (pH 9.6, 0.05 mol/L carbonate buffer) and substrate developing solution. Sealing solution: 3% skim milk (3 g skim milk powder/100 ml PBS).

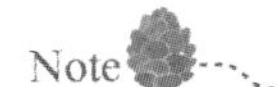

Mouse antiserum (obtained by animal experiment of schistosomiasis, frozen at −20 ℃ for use), goat anti-mouse IgG-HRP, adult *S. japonicum* antigen, etc.

3. Main steps

(1)Coating: dilute the antigen with the coated solution into 5 μg/ml, 100 μl/well, and incubate in the wet box at 4 ℃ overnight.

(2)Washing: wash with PBST 5 times.

(3)Sealing: it is sealed with 3% skim milk, 300 μl/well, at room temperature for 1 h.

(4)Reaction with antiserum: add mouse antiserum (1 : 100), 100 μl/well, at room temperature for 1 h.

(5)Wash 6 times as above.

(6)Reaction with enzyme-conjugate secondary antibody: add goat anti-mouse IgG-HRP (1 : 500), 100 μl/well, at room temperature for 1 h.

(7)Wash 6 times as above.

(8)Color development: add substrate developing solution, 200 μl/well, and let it sit at room temperature for 0.5 h, avoiding light.

(9)Termination: terminate the reaction with 50 μl 1 mol/L H_2SO_4.

4. Observation and analysis of experimental results

Read results at 490 nm (positive reactions are brown or brownish yellow).

5. Attentions

(1) Strictly observe the rules of experimental operation to prevent cross-contamination between wells.

(2)Blank control without antigen, positive control and negative control should be set in the experiment.

[Questions]

According to the experimental results, please analyze the significance of the antibody detection results of schistosomiasis japonica.

(Fang Tian)

Note

附录 A　常用染色液和试剂的配制

1. 革兰染色液

(1)结晶紫液:取 2 g 结晶紫溶于 20 ml 95%酒精中;取 0.8 g 草酸铵溶于 80 ml 蒸馏水中。两液混合,静置 48 h,过滤后使用。

(2)鲁氏碘液:先将 2 g 碘化钾溶于少量水中,再将 1 g 碘溶于上述溶液中,加蒸馏水至 300 ml,保存于棕色瓶中。

(3)石炭酸复红稀释液:按 10 ml 石炭酸复红原液(10 g 复红溶于 100 ml 95%酒精)加 90 ml 蒸馏水的比例混合后存放于瓶内,临用前过滤。

2. 抗酸染色液

(1)取 4 g 碱性复红溶于 100 ml 95%酒精,再与 900 ml 5%石炭酸水溶液混合。

(2)3%盐酸酒精:取 3 ml 浓盐酸加入 97 ml 95%酒精中。

(3)吕氏美蓝溶液:取 30 ml 美蓝酒精饱和液,加入 1 ml 1%氢氧化钾溶液和 100 ml 蒸馏水。临用前过滤。

3. 乳酸酚棉蓝染色液　取 0.125 g 棉蓝(苯胺蓝)溶于 50 ml 蒸馏水,放置过夜等待溶解。第 2 天取 50 g 碳酸晶体加入盛有 50 ml 乳酸的烧杯中,并用磁力搅拌器搅拌。在上述乳酸溶液中加入 100 ml 甘油,并将第 1 天配制且过滤后的棉蓝溶液加入其中,存放于室温,待用。

4. 吉姆萨(Giemsa)染色液

(1)取 0.5 g Giemsa 粉末加入 33 ml 甘油,于研钵中研细,置于 56 ℃孵育 90 min 后,加入 33 ml甲醇,混匀后过滤,装入棕色瓶中备用。

(2)上述 Giemsa 原液用 0.1 mol/L 磷酸缓冲液稀释 20 倍或 50 倍后使用。

5. Fontana 镀银染色剂

(1)固定液:取 1 ml 冰醋酸、2 ml 甲醛,加蒸馏水至 100 ml。

(2)媒染液:取 5 g 鞣酸、1 g 石炭酸,加蒸馏水至 100 ml。

(3)硝酸银溶液:取 5 g 硝酸银加入 100 ml 蒸馏水中。

用前取硝酸银溶液 20 ml,逐滴加入 100 g/L 氢氧化铵溶液直至产生棕色沉淀,轻摇后沉淀溶解,微呈乳白色。

6. 吲哚试剂(柯氏试剂)　取 5.0 g 对二甲氨基苯甲醛,溶于 75 ml 正戊醇中,再徐徐加入 25 ml浓盐酸。

7. 甲基红试剂　取 100 mg 甲基红,加 7.4 ml 0.05 mol/L NaOH 溶液使其溶解,再加蒸馏水稀释至 200 ml 并转移到指示剂瓶中即可。颜色变化范围为红色到黄色(pH 4.2～6.3)。

8. VP 试剂　50 g/L α-萘酚溶液:取 0.5 g α-萘酚溶于 10 ml 95%酒精中。

9. 枸橼酸盐试验试剂　溴麝香草酚蓝指示液:取 0.1 g 溴麝香草酚蓝,加入 3.2 ml 0.05 mol/L NaOH 溶液,再加蒸馏水至 200 ml。

10. 1%盐酸四甲基对苯二胺溶液　取 1 g 盐酸四甲基对苯二胺溶于 100 ml 蒸馏水中,储存于棕色瓶,并置于冰箱冷藏待用。

11. 硝酸盐还原试验试剂

(1)甲液:于 100 ml 5 mol/L 醋酸中加入 0.8 g 对氨基苯磺酸。

(2)乙液:于 100 ml 5 mol/L 醋酸中加入 0.5 g α-萘胺。

12. 过氧化氢酶试验试剂 0.3% H_2O_2溶液:吸取 0.5 ml 30% H_2O_2溶液并加入 pH 7.0 磷酸缓冲液至 50 ml。

13. 碘染色试剂 取 2 g 碘化钾溶于少量蒸馏水中,待完全溶解后加入 1 g 碘,搅拌溶解后加入蒸馏水至 300 ml,保存于棕色瓶内待用。

附录B　常用培养基的配制

1. SS培养基　取48 g SS琼脂培养基干粉置于烧杯中，加入1000 ml蒸馏水，将烧杯置于微波炉中加热1～2 min(注意不要煮沸)。取出烧杯用玻璃棒搅拌后放回微波炉继续加热，重复上述操作直至培养基干粉完全溶解。将完全溶解的培养基放于室温中稍冷后，倾注于无菌平板中(每个平板15～20 ml)，待琼脂凝固后即可用于细菌的分离和培养。

2. 沙氏培养基　取1.8 g琼脂、1 g蛋白胨、4 g葡萄糖或麦芽糖溶于100 ml蒸馏水中，加热使之溶解，调节pH至5.5～6.0，分装于试管中并于112 ℃高压灭菌15 min后，制成高层斜面备用。将上述组分改为1 g蛋白胨、1.2 g琼脂及100 ml蒸馏水，可供真菌缓慢生长，适用于菌种保存。

3. 庖肉培养基　取0.5 g牛肉渣，装于15 mm×150 mm的试管中，加入7 ml pH 7.6的肉汤培养基，再在上面加入3～4 mm厚的熔化的凡士林，高压灭菌后备用。

4. 葡萄糖发酵管

(1)配制浓度为20%的葡萄糖溶液，于112 ℃高压灭菌15 min。

(2)取1000 ml pH 7.6的蛋白胨水培养基，加入1 ml 1.6%溴甲酚紫溶液，分装于内有小导管的试管(10 mm×100 mm)中，121 ℃高压灭菌20 min。

(3)采用无菌操作加入0.25 ml 20%无菌葡萄糖溶液，使终浓度为1%。

5. 乳糖发酵管

(1)配制浓度为20%的乳糖溶液，于112 ℃高压灭菌15 min。

(2)取1000 ml pH 7.6的蛋白胨水培养基，加入1 ml 1.6%溴甲酚紫溶液，分装于内有小导管的试管中，121 ℃高压灭菌20 min。

(3)采用无菌操作加入0.25 ml 20%无菌乳糖溶液，使终浓度为1%。

6. 蛋白胨水培养基　取10 g蛋白胨、5 g氯化钠溶于1000 ml蒸馏水中，调节pH为7.6，121 ℃高压灭菌20 min后备用。

7. 醋酸铅培养基

(1)取0.5 g醋酸铅、0.25 g硫代硫酸钠，加入500 ml蒸馏水中混匀后，置于灭菌器内灭菌15 min。

(2)灭菌后加入500 ml营养琼脂，混匀后分装于试管(10 mm×100 mm)内，每管约3 ml。

(3)115 ℃高压灭菌10 min后备用。

8. 尿素培养基　取0.1 g蛋白胨、0.5 g氯化钠、0.2 g磷酸二氢钾溶于100 ml蒸馏水中，调节pH为7.4，过滤，加入0.2 ml 0.6% 酚红溶液混匀，112 ℃高压灭菌15 min，冷却后加入1 ml 10%无菌葡萄糖溶液和经过滤除菌的2 ml 10%尿素溶液，混匀后分装于小试管中备用。

9. 克氏双糖铁琼脂(KIA)培养基

(1)成分：蛋白胨20 g、牛肉膏3 g、酵母膏3 g、乳糖10 g、葡萄糖1 g、氯化钠5 g、枸橼酸铁铵0.5 g、硫代硫酸钠0.5 g、琼脂10 g、酚红0.025 g。

(2)将除琼脂和酚红以外的各成分溶解于1000 ml蒸馏水中，调节pH至7.2。

(3)加入琼脂，加热至全部溶解后加入12.5 ml 0.2%酚红溶液混匀，分装于试管(10 mm×

100 mm)中(每管约 4 ml),121 ℃高压灭菌 15 min 后,制成高层斜面备用。

10. 麦康凯琼脂培养基 取 20 g 蛋白胨,5 g 氯化钠,10 g 乳糖,13 g 琼脂,1.5 g 胆盐(3 号),0.03 g 中性红,0.001 g 结晶紫溶于 1000 ml 蒸馏水中,调节 pH 为 7.4±0.2,121 ℃高压灭菌 15 min后备用。

11. 血琼脂培养基

(1)取 3.3 g 营养琼脂,加 100 ml 蒸馏水,加热至完全溶解,121 ℃高压灭菌 20 min。

(2)冷却至 50～55 ℃时,采用无菌操作加入 8～10 ml 无菌脱纤维羊血(或兔血)。

(3)轻轻摇匀(注意不要产生气泡)后,倒入无菌培养皿或制成斜面。完全凝固后随机取部分于 37 ℃培养箱培养 18～24 h,无细菌生长则可使用或于 4 ℃冷藏备用。

12. 科玛嘉念珠菌显色培养基 琼脂 15.0 g/L、蛋白胨 10.2 g/L、氯霉素 0.5 g/L、色素 22.0 g/L,调节 pH 至 6.1。

13. 缓冲炭酵母提取物琼脂基础(buffered charcoal yeast extract agar base) 简称军团菌 BCYE 琼脂基础(legionella BCYE agar base),加入添加剂后用于选择性培养军团菌。取 10 g 酵母提取物,2 g 活性炭,1 g α一酮戊二酸单钾盐,10 g N一(2一乙酰胺基)一2一氨基乙烷磺酸(ACES 缓冲剂),17 g 琼脂,溶解于 1 L 蒸馏水中,调节 pH 为 6.9 ± 0.2。军团菌添加剂配方如下:L一半胱氨酸盐酸盐 400 mg,焦磷酸铁 250 mg。

14. 伊红美蓝(EMB)培养基 蛋白胨 10 g、乳糖 10 g、磷酸氢二钾 2 g、琼脂 25 g、2%伊红 Y(曙红)溶液 20 ml、0.5%美蓝(亚甲蓝)溶液 13 ml,pH 7.4。

15. 动力-吲哚-脲酶(MIU)培养基 胰蛋白胨 1 g、氯化钠 0.75 g、磷酸氢二钾 0.2 g、葡萄糖 0.1 g、琼脂 0.4 g、蒸馏水 100 ml、20%尿素溶液 10 ml。将上述成分(20%尿素溶液除外)溶于蒸馏水,加适量 0.4%酚红溶液,116 ℃高压灭菌 20 min,然后将过滤除菌后的 20%尿素溶液加入灭菌后的培养基中,分装、备用。

16. GN 增菌液 简称 GN 肉汤(Gram-negative bacteria broth,即革兰阴性菌肉汤),用于革兰阴性菌的选择性培养,特别是志贺菌和沙门菌的增菌培养。取 20 g 胰蛋白胨,1 g 葡萄糖,2 g 甘露醇,5 g 柠檬酸钠,0.5 g 去氧胆酸钠,4 g 磷酸氢二钠,1.5 g 磷酸氢二钾,5 g 氯化钠,溶于 1 L 蒸馏水,加热使溶解,调节 pH 为 7.0。

17. 碱性蛋白胨水 蛋白胨 20 g、氯化钠 5 g、硝酸钾 0.1 g、结晶碳酸钠($Na_2CO_3 \cdot 12H_2O$) 0.2 g、蒸馏水 1000 ml。调节 pH 至 8.4 后于 121 ℃高压灭菌 15 min,备用。

18. TCBS 琼脂平板 酵母粉 5 g、蛋白胨 10 g、硫代硫酸钠 10 g、枸橼酸钠 10 g、牛胆粉 5 g、牛磺胆酸钠 3 g、蔗糖 20 g、氯化钠 10 g、枸橼酸铁 1 g、溴麝香草酚蓝(指示剂)0.04 g、琼脂 15 g、蒸馏水 1000 ml。

19. 罗氏培养基 磷酸二氢钾 2.4 g、一水硫酸镁 0.24 g、枸橼酸镁 0.6 g、天冬酰胺 3.6 g、马铃薯淀粉 30 g、2%孔雀绿溶液 20 ml、蒸馏水 600 ml、甘油 12 ml、新鲜鸡蛋液 1000 ml。

Appendix A Preparation of Common Staining Solution and Reagents

1. Gram staining solution

(1)Crystal violet solution: 2 g of crystal violet was dissolved in 20 ml of 95% ethanol, and 0.8 g of ammonium oxalate was dissolved in 80 ml distilled water. The two solutions described above were mixed and filtered after staying for 48 h.

(2)Lugol's iodine solution: first, 2 g of potassium iodide was dissolved in a small amount of water, and then 1 g of iodine was dissolved in the above solution. Distilled water was added to 300 ml and the solution was stored in a brown bottle.

(3)Carbolfuchsin dilution: 10 ml of carbolfuchsin stock solution (10 g of carbolfuchsin was dissolved in 100 ml of 95% ethanol) was mixed with 90 ml of distilled water and filtered before use.

2. Acid-fast staining solution

(1)4 g of basic fuchsin was dissolved in 100 ml of 95% ethanol and mixed with 900 ml of 5% carbolic acid solution.

(2)3% hydrochloric acid ethanol solution: 3 ml of concentrated hydrochloric acid was added to 97 ml of 95% ethanol.

(3)Loeffler methylene blue solution: 30 ml of methylene blue ethanol saturated solution, 1 ml of 1% potassium hydroxide, and 100 ml of distilled water were mixed and filtered before use.

3. Lactophenol cotton blue staining solution

On the first day, dissolve 0.125 g of cotton blue (aniline blue) in 50 ml of distilled water and leave it overnight. On the second day, add 50 g of carbonic acid crystals to containing a glass beaker and stir it with a magnetic stirrer. Add 100 ml of glycerin to the lactic acid solution. Mix the filtered cotton blue solution from the first day into the phenol, glycerin, and lactic acid solution. Store at room temperature for use.

4. Giemsa staining solution

(1)Preparation of Giemsa stock solution: 0.5 g of Giemsa powder was added to 33 ml of glycerin, ground in a mortar, and after incubating at 56 ℃ for 90 min, 33 ml of methanol was added, mixed well and filtered, then placed in a brown bottle for later use.

(2)The Giemsa stock solution was diluted 20-fold or 50-fold with 0.1 mol/L phosphate buffer when use.

5. Fontana silver plating staining solution

(1)Fixed solution: take 1 ml of glacial acetic acid and 2 ml of formaldehyde and add distilled water to 100 ml.

(2)Mordant solution: take 5 g of tannic acid and 1 g of carbolic acid and add distilled water to 100 ml.

(3)Silver nitrate solution: take 5 g of silver nitrate into 100 ml of distilled water.

Before use, take 20 ml of silver nitrate solution and add 100 g/L of ammonium hydroxide dropwise until a brown precipitate is formed. Shake gently and dissolve until the liquid is slightly milky white.

6. Indole reagent (Kovac's reagent)

Take 5.0 g of *p*-dimethylaminobenzaldehyde and dissolve it in 75 ml of *n*-pentanol, then slowly add 25 ml of concentrated hydrochloric acid.

7. Methyl red reagent

Take 100 mg of methyl red, dissolve it in 7.4 ml of 0.05 mol/L NaOH solution, and dilute it with distilled water to 200 ml before transferring it to an indicator bottle. The color change range is red to yellow (pH 4.2 to 6.3).

8. VP reagent

50 g/L α-naphthol solution: take 0.5 g of α-naphthol and dissolve it in 10 ml of 95% ethanol.

9. Citrate test reagent

Bromothymol blue indicator solution: take 0.1 g of bromothymol blue, add 3.2 ml of 0.05 mol/L NaOH solution, and then add distilled water to 200 ml.

10. 1% tetramethyl-*p*-phenylenediamine hydrochloride

1 g of tetramethyl-*p*-phenylenediamine hydrochloride is added to 100 ml of distilled water, store it in brown bottles and refrigerate for future use.

11. Nitrate reduction test reagent

(1) Solution A: add 0.8 g of *p*-aminobenzene sulfonic acid to 100 ml of 5 mol/L acetic acid.

(2) Solution B: add 0.5 g of α-naphthylamine to 100 ml of 5 mol/L acetic acid.

12. Catalase test reagent

0.3% H_2O_2 solution: suck 0.5 ml of 30% H_2O_2 solution and add pH 7.0 phosphate buffer to 50 ml.

13. Iodine staining reagent

Dissolve 2 g of potassium iodide in a small amount of distilled water, add 1 g of iodine after complete dissolution, stir and dissolve, add distilled water to 300 ml, and store in a brown bottle for use.

Appendix B Preparation of Common Culture Medium

1. SS medium

Place 48 g of SS agar medium dry powder in a beaker, add 1000 ml of distilled water, and heat the beaker in a microwave oven for 1-2 min (be careful not to boil). Remove the beaker and stir with a glass rod before returning it to the microwave oven for further heating. Repeat the above operation until the medium dry powder is completely dissolved. Place the completely dissolved medium at room temperature and cool it slightly before pouring it into a sterile plate (15-20 ml per plate). After the agar solidifies, it can be used for bacterial isolation and cultivation.

2. Sabouraud medium

Dissolve 1.8 g of agar, 1 g of peptone, and 4 g of glucose or maltose in 100 ml of distilled water. Dissolve it at high temperature, adjust the pH to 5.5-6.0, and divide it into test tubes. After 15 min of high-pressure sterilization at 112 ℃, the culture medium was prepared as a slope with a relatively large inclination for future use. The above components were changed to 1 g of peptone, 1.2 g of agar and 100 ml of distilled water for slow growth of fungi and strain preservation.

3. Cooked meat medium

Take 0.5 g of beef residue and pack it in 15 mm×150 mm test tubes. Add 7 ml of broth medium with a pH of 7.6, and add 3-4 mm thick melted vaseline on the top. Set aside after high-pressure sterilization.

4. Glucose fermentation tube

(1) Prepare an glucose solution with a concentration of 20% and sterilize it with high-pressure at 112 ℃ for 15 min.

(2) Take 1000 ml of peptone water medium with a pH of 7.6, add 1 ml of 1.6% bromocresol purple solution, and divide into test tubes (10 mm×100 mm) with small tubes. Sterilize under high-pressure at 121 ℃ for 20 min.

(3) Aseptically add 0.25 ml of 20% sterile glucose solution to a final concentration of 1%.

5. Lactose fermentation tube

(1) Prepare an lactose solution with a concentration of 20% and sterilize it with high-pressure at 112 ℃ for 15 min.

(2) Take 1000 ml of peptone water medium with a pH of 7.6, add 1 ml of 1.6% bromocresol purple solution, and divide into test tubes with small tubes. Sterilize under high-pressure at 121 ℃ for 20 min.

(3) Aseptically add 0.25 ml of 20% sterile lactose solution to a final concentration of 1%.

6. Peptone water medium

Dissolve 10 g of peptone and 5 g of sodium chloride in 1000 ml of distilled water, adjust the pH to 7.6, and sterilize under high-pressure at 121 ℃ for 20 min for later use.

7. Lead acetate medium

(1)Mix 0.5 g of lead acetate, 0.25 g of sodium thiosulfate, and 500 ml of distilled water, and sterilize in a sterilizer for 15 min.

(2)After sterilization, add 500 ml of nutrient agar, mix well, and then divide into test tubes (10 mm×100 mm), with approximately 3 ml per tube.

(3)Sterilize under high-pressure at 115 ℃ for 10 min for later use.

8. Urea medium

Dissolve 0.1 g of peptone, 0.5 g of sodium chloride, and 0.2 g of potassium dihydrogen phosphate in 100 ml of distilled water, adjust the pH to 7.4, filter, add 0.2 ml of 0.6% phenol red solution, mix well, and sterilize under high-pressure at 112 ℃ for 15 min. After cooling, add 1 ml of 10% sterile glucose solution and 2 ml of filtered 10% urea solution. After mixing, divide into small test tubes for later use.

9. KIA medium

(1)Components: 20 g of peptone, 3 g of beef extract, 3 g of yeast extract, 10 g of lactose, 1 g of glucose, 5 g of sodium chloride, 0.5 g of ammonium ferric citrate, 0.5 g of sodium thiosulfate, 10 g of agar, 0.025 g of phenol red.

(2)Dissolve all components except agar and phenol red in 1000 ml of distilled water and adjust pH to 7.2.

(3)Add agar and heat until completely dissolved. Then, add 12.5 ml of 0.2% phenol red solution and mix well. Divide into test tubes (10 mm×100 mm) with about 4 ml each. After 15 min of high-pressure sterilization at 121 ℃, the culture medium was prepared as a slope with a relatively large inclination for later use.

10. MacConkey agar medium

Dissolve 20 g of peptone, 5 g of sodium chloride, 10 g of lactose, 13 g of agar, 1.5 g of bile salt (No. 3), 0.03 g of neutral red, and 0.001 g of crystal violet in 1000 ml of distilled water; adjust the pH to 7.4±0.2 and sterilize under high-pressure at 121 ℃ for 15 min before use.

11. Blood agar medium

(1)Take 3.3 g of nutrient agar, add 100 ml of distilled water, heat until completely dissolved, and sterilize under high-pressure at 121 ℃ for 20 min.

(2)When cooled to 50-55 ℃, aseptically add 8-10 ml of sterile defibrinated sheep blood (or rabbit blood).

(3)After gently shaking (be careful not to produce bubbles), pour into a sterile culture dish or make a slant surface. After completely solidified, randomly take a portion and incubate it in a 37 ℃ incubator for 18-24 h. If there is no bacterial growth, use it or refrigerate it at 4 ℃ for later use.

12. CHROMagar candida coloring medium

Agar 15.0 g/L, peptone 10.2 g/L, chloramphenicol 0.5 g/L, and pigment 22.0 g/L. Adjust the pH to 6.1.

13. Buffered charcoal yeast extract agar base

Buffered charcoal yeast extract agar base, abbreviated as legionella BCYE agar base, is used to selectively culture legionella after adding additives. 10 g of yeast extract, 2 g of activated carbon, 1 g of α-ketoglutarate monopotassium salt, 10 g of N-(2- acetamido) -2-aminoethane sulfonic acid (ACES buffer), 17 g of agar were dissolved in 1 L distilled water, and adjusted the pH to 6 . 9±0. 2. Legionella supplement is formulated as follows: L-cysteine hydrochloride 400 mg, iron pyrophosphate 250 mg.

14. Eosin methylene blue (EMB) medium

10 g of peptone, 10 g of lactose, 2 g of dipotassium phosphate, 25 g of agar, 20 ml of 2% eosin Y solution, 13 ml of 0. 5% methylene blue solution. Adjust the pH to 7. 4.

15. MIU medium

1 g of tryptone, 0. 75 g of sodium chloride, 0. 2 g of dipotassium phosphate, 0.1 g of glucose, 0. 4 g of agar, 100 ml of distilled water, and 10 ml of 20% urea solution. Dissolve the above ingredients (excluding 20% urea solution) in distilled water, add an appropriate amount of 0. 4% phenol red solution, and sterilize under high pressure at 116 ℃ for 20 min; the filtered and sterilized 20% urea solution is added to the sterilized medium for further packaging and use.

16. GN enrichment solution

GN enrichment solution, also known as Gram-negative bacteria broth, is used for the selective culture of Gram-negative bacteria, particularly for the enrichment of *Shigella* and *Salmonella*. Take 20 g of casein peptone, 1 g of glucose, 2 g of mannitol, 5 g of sodium citrate, 0. 5 g of deoxysodium cholate, 4 g of sodium hydrogen phosphate, 1. 5 g of potassium hydrogen phosphate, and 5 g of sodium chloride, dissolve them in 1 L of distilled water, heat to dissolve, and adjust the pH to 7. 0.

17. Alkaline peptone water

20 g of peptone, 5 g of sodium chloride, 0. 1 g of potassium nitrate, 0. 2 g of crystalline sodium carbonate ($Na_2CO_3 \cdot 12H_2O$), and 1000 ml of distilled water. After adjusting the pH to 8. 4, autoclave at 121 ℃ for 15 min for use.

18. TCBS agar tablet

5 g of yeast powder, 10 g of peptone, 10 g of sodium thiosulfate, 10 g of sodium citrate, 5 g of bovine bile powder, 3 g of sodium taurocholate, 20 g of sucrose, 10 g of sodium chloride, 1 g of ferric citrate, 0. 04 g of bromothymol blue (indicator), 15 g of agar, 1000 ml distilled water.

19. Lowenstein-Jensen medium

2. 4 g of potassium dihydrogen phosphate, 0. 24 g of magnesium sulfate monohydrate, 0. 6 g of magnesium citrate, 3. 6 g of asparagine, 30 g of potato starch, 20 ml of 2% peacock green solution, 600 ml of distilled water, 12 ml of glycerin, and 1000 ml of fresh egg liquid.

部分实验结果的彩图
Color Figures of Some Experimental Results

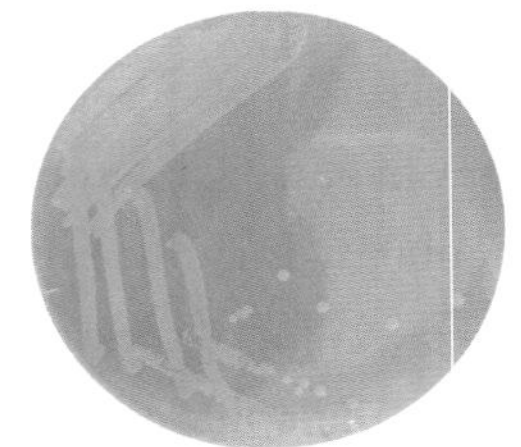
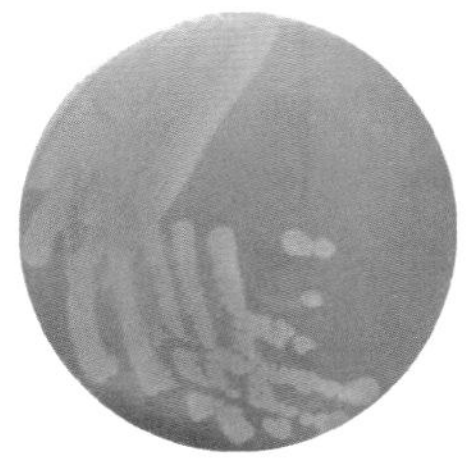

左—金黄色葡萄球菌；右—铜绿假单胞菌
Left — *Staphylococcus aureus*; right — *Pseudomonas aeruginosa*

彩图 1　平板四区划线结果
Color fig. 1　Plate four-zone delineation results

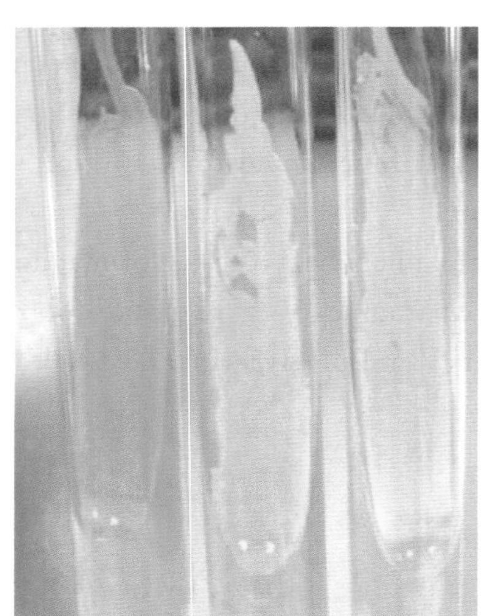

左—金黄色色素；中—柠檬色色素；右—白色色素
Left — golden yellow pigment; middle — lemon pigment; right — white pigment

彩图 2　不同细菌在斜面培养基上的色素产生情况
Color fig. 2　Pigment production by different bacteria on slant media

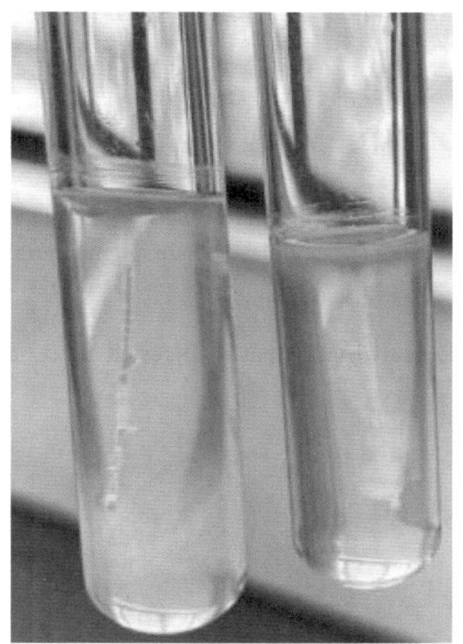

左—无动力；右—有动力

Left — undynamic; right — dynamic

彩图 3　不同细菌在半固体培养基中的运动能力

Color fig. 3　Motility of different bacteria in semi-solid media

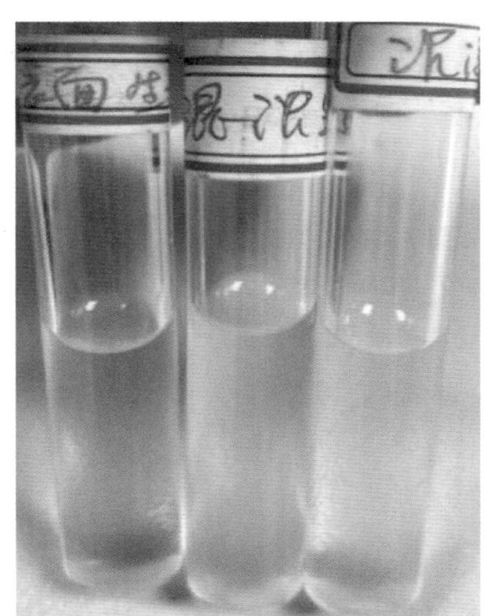

左—表面生长；中—混浊生长；右—沉淀生长

Left — surface growth; middle — turbid growth; right — sedimentation growth

彩图 4　不同细菌在液体培养基中的生长情况

Color fig. 4　The growth of different bacteria in liquid media

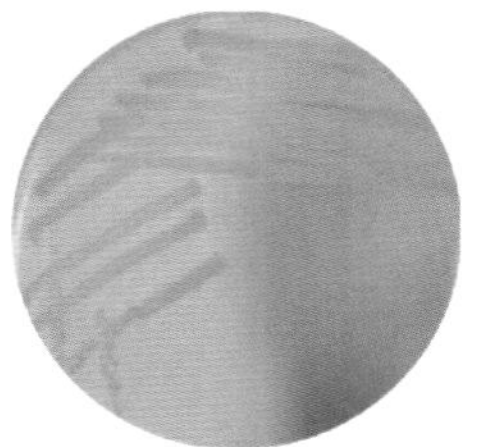
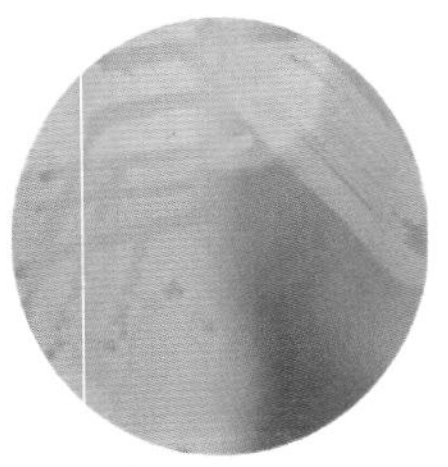
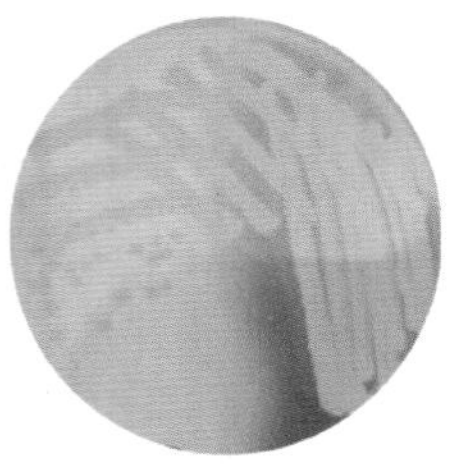

左—金黄色色素；中—柠檬色色素；右—白色色素
Left — golden yellow pigment; middle — lemon pigment; right — white pigment

彩图 5　不同细菌在固体培养基上的色素产生情况

Color fig. 5　Pigment production by different bacteria on solid media

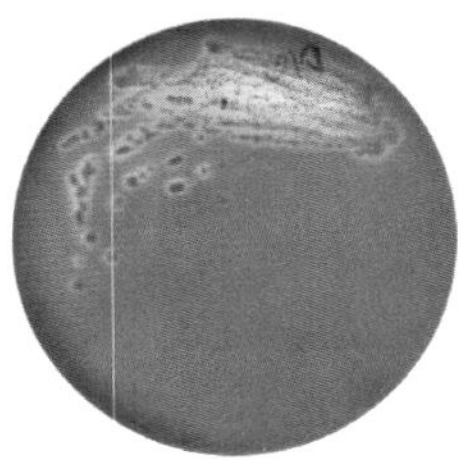

彩图 6　咽喉部微生物在血平板上的溶血现象

Color fig. 6　Hemolysis of pharyngeal microorganisms on a blood agar plate

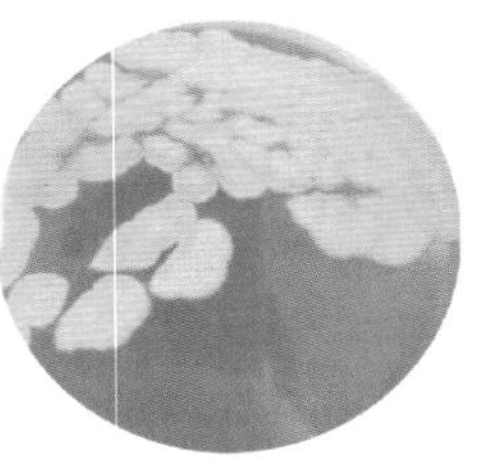

彩图 7　粗糙型菌落(枯草芽孢杆菌)

Color fig. 7　Rough-type colonies (*Bacillus subtilis*)

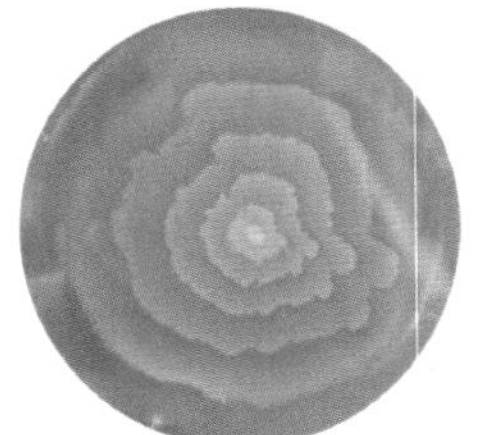
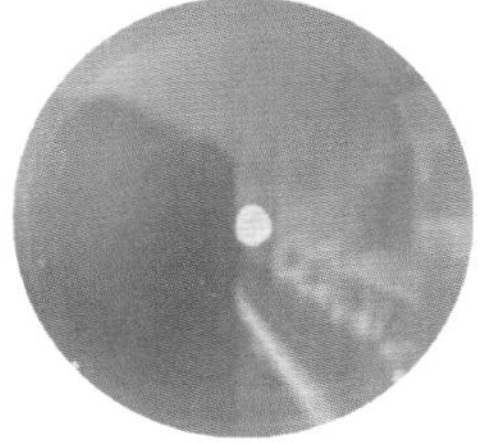

左—迁徙现象，有鞭毛(H)；右—无鞭毛(O)
Left — migration phenomenon with flagella (H); right — no flagella (O)

彩图 8　不同细菌在固体培养基上的运动情况

Color fig. 8　Mobility of different bacteria on solid media

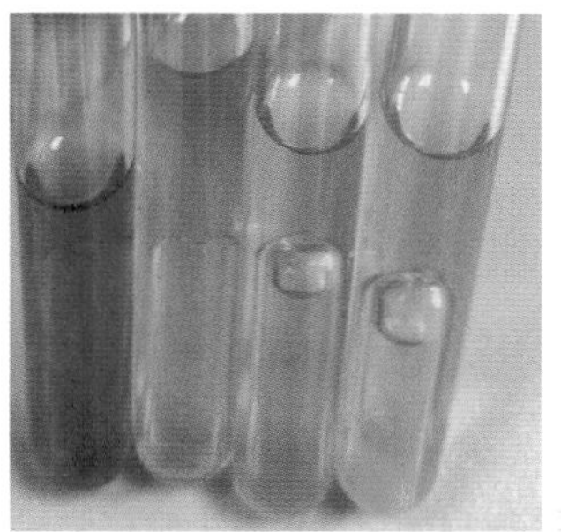

左一，伤寒杆菌，不发酵乳糖（－）；左二，伤寒杆菌，发酵葡萄糖，产酸不产气（＋）；右二，大肠埃希菌，发酵葡萄糖，产酸产气（⊕）；右一，大肠埃希菌，发酵乳糖，产酸产气（⊕）

First left, *S. typhi*, no lactose fermentation (−); second left, *S. typhi*, fermentation of glucose for acid production and no gas production (+); second right, *E. coli*, fermentation of glucose for acid production and gas production (⊕); first right, *E. coli*, fermentation of lactose for acid production and gas production (⊕)

彩图 9　糖发酵试验

Color fig. 9　Carbohydrate fermentation test

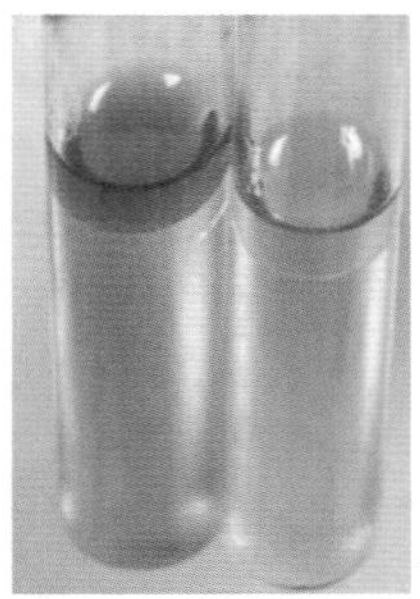

左—大肠埃希菌（＋）；右—伤寒杆菌（－）

Left — *E. coli* (+); right — *S. typhi* (−)

彩图 10　吲哚试验

Color fig. 10　Indole test

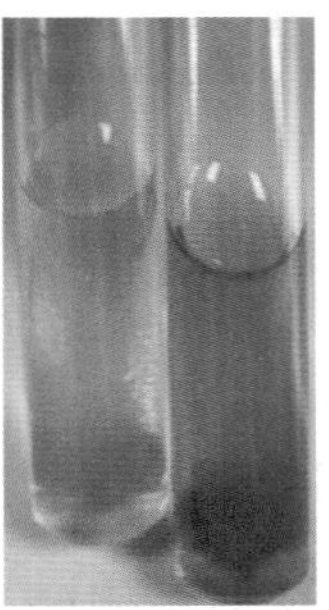

左—大肠埃希菌（－）；右—普通变形杆菌（＋）

Left — *E. coli* (−); right — *P. vulgaris*(+)

彩图 11　尿素酶试验

Color fig. 11　Urease test

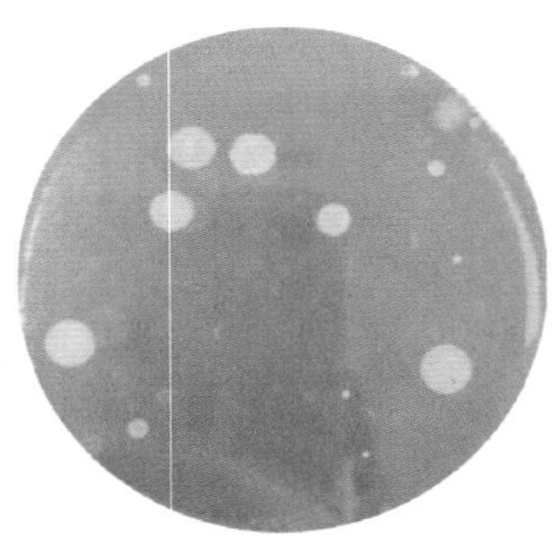

彩图 12　空气中微生物检测结果

Color fig. 12　Airborne microbiological test results

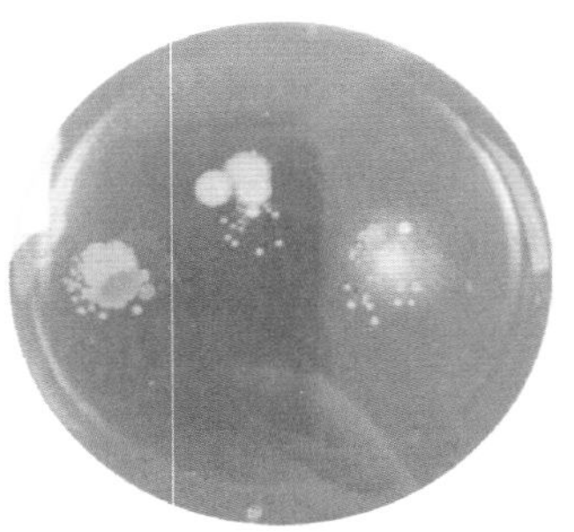

彩图 13　手指部微生物检测结果

Color fig. 13　Finger microbiological test results

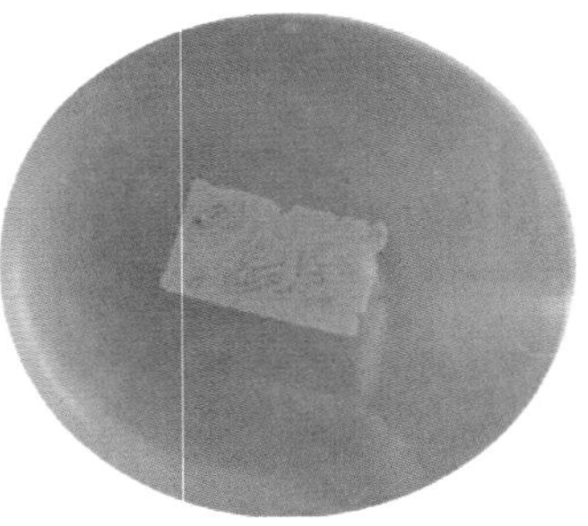

彩图 14　紫外线杀菌试验结果(金黄色葡萄球菌)

Color fig. 14　Results of UV sterilization test (*Staphylococcus aureus*)

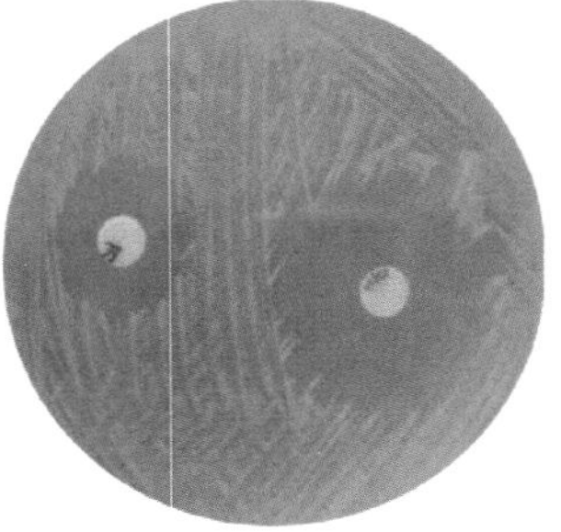

彩图 15　药敏纸片试验结果(金黄色葡萄球菌)

Color fig. 15　Drug sensitive paper test results (*Staphylococcus aureus*)

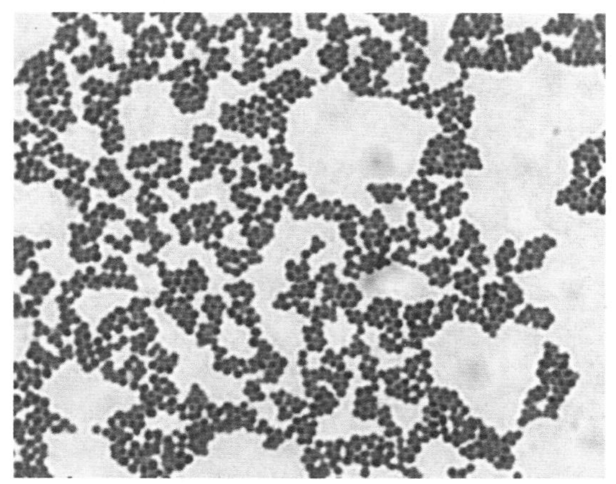

彩图 16　葡萄球菌(革兰染色,1000×)

Color fig. 16　*Staphylococcus* (Gram staining,1000×)

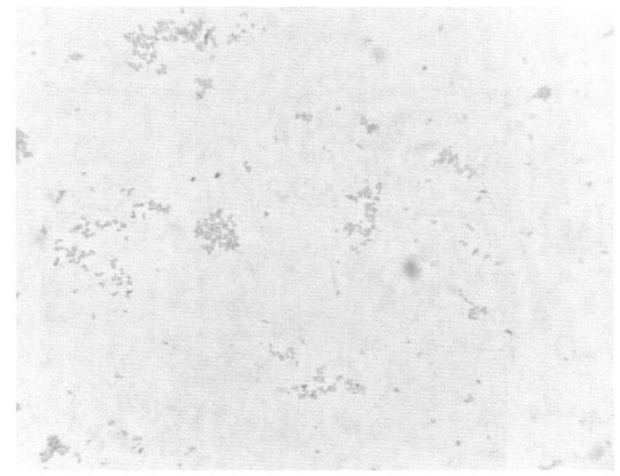

彩图 17　淋病奈瑟球菌(革兰染色,1000×)

Color fig. 17　*Neisseria gonorrhoeae* (Gram staining,1000×)

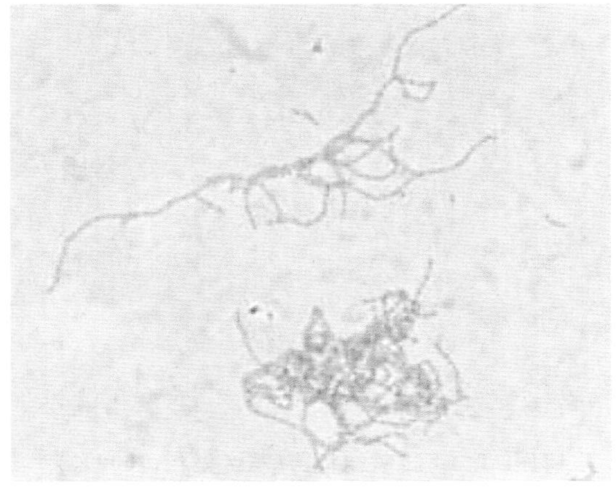

彩图 18　链球菌(革兰染色,1000×)

Color fig. 18　*Streptococcus* (Gram staining,1000×)

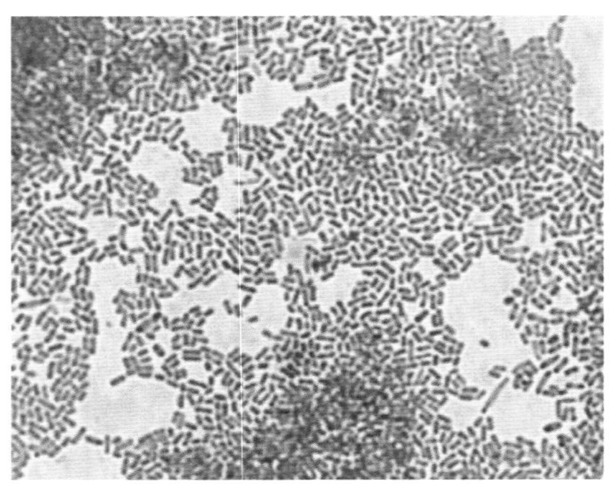

彩图 19 大肠埃希菌(革兰染色,1000×)

Color fig. 19 *E. coli* (Gram staining,1000×)

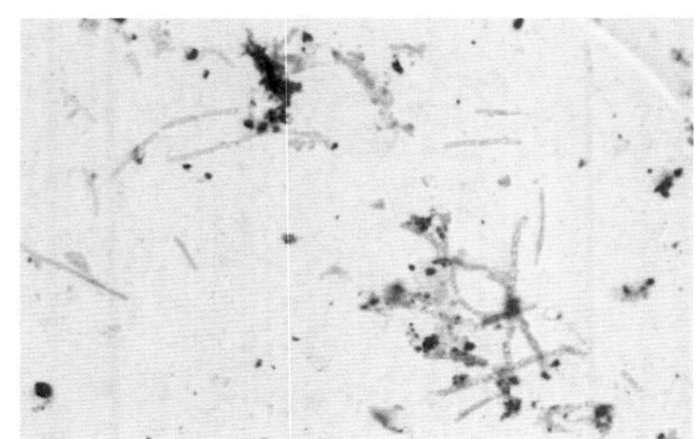

彩图 20 炭疽芽孢杆菌(革兰染色,1000×)

Color fig. 20 *Bacillus anthracis* (Gram staining,1000×)

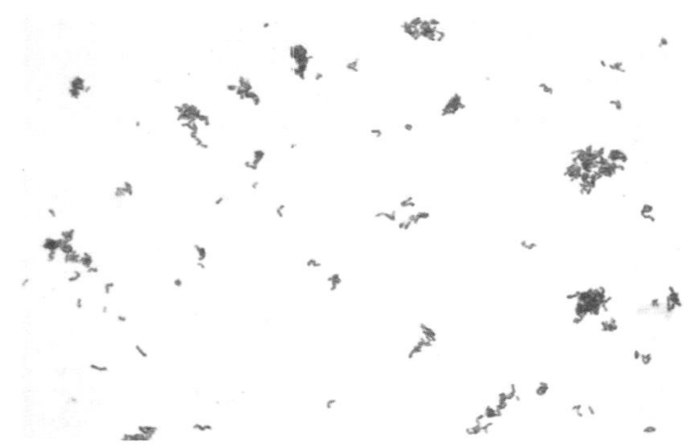

彩图 21 百日咳鲍特菌(革兰染色,1000×)

Color fig. 21 *Bordetella pertussis* (Gram staining,1000×)

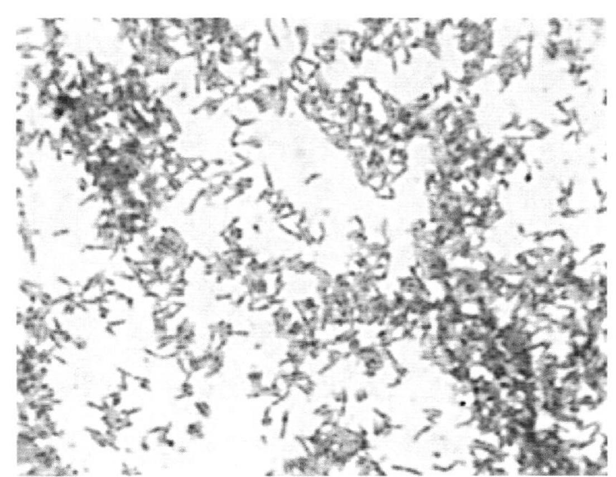

彩图 22　白喉棒状杆菌(革兰染色,1000×)

Color fig. 22　*Corynebacterium diphtheriae* (Gram staining,1000×)

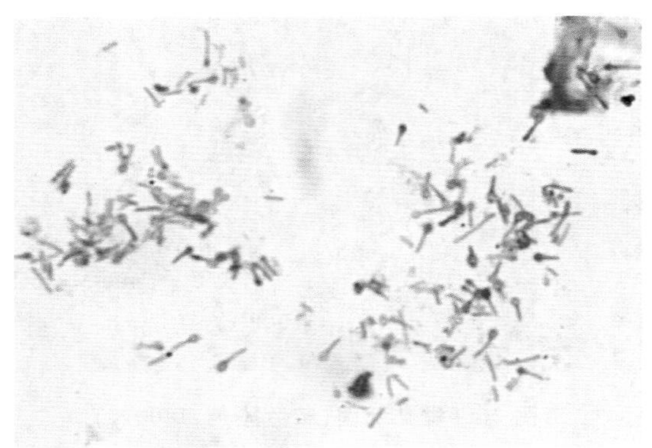

彩图 23　破伤风梭菌(革兰染色,1000×)

Color fig. 23　*Clostridium tetani* (Gram staining,1000×)

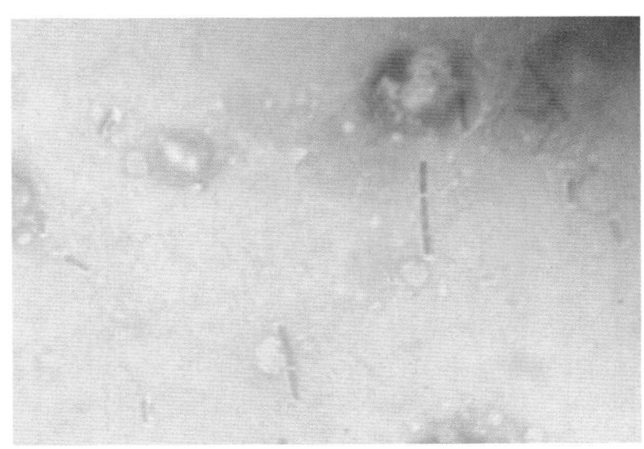

彩图 24　产气荚膜梭菌(革兰染色,1000×)

Color fig. 24　*Clostridium perfringens* (Gram staining,1000×)

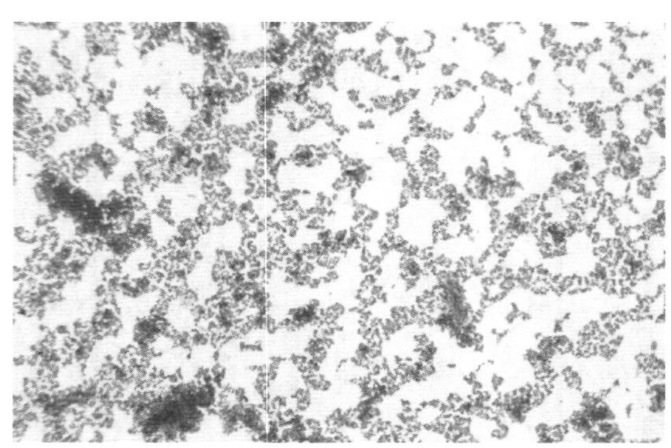

彩图 25　结核分枝杆菌(抗酸染色,1000×)

Color fig. 25　*Mycobacterium tuberculosis* (acid-fast staining,1000×)

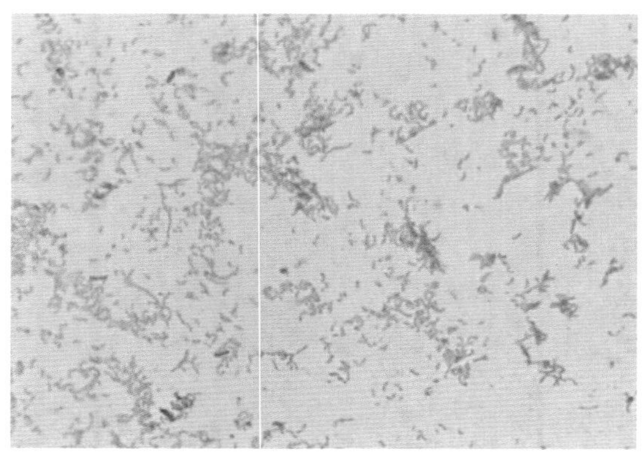

彩图 26　霍乱弧菌(革兰染色,1000×)

Color fig. 26　*Vibrio cholerae* (Gram staining,1000×)

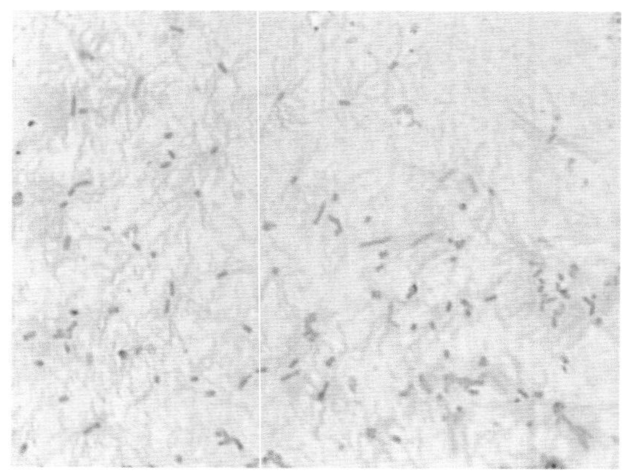

彩图 27　细菌鞭毛(结晶紫染色,1000×)

Color fig. 27　Bacterial flagella (crystal violet staining,1000×)

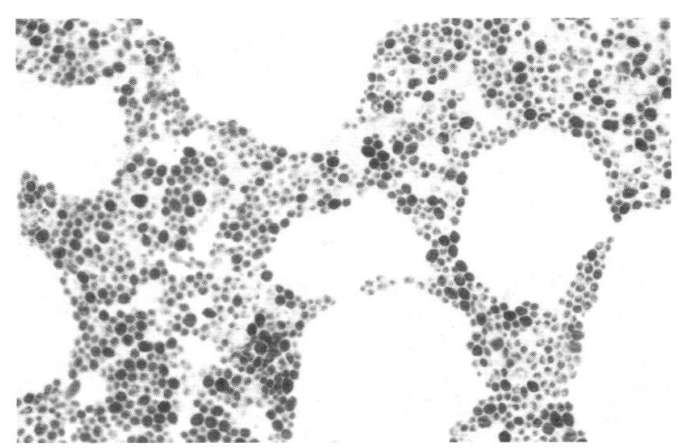

彩图 28　白念珠菌

Color fig. 28　*Candida albicans*

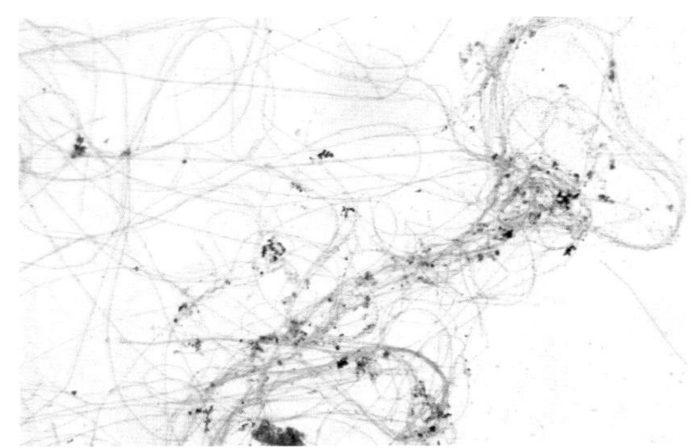

彩图 29　红色毛藓菌

Color fig. 29　*Trichophyton rubrum*

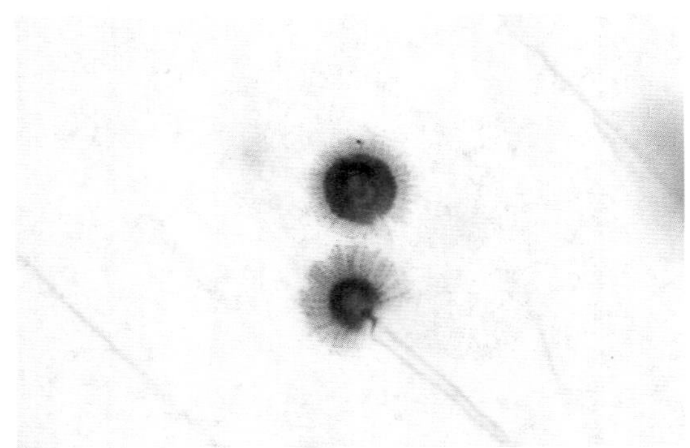

彩图 30　真菌孢子囊

Color fig. 30　Fungal sporangia

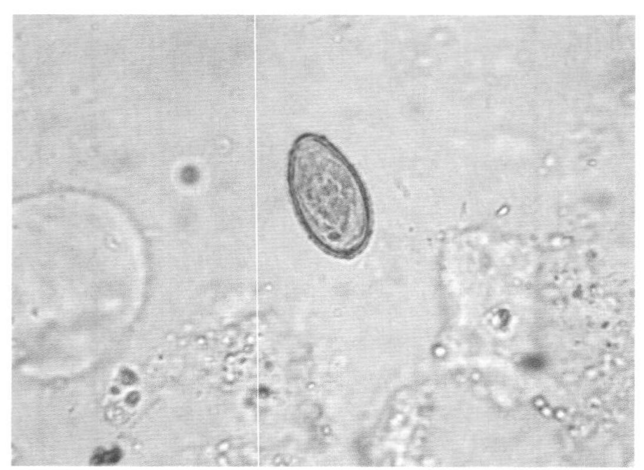

彩图 31　华支睾吸虫虫卵(400×)

Color fig. 31　Egg of *Clonorchis sinensis* (400×)

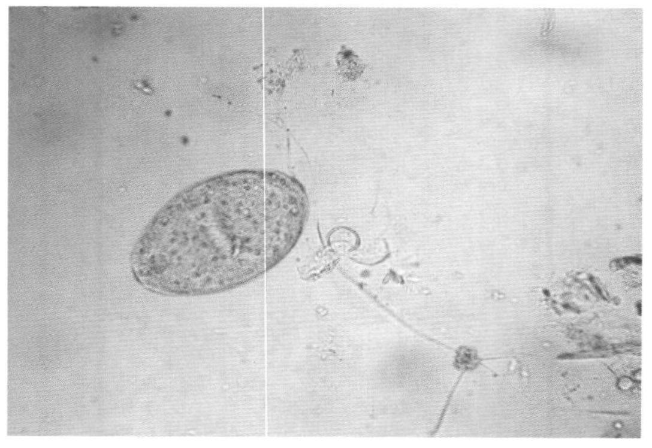

彩图 32　布氏姜片吸虫虫卵(100×)

Color fig. 32　Egg of *Fasciolopsis buski* (100×)

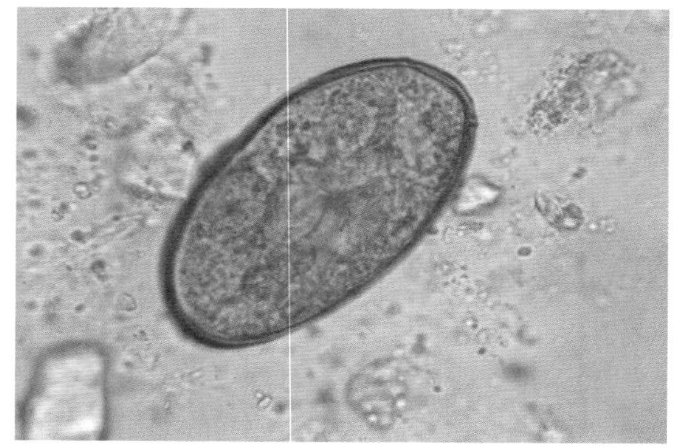

彩图 33　卫氏并殖吸虫虫卵(400×)

Color fig. 33　Egg of *Paragonimus westermani* (400×)

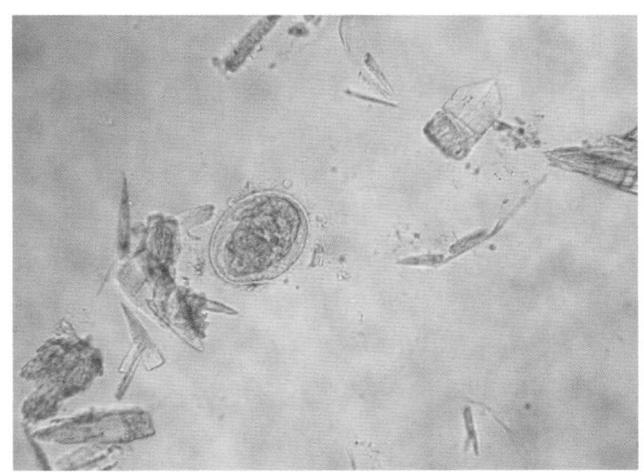

彩图 34　日本血吸虫虫卵(400×)

Color fig. 34　Egg of *Schistosoma japonicum* (400×)

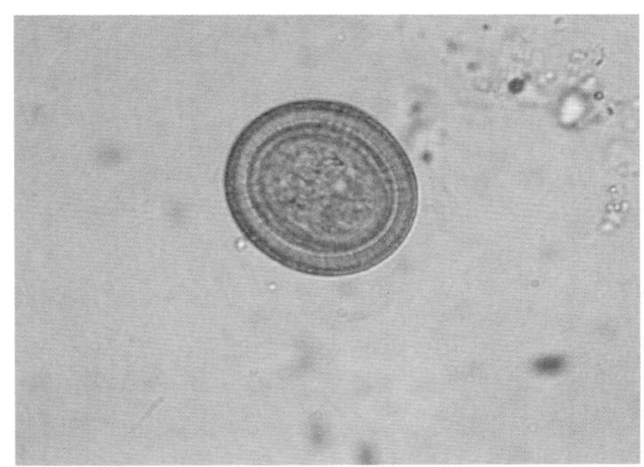

彩图 35　带绦虫虫卵(400×)

Color fig. 35　Egg of *Taenia solium or Taenia saginata* (400×)

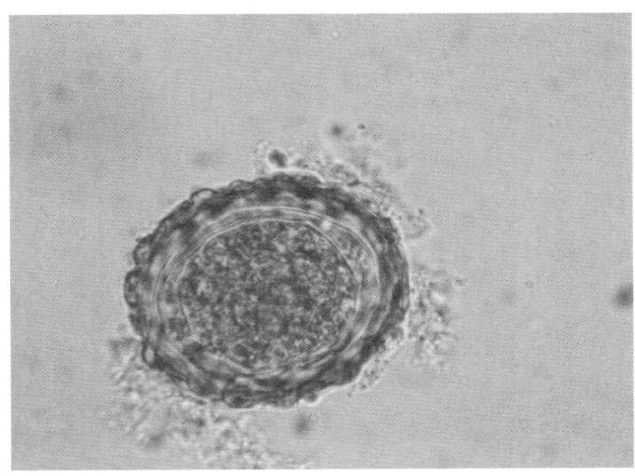

彩图 36　蛔虫受精卵(400×)

Color fig. 36　Fertilized egg of *Ascaris lumbricoides* (400×)

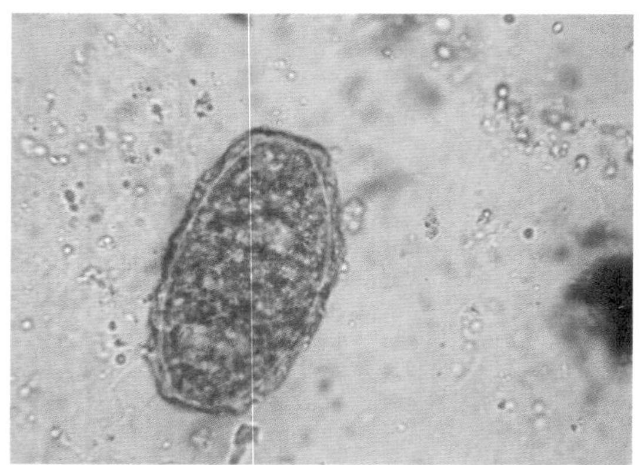

彩图 37　蛔虫未受精卵(400×)

Color fig. 37　Unfertilized egg of *Ascaris lumbricoides* (400×)

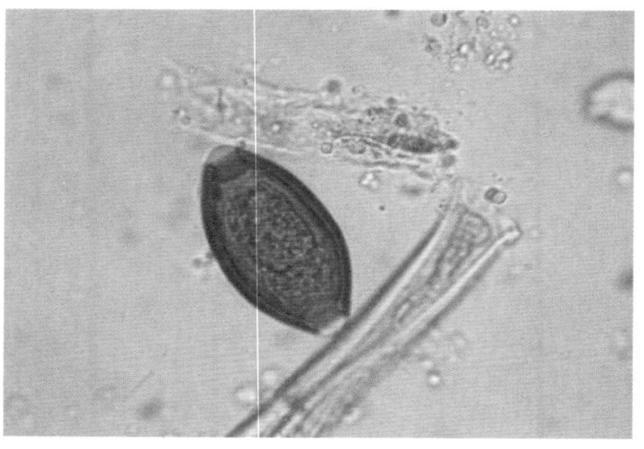

彩图 38　毛首鞭形线虫虫卵(400×)

Color fig. 38　Egg of *Trichuris trichiura* (400×)

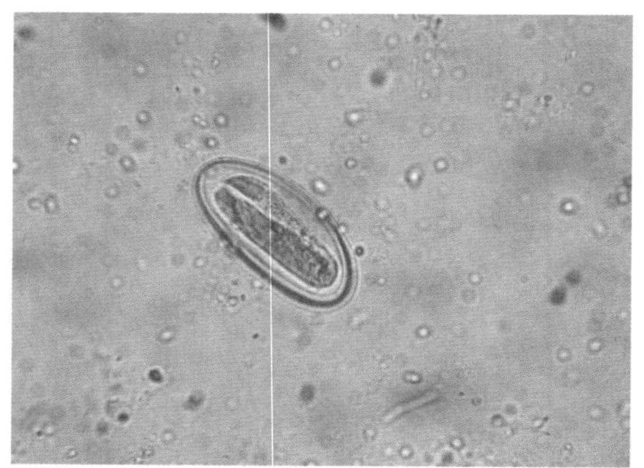

彩图 39　蠕形住肠线虫虫卵(400×)

Color fig. 39　Egg of *Enterobius vermicularis* (400×)

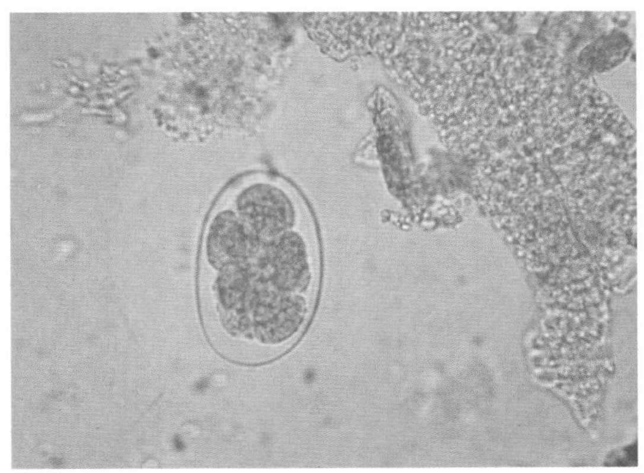

彩图 40　钩虫虫卵(400×)
Color fig. 40　Egg of hookworm (400×)

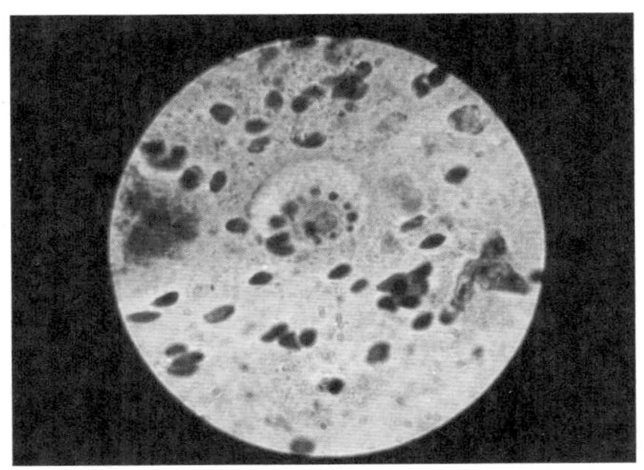

彩图 41　溶组织内阿米巴滋养体(1000×)
Color fig. 41　Trophozoite of *Entamoeba histolytica* (1000×)

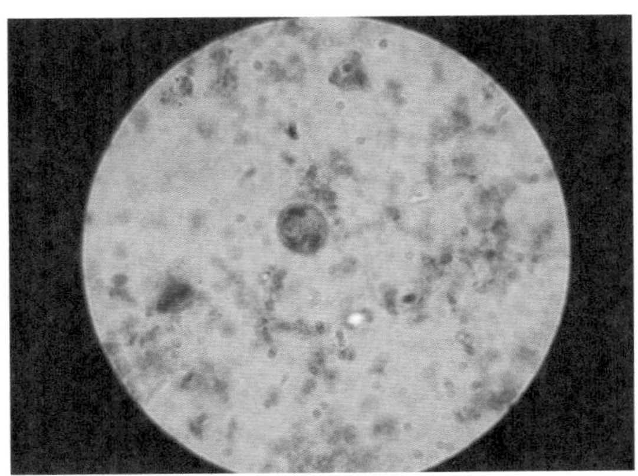

彩图 42　溶组织内阿米巴包囊(1000×)
Color fig. 42　Cyst of *Entamoeba histolytica* (1000×)

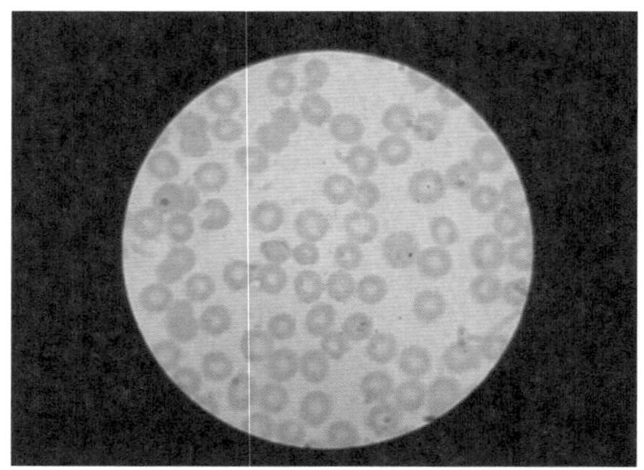

彩图 43　间日疟原虫环状体(1000×)

Color fig. 43　Ring form of *Plasmodium vivax* (1000×)

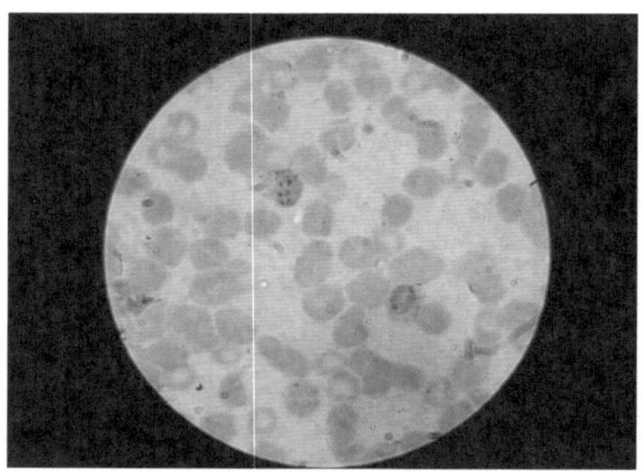

彩图 44　间日疟原虫未成熟裂殖体(1000×)

Color fig. 44　Immature schizont of *Plasmodium vivax* (1000×)

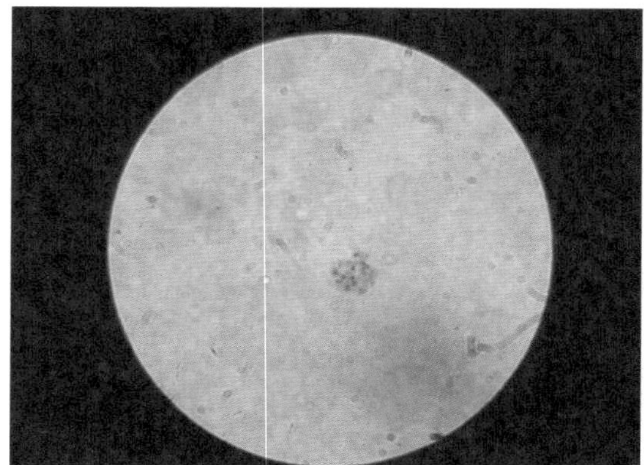

彩图 45　间日疟原虫成熟裂殖体(1000×)

Color fig. 45　Mature schizont of *Plasmodium vivax* (1000×)

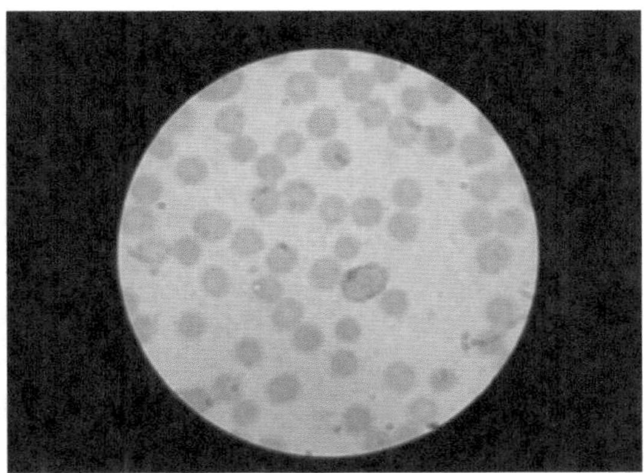

彩图 46　间日疟原虫雌配子体(1000×)

Color fig. 46　Female gametophyte of *Plasmodium vivax* (1000×)

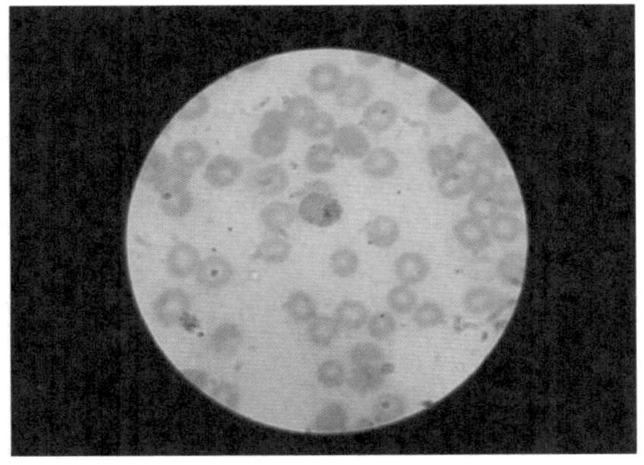

彩图 47　间日疟原虫雄配子体(1000×)

Color fig. 47　Male gametophyte of *Plasmodium vivax* (1000×)

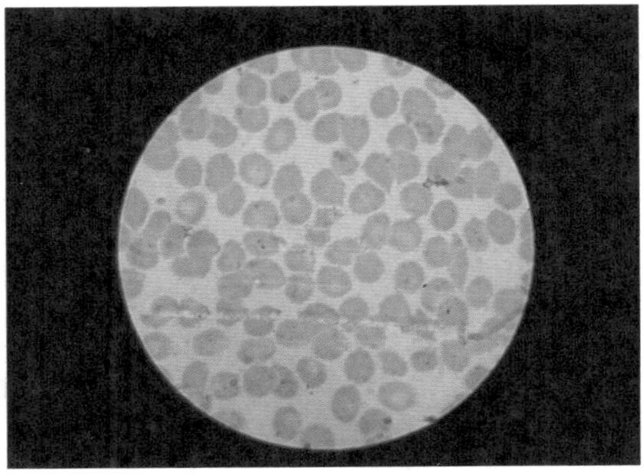

彩图 48　恶性疟原虫环状体(1000×)

Color fig. 48　Ring form of *Plasmodium falciparum* (1000×)

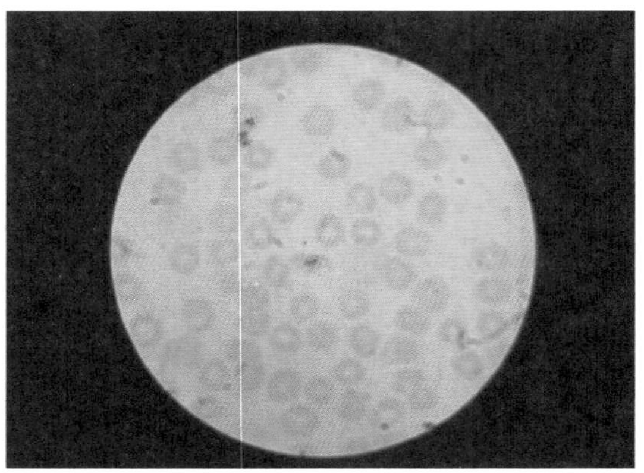

彩图 49　恶性疟原虫配子体(1000×)

Color fig. 49　Gametophyte of *Plasmodium falciparum* (1000×)

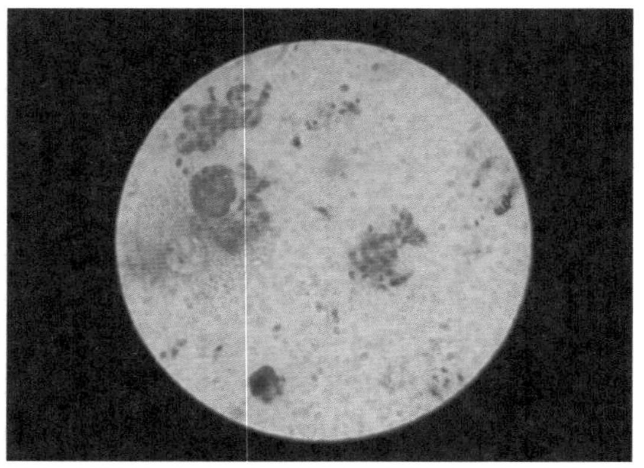

彩图 50　弓形虫滋养体(1000×)

Color fig. 50　Trophozoite of *Toxoplasma gondii* (1000×)

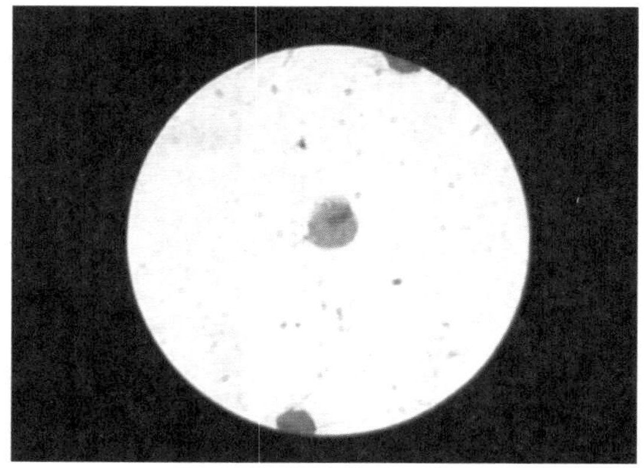

彩图 51　阴道毛滴虫(1000×)

Color fig. 51　*Trichomonas vaginalis* (1000×)

参考文献

[1] 赵飞骏,李忠玉.病原生物学实验(医学微生物学分册)[M].2版.北京:科学出版社,2017.

[2] 袁树民,康曼,周亚莉.医学微生物学实验指导及习题集[M].北京:电子工业出版社,2021.

[3] 杨健,胡为民,杨继文.病原生物学与医学免疫学实验[M].4版.北京:科学出版社,2015.

[4] 吴高莉.病原生物学与免疫学实验教程[M].北京:人民卫生出版社,2017.

[5] 汤仁仙.病原生物学与医学免疫学实验[M].北京:科学出版社,2018.

[6] 李士根,陈盛霞,李晓霞.人体寄生虫学实验与学习指导[M].北京:人民卫生出版社,2019.

[7] 史丽云.医学免疫和病原生物实验学[M].2版.北京:人民卫生出版社,2022.

[8] 沈晓玲,木兰,王利.病原生物学与免疫学实验指导[M].南京:江苏凤凰科学技术出版社,2022.

[9] 彭鸿娟,夏超明,周怀瑜.医学寄生虫学实验指导[M].郑州:郑州大学出版社,2020.

[10] 潘渠,张宗诚.病原生物与免疫学实验[M].北京:科学出版社,2018.

[11] 苗旭欣,李丽.病原生物与免疫学实验及学习指导[M].北京:人民卫生出版社,2020.

[12] 马海梅,张春桃.医学微生物学实验教程[M].2版.北京:科学出版社,2020.

[13] 刘荣臻,曹元应,张晓延.病原生物与免疫学实验及学习指导[M].北京:人民卫生出版社,2019.

[14] 李楠,徐晓可.病原生物学与免疫学实验及学习指导[M].武汉:华中科技大学出版社,2020.

[15] 管俊昌,刘勇.医学微生物学实验指导[M].2版.北京:中国科学技术大学出版社,2021.

[16] 单颖,张轶博.医学免疫学与病原生物学实验[M].2版.北京:科学出版社,2018.

[17] Garcia L S. Diagnostic medical parasitology [M]. 6th ed. Washington DC: American Society for Microbiology Press,2017.

[18] 张力平.病原生物学与免疫学实验[M].北京:高等教育出版社,2012.

[19] 曹虹,彭宜红,金成允,等.医学微生物学实验指导[M].郑州:郑州大学出版社,2019.